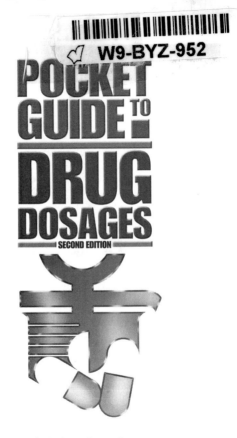

POCKET GUIDE TO DRUG DOSAGES

SECOND EDITION

Springhouse Corporation
Springhouse, Pennsylvania

Staff

Publisher
Donna O. Carpenter, ELS

Editorial Director
William J. Kelly

Clinical Director
Ann M. Barrow, RN, MSN, CCRN

Design Director
John Hubbard

Art Director
Elaine Kasmer Ezrow

Drug Information Editor
Lisa Truong, RPh, PharmD

Senior Associate Editor
Karen C. Comerford

Clinical Project Editor
Eileen Cassin Gallen, RN, BSN

Editor
Kevin Dodds

Clinical Editor
Margaret Friant Cramer, RN, MSN

Copy Editors
Colleen P. Coady, Leslie Dworkin, Dolores Matthews

Designers
Arlene Putterman (Associate Design Director), Joseph John Clark, Jackie Facciolo, Donald G. Knauss

Typographers
Diane Paluba (manager), Joyce Rossi Biletz

Manufacturing
Deborah Meiris (director), Patricia K. Dorshaw (manager), Otto Mezei (book production manager)

Editorial Assistants
Carol A. Caputo, Arlene P. Claffee

Indexer
Barbara Hodgson

Visit our Web site at www.NDHnow.com

R A member of the Reed Elsevier plc group

ISBN 1-58255-045X
ISSN 1096-7044
NDHPGDD—D N O S A J J M A M F
03 02 01 00 10 9 8 7 6 5 4 3 2 1

Contents

Clinical consultants iv

How to use this book v

Abbreviations vi

Generic drugs in alphabetical order 2

Appendices

Selected narcotic analgesic combination
products 317

Drugs that shouldn't be crushed 321

Dangerous drug interactions 325

Table of equivalents 328

Managing anaphylaxis 330

Index 331

Clinical consultants

David M. DiPersio, BS, PharmD
Clinical Pharmacist, Critical Care
Vanderbilt University Medical Center
Nashville, Tenn.

Barbara S. Kannewurf, PharmD
Clinical Fellow
Virginia Commonwealth University
Medical College of Virginia Campus
Richmond, Va.

Tamara Luedtke, RN, MSN, CCRN
Nurse Manager, Critical Care Unit
Hendrick Medical Center
Abilene, Tex.

Randall A. Lynch, RPh, PharmD
Assistant Director, Pharmacy Services
Presbyterian Medical Center, University of
Pennsylvania Health System
Philadelphia

Dawna Martich, RN, MSN
Clinical Trainer
Diabetes Treatment Centers of America
Liberty Technology Center
Pittsburgh

Larry A. Pfeifer, RPh, MApSt
Chief, Pharmacy Services
Gillis W. Long Hansen's Disease Center
Carville, La.

Ruthie Robinson, RN, MSN, CEN, CCRN
Adjunct Professor, ER Staff Nurse
Lamar University
Beaumont, Tex.

Carla M. Roy, RN, BSN, CCRN
Staff Nurse
Our Lady of Lourdes Medical Center
Camden, N.J.

C. Robin Twigg, RN, BSN
Registered Nurse
Susquehanna Health System
Williamsport, Pa.

Theresa M. Wadas, RN, MSN, CCRN, CRNP
Nurse Practitioner
Heart Failure, Heart Transplant Service
University of Alabama Hospital
Birmingham, Ala.

Kimberly A. Zalewski, RN, MSN, CEN
Registered Nurse
St. Luke's Hospital
Bethlehem, Pa.

How to use this book

NDH Pocket Guide to Drug Dosages, Second Edition offers comprehensive dosage information in a unique, quick-scan format. The book opens with a list of abbreviations used in the entries. Then, organized alphabetically by generic name, each drug entry covers generic and common trade names, pharmacologic and therapeutic classes, pregnancy risk category, controlled substance schedule (where appropriate), common indications and dosages, and key nursing considerations. Information is divided into columns for quick reference.

The first column shows the generic name in boldface, followed by trade names. Canadian and Australian brand-name drugs are denoted by a dagger (†) and a double-dagger (‡), respectively. Below the list of trade names are the drug's pharmacologic class and then its therapeutic class. Pregnancy risk category and, where applicable, controlled substance schedule are listed next.

Pregnancy risk categories parallel those assigned by the Food and Drug Administration to reflect a drug's potential to cause birth defects.

- A: Adequate studies in pregnant women have failed to show a risk to the fetus.
- B: Animal studies have not shown a risk to the fetus, but controlled studies have not been conducted in pregnant women; or animal studies have shown an adverse effect on the fetus, but adequate studies in pregnant women have not shown a fetal risk.
- C: Animal studies have shown an adverse effect on the fetus, but adequate studies have not been conducted in humans. The benefits may be acceptable despite potential risks.
- D: The drug may pose risks to the human fetus, but potential benefits may be acceptable despite the risks.
- X: Studies in animals or humans show fetal abnormalities, or reports of adverse reactions indicate evidence of fetal risk. The risks involved clearly outweigh the potential benefits.
- NR: Not rated.

Drugs regulated under the Controlled Substances Act of 1970 are divided into the following schedules:

- I: high abuse potential, no accepted medical use
- II: high abuse potential, severe dependence liability
- III: less abuse potential than schedule II drugs, moderate dependence liability
- IV: less abuse potential than schedule III drugs, limited dependence liability
- V: limited abuse potential.

The second column covers major indications and the most common dosages ordered for a particular drug. The third column lists the important nursing considerations, including those related to monitoring, drug administration, and patient teaching.

Appendices include selected narcotic analgesic combination products, drugs that shouldn't be crushed, dangerous drug interactions, a table of equivalents, and managing anaphylaxis.

The index is organized by generic name, trade name, and disease.

Abbreviations

ABG	arterial blood gas	ET	endotracheal
ACE	angiotensin-converting enzyme	Fio$_2$	forced inspiratory oxygen
ADH	antidiuretic hormone	G	gauge
AIDS	acquired immunodeficiency syndrome	g	gram
		GI	gastrointestinal
ALT	alanine aminotransferase	GU	genitourinary
AST	aspartate aminotransferase	H	histamine
AV	atrioventricular	Hct	hematocrit
b.i.d.	twice a day	Hgb	hemoglobin
BP	blood pressure	HIV	human immunodeficiency
BPH	benign prostatic hyperplasia		virus
BUN	blood urea nitrogen	HR	heart rate
CABG	coronary artery bypass graft	hr	hour
CAD	coronary artery disease	h.s.	at bedtime
CBC	complete blood count	I&O	intake and output
CDC	Centers for Disease Control and Prevention	I.M.	intramuscular
		INR	international normalized ratio
CK	creatinine kinase	IOP	intraocular pressure
cm	centimeter	IPPB	intermittent positive-pressure breathing
CMV	cytomegalovirus		
CNS	central nervous system	IU	international unit
COPD	chronic obstructive	I.V.	intravenous
CSF	cerebrospinal fluid	kg	kilogram
CV	central venous	L	liter
CVA	cerebrovascular accident	lb	pound
CVP	central venous pressure	LDL	low-density lipoprotein
D$_5$W	dextrose 5% in water	M	molar
dl	deciliter	m^2	square meter
DTP	diphtheria, tetanus, and pertussis	MAC	Mycobacterium avium complex
		MAO	monoamine oxidase
ECG	electrocardiogram	mcg	microgram
EEG	electroencephalogram	mEq	milliequivalent

Abbreviations

mg	milligram	q.i.d.	four times a day
MI	myocardial infarction	q.o.d.	every other day
min	minute	RBC	red blood cell
ml	milliliter	RDA	recommended daily allowance
mm^3	cubic millimeter	RSV	respiratory syncytial virus
mo	month	SaO$_2$	oxygen saturation
NaCl	sodium chloride	S.C.	subcutaneous
NG	nasogastric	sec	second
NSAID	nonsteroidal anti-inflammatory drug	S.L.	sublingual
		T$_3$	triiodothyronine
O$_2$	oxygen	T$_4$	thyroxine
OTC	over-the-counter	TB	tuberculosis
oz	ounce	TCA	tricyclic antidepressant
PacO$_2$	partial pressure of arterial carbon dioxide	t.i.d.	three times a day
		TPN	total parenteral nutrition
PaO$_2$	partial pressure of arterial oxygen	tsp	teaspoon
		U	unit
PAWP	pulmonary artery wedge pressure	USP	United States Pharmacopeia
		UTI	urinary tract infection
P.O.	by mouth	w	with
P.R.	per rectum	WBC	white blood cell
p.r.n.	as needed	wk	week
PSVT	paroxysmal supraventricular tachycardia	yr	year
PT	prothrombin time		
PTCA	percutaneous transluminal coronary angioplasty		
PTT	partial thromboplastin time		
PVD	peripheral vascular disease		
q	every		
q.d.	once a day		

DRUG / CLASS / CATEGORY	INDICATIONS / DOSAGES	KEY NURSING CONSIDERATIONS
abacavir sulfate Ziagen *Antiviral (antiretroviral)* *Nucleoside analogue reverse transcriptase inhibitor* Pregnancy Risk Category: C	*Treatment of patients with HIV type 1 infection* — **Adults:** 300 mg P.O. b.i.d. in combination with other antiretroviral agent.	• Always use with other antiretroviral agents. Don't add as a single agent when antiretroviral regimens are changed because of loss of virologic response. • Fatal hypersensitivity reactions have been associated with drug therapy.
abciximab ReoPro *Antiplatelet aggregate* *Platelet aggregation inhibitor* Pregnancy Risk Category: C	*Adjunct to PTCA or atherectomy to prevent acute cardiac ischemic complications in patients at high risk for abrupt closure of treated coronary vessel* — **Adults:** 0.25 mg/kg I.V. bolus 10 to 60 min before start of PTCA or atherectomy; then continuous I.V. infusion of 10 mcg/min for 12 hr.	• Give in separate I.V. line; don't add other drug to solution. • Institute bleeding precautions. Keep on bed rest for 6 to 8 hr after sheath removal or drug discontinuation, whichever is later. Minimize punctures and invasive procedures. • Intended for use with aspirin and heparin.
acarbose Precose *Alpha-glucosidase inhibitor* *Antidiabetic* Pregnancy Risk Category: B	*Adjunct to diet to lower blood glucose in type 2 diabetes mellitus. May be used as monotherapy or in combination when hyperglycemia can't be managed by diet alone* — **Adults:** Individualized. 25 mg P.O. t.i.d. at start of main meals; then adjust q 4 to 8 wk. Maintenance: 50 to 100 mg P.O. t.i.d.; don't exceed 50 mg t.i.d. in patients < 60 kg (132 lb) or 100 mg t.i.d. in patients > 60 kg.	• May increase hypoglycemic potential of sulfonylureas. Closely monitor patient. • Don't use in patients with severe liver impairment. • Patient may need insulin during increased stress. Monitor for hyperglycemia. • Monitor 1-hr postprandial plasma glucose.

acebutolol hydrochloride
Sectral
Beta blocker
Antihypertensive/antiarrhythmic
Pregnancy Risk Category: B

Hypertension — **Adults:** 400 mg P.O. as 1 daily dose or in divided doses b.i.d. to maximum 1,200 mg q.d.
Ventricular arrhythmias — **Adults:** 400 mg P.O. daily divided b.i.d.; increase p.r.n. Usual dose 600 to 1,200 mg.
Adjust-a-dose: In patients with creatinine clearance of 25 to 50 ml/min, reduce dose by 50%; if < 25 ml/min, reduce dose by 75%.

- Check apical pulse before giving; if < 60, withhold drug and call doctor. Monitor BP.
- Before surgery, tell anesthesiologist that patient is taking drug.
- Drug may mask hyperthyroidism signs.
- Don't discontinue drug abruptly.

---

acetaminophen (APAP, paracetamol)
Acephen, Aceta, Anacin (aspirin free), Apacet, Dapacin, Feverall, Neopap, Panadol, Tempra, Tylenol
Para-aminophenol derivative
Nonnarcotic analgesic/antipyretic
Pregnancy Risk Category: B

Mild pain or fever — **Adults and children >11 yr:** 325 to 650 mg P.O. q 4 to 6 hr; or 1 g P.O. t.i.d. or q.i.d. or P.R. Maximum 4 g q.d. For long-term use, maximum 2.6 g q.d. Or 2 extended-release capsules P.O. q 8 hr. Maximum 4 g q.d. **Children 11 yr:** 480 mg P.O. or P.R. q 4 to 6 hr. **Children 9 to 10 yr:** 400 mg P.O. or P.R. q 4 to 6 hr. **Children 6 to 8 yr:** 320 mg P.O. or P.R. q 4 to 6 hr. **Children 4 to 5 yr:** 240 mg P.O. or P.R. q 4 to 6 hr. **Children 2 to 3 yr:** 160 mg P.O. or P.R. q 4 to 6 hr. **Children 12 to 23 mo:** 120 mg P.O. q 4 to 6 hr. **Children 4 to 11 mo:** 80 mg P.O. q 4 to 6 hr. **Children < 3 mo:** 40 mg P.O. q 4 to 6 hr.

- Warn that high doses or unsupervised long-term use can cause liver damage.
- Caution that excessive alcohol use may increase risk of liver toxicity.
- Warn not to take for marked fever (> 103.1° F [39.5° C]), fever lasting > 3 days, or recurrent fever, unless directed by doctor.
- May cause false-positive blood glucose decrease in home monitoring systems.
- Don't give to children < 2 yr without consulting doctor.

DRUG/CLASS/ CATEGORY	INDICATIONS/ DOSAGES	KEY NURSING CONSIDERATIONS
acetazolamide Acetazolam†, AK-Zol, Dazamide, Diamox, Diamox Sequels **acetazolamide sodium** Diamox Parenteral *Carbonic anhydrase inhibitor* *Antiglaucoma agent/diuretic* Pregnancy Risk Category: C	*Secondary glaucoma and preoperative treatment of acute angle-closure glaucoma* — **Adults:** 250 mg P.O. q 4 hr; or 250 mg P.O. b.i.d. for short-term therapy. For extended-release capsules, 500 mg P.O. q.d. or b.i.d. To rapidly lower IOP, 500 mg I.V.; then 125 to 250 mg I.V. q 4 hr. *Edema in heart failure* — **Adults:** 250 to 375 mg P.O. or I.V. q morning. **Children:** 5 mg/kg P.O. or I.V. q morning. *Chronic open-angle glaucoma* — **Adults:** 250 mg to 1 g P.O. daily in divided doses q.i.d., or 500 mg (extended-release) P.O. b.i.d. **Children:** 8 to 30 mg/kg P.O. in 3 divided doses.	▪ Monitor I&O, glucose, and electrolytes. When drug used as diuretic, consult doctor and dietitian about high-potassium diet. ▪ Elderly patients are especially susceptible to excessive diuresis; monitor closely. ▪ Weigh patient daily; rapid fluid loss may cause weight loss and hypotension. ▪ *I.V. use:* Inject 100 to 500 mg/min into large vein using 21G or 23G needle.
acetylcholine chloride Miochol *Cholinergic agonist* *Miotic* Pregnancy Risk Category: NR	*Anterior segment surgery* — **Adults and children:** during surgery, 0.5 to 2 ml instilled gently into anterior chamber.	▪ Reconstitute immediately before using, shaking vial gently until solution is clear. Discard unused portion. ▪ Don't gas-sterilize vial. ▪ Don't use solution if discolored.

acetylcysteine
Airbront, Mucomyst,
Mucomyst 10, Mucosil-10,
Mucosil-20
*Amino acid (L-cysteine)
derivative*
*Mucolytic agent/antidote for
acetaminophen overdose*
Pregnancy Risk Category: B

*Adjuvant therapy for abnormal viscid or in-
spissated mucus secretions in pneumonia,
bronchitis, TB, cystic fibrosis, emphysema,
atelectasis (adjunct), pulmonary complications of thoracic and CV surgery* — **Adults
and children:** 1 to 2 ml of 10% or 20% solution by direct instillation into trachea up to
q hr; or 1 to 10 ml of 20% solution or 2 to
20 ml of 10% solution by nebulization q 2 to
6 hr, p.r.n.

Acetaminophen toxicity — **Adults and children:** initially, 140 mg/kg P.O.; then 70 mg/
kg P.O. q 4 hr for 17 doses.

- Start treatment immediately; don't wait for
  blood drug levels. Drug can't be administered if > 24 hr has elapsed since ingestion.
- To use orally for acetaminophen overdose,
  dilute with cola, fruit juice, or water. Add 3
  ml diluent to each ml acetylcysteine. Use
  diluted oral solutions within 1 hr. If given by
  NG tube, water may be used as diluent.
- Repeat dose if patient vomits within 1 hr of
  loading or maintenance dose.
- Use plastic, glass, stainless steel, or other
  nonreactive metal when giving by nebulization. Hand-bulb nebulizer not recommended.

activated charcoal
Actidose, Actidose-Aqua,
Charcoaid, Charcocaps,
Liqui-Char
Adsorbent
*Antidote/antidiarrheal/anti-
flatulent*
Pregnancy Risk Category: C

Flatulence; dyspepsia — **Adults:** 600 mg to
5 g P.O. as single dose or 0.975 to 3.9 g
P.O. t.i.d. after meals.

Poisoning — **Adults and children:** initially,
1 to 2 g/kg (30 to 100 g) P.O. or 10 times
amount of poison ingested, given as suspension in 120 to 240 ml of water. Check
with poison control center for specific uses
in poisonings or overdoses.

- Inactivates ipecac syrup; give after emesis.
- Mix powder form with water to form thick
  consistency. May add small amount of
  fruit juice. Give by large-bore NG tube after lavage, if necessary.
- Space doses at least 1 hr apart from other
  drugs when giving for indications other
  than poisoning.

acyclovir
Zovirax
Synthetic purine nucleoside
Antiviral
Pregnancy Risk Category: C

*Initial herpes genitalis; limited, non-life-
threatening mucocutaneous herpes simplex
virus infections in immunocompromised
patients* — **Adults and children:** cover all
lesions q 3 hr, 6 times daily for 7 days.

- As ordered, start therapy as soon as possible after symptom onset.
- Apply with finger cot or rubber glove.
- For cutaneous use only; don't apply to
  eye.

†Canadian. ‡Australian

DRUG/CLASS/CATEGORY	INDICATIONS/DOSAGES	KEY NURSING CONSIDERATIONS
acyclovir sodium Aviraxt, Zovirax *Synthetic purine nucleoside* *Antiviral* Pregnancy Risk Category: C	*Mucocutaneous herpes simplex virus infections in immunocompromised patients; genital herpes in immunocompetent patients* — **Adults and children ≥ 12 yr:** 5 mg/kg I.V. q 8 hr for 7 to 14 days (5 to 7 days for severe initial genital episode). **Children < 12 yr:** 250 mg/m² I.V. q 8 hr for 7 days. *Initial genital herpes* — **Adults:** 200 mg P.O. q 4 hr while awake (total 5 capsules daily); or 400 mg P.O. q 8 hr. Continue 7 to 10 days. *Chronic suppression therapy for recurrent genital herpes* — **Adults:** 400 mg P.O. b.i.d. for up to 12 mo. *Varicella (chickenpox) infections in immunocompromised patients* — **Adults and children ≥ 12 yr:** 10 mg/kg I.V. q 8 hr for 7 days. **Children < 12 yr:** 500 mg/m² I.V. q 8 hr for 7 to 10 days. *Adjust-a-dose:* Dosage adjustments required in patients with renal failure.	▪ *I.V. use:* Give infusion over at least 1 hr. ▪ Don't give by bolus injection or by I.M. or S.C. injection. ▪ As ordered, start therapy as soon as possible after symptom onset. ▪ Encourage adequate fluid intake. ▪ Encephalopathic changes more likely in neurologic disorders and in history of neurologic reactions to cytotoxic drugs. ▪ Dosage for obese patients based on ideal weight.
adenosine Adenocard *Nucleoside* *Antiarrhythmic* Pregnancy Risk Category: C	*Conversion of PSVT to sinus rhythm* — **Adults:** 6 mg rapid I.V. push over 1 to 2 sec. If PSVT persists after 1 to 2 min, give 12 mg by rapid I.V. push and repeat if needed. Single doses > 12 mg not recommended.	▪ Use cautiously in asthma. ▪ *I.V. use:* Administer directly into vein if possible; use port closest to patient and flush immediately and rapidly with 0.9% NaCl. ▪ Monitor ECG for arrhythmias.

albumin 5%
Albuminar 5, Albutein 5%

albumin 25%
Albuminar 25, Albutein 25%

Blood derivative

Plasma protein

Pregnancy Risk Category: C

Hypovolemic shock — Adults: initially, 500 to 750 ml of 5% solution by I.V. infusion. In children: re- peat q 30 min, p.r.n. Or, 100 to 200 ml I.V. of 25% solution; repeat in 10 to 30 min, if needed. **Children:** 12 to 20 ml 5% solution/ kg by I.V. infusion; repeat in 15 to 30 min if response inadequate. Or, 2.5 to 5 ml I.V. of 25% solution/kg; repeat in 10 to 30 min if needed.

Hypoproteinemia — Adults: 200 to 300 ml of 25% albumin.

Hyperbilirubinemia — Infants: 1 g/kg albu- min (4 ml/kg of 25% solution) 1 to 2 hr be- fore transfusion.

- Ensure proper hydration before infusion.
- ▪ **I.V. use:** Specific dosage and rate varies with condition. 5% albumin infused undi- luted or undiluted or diluted with 0.9% NaCl solution or D₅W. Don't give > 250 ml in 48 hr.
- Watch for hemorrhage or shock after surgery or injury.
- Watch for signs of vascular overload.
- Monitor I&O, Hgb, Hct, serum protein, and electrolytes.

albuterol (salbutamol)
Asmol‡, Proventil, Ventolin

albuterol sulfate (salbutamol sulfate)
Proventil, Proventil Repetabs, Respolin In- haler‡, Respolin Respirator Solution‡, Ventolin

Adrenergic

Bronchodilator

Pregnancy Risk Category: C

To prevent or treat bronchospasm in re- versible obstructive airway disease or to prevent exercise-induced bronchospasm — Adults and children ≥ 12 yr: *Aerosol in- halation:* 1 to 2 inhalations q 4 to 6 hr. *Solu- tion for inhalation:* 2.5 mg t.i.d. or q.i.d. by nebulizer. *Capsule for inhalation:* 200 to 400 mcg inhaled q 4 to 6 hr using Rotahaler. *Oral tablet:* 2 to 4 mg P.O. t.i.d. or q.i.d.; maximum 8 mg q.i.d. *Extended-release tablet:* 4 to 8 mg P.O. q 12 hr; maximum 16 mg b.i.d. **Children 6 to 13 yr:** 2 mg (1 tsp) P.O. t.i.d. or q.i.d. **Children 2 to 5 yr:** 0.1 mg/kg P.O. t.i.d., up to 2 mg (1 tsp) t.i.d. or q.i.d. **Adults > 65 yr:** 2 mg P.O. t.i.d. or q.i.d.

- Use extended-release tablets cautiously in preexisting GI narrowing.
- Pleasant-tasting syrup may be taken by children as young as 2 yr. Contains no al- cohol or sugar.
- Aerosol form may be used 15 min before exercise.
- May use tablets and aerosol concomitant- ly. Monitor closely for toxicity.
- ▪ If doctor orders >1 inhalation, instruct pa- tient to wait at least 2 min between inhala- tions.

(continued)

‡Canadian, †Australian

7

DRUG/CLASS/ CATEGORY	INDICATIONS/ DOSAGES	KEY NURSING CONSIDERATIONS
albuterol *(continued)*	*Prevention of exercise-induced broncho-spasm —* **Adults and children > 12 yr:** 2 inhalations 15 min before exercise.	• If patient also uses steroid inhaler, advise him to use steroid 5 min after taking albuterol.
aldesleukin (interleukin-2, IL-2) Proleukin Lymphokine Immunoregulatory agent Pregnancy Risk Category: C	*Metastatic renal cell carcinoma —* **Adults:** 600,000 IU/kg (0.037 mg/kg) I.V. q 8 hr for 5 days (total of 14 doses). Repeat sequence for another 14 doses. May give repeat courses after rest period of ≥ 7 wk.	• Monitor CBC, serum electrolytes, and renal and liver function tests. • Monitor vital signs closely. • Withhold dose if moderate lethargy occurs. • Add ordered dose of reconstituted drug to 50 ml D_5W and infuse over 15 min. Don't use in-line filter.
alendronate sodium Fosamax *Osteoclast-mediated bone resorption inhibitor Antiosteoporotic agent* Pregnancy Risk Category: C	*Osteoporosis in postmenopausal women —* **Adults:** 10 mg P.O. q.d. taken with a full glass of plain water only, ≥ 30 min before first food, beverage, or medication of day. *Paget's disease of bone —* **Adults:** 40 mg P.O. q.d. for 6 mo, taken with plain water only, ≥ 30 min before first food, beverage, or medication of day.	• Correct hypocalcemia and other disturbances of mineral metabolism before therapy begins. • Patients should remain in upright position for at least 30 min after ingesting drug.

alfentanil hydrochloride

Alfenta

Opioid

Analgesic/adjunct to anesthesia/anesthetic

Pregnancy Risk Category: C

Controlled Substance

Schedule: II

Adjunct to general anesthetic — **Adults:** 8 to 50 mcg/kg I.V.; then increments of 3 to 15 mcg/kg I.V. q 5 to 20 min.
As primary anesthetic — **Adults:** initially, 130 to 245 mcg/kg I.V.; then 0.5 to 1.5 mcg/kg/min I.V.
Adjust-a-dose: In patients with renal or hepatic impairment, increase dosage interval to 6 to 8 hr.

- Should be administered only by persons specifically trained in I.V. anesthetic use.
- Use tuberculin syringe to give small volumes accurately.
- Monitor Sao₂.
- Keep narcotic antagonist and resuscitation equipment available when giving I.V.

alitretinoin

Panretin

Antikeratinizing agent (retinoid analogue)

Antineoplastic

Pregnancy Risk Category: D

Topical treatment of cutaneous lesions in patients with Kaposi's sarcoma related to AIDS — **Adults:** initially, apply generous coating of gel b.i.d. to lesions only. May increase to t.i.d. to q.i.d. If site toxicity occurs, may need to reduce frequency. If severe irritation occurs, drug may be stopped for a few days.

- Use sufficient gel to cover lesion with generous coating. Allow to dry for 3 to 5 min before covering with clothing.
- Avoid applying gel to normal skin surrounding lesions; don't apply gel on or near mucosal surfaces of body.
- Don't use occlusive dressings.

allopurinol

Lopurin, Purinol†, Zyloprim

Xanthine oxidase inhibitor

Antigout agent

Pregnancy Risk Category: C

Gout — Dosage varies with disease severity; divide doses > 300 mg. **Adults:** mild gout, 200 to 300 mg P.O. q.d.; severe gout, 400 to 600 mg P.O. q.d. Same dosage for maintenance in secondary hyperuricemia, up to 800 mg/day.
Hyperuricemia secondary to malignancies — **Children < 6 yr:** 50 mg P.O. t.i.d. **Children 6 to 10 yr:** 300 mg P.O. q.d. or divided t.i.d.
Prevention of acute gouty attacks — **Adults:** 100 mg P.O. q.d.; increase q wk by 100 mg up to maximum of 800 mg until serum uric acid ≤ 6 mg/dl.

- Monitor serum uric acid.
- Monitor I&O; daily output of ≥ 2 L and maintenance of neutral or slightly alkaline urine desirable.
- Periodically monitor CBC and hepatic and renal function.
- If renal insufficiency occurs, be prepared to reduce dosage.
- Optimal benefits may require 2 to 6 wk of therapy. Concurrent colchicine may be prescribed prophylactically for acute gouty attacks.

DRUG/CLASS/ CATEGORY	INDICATIONS/ DOSAGES	KEY NURSING CONSIDERATIONS
alprazolam Apo-Alprazt, Novo-Alprazlt, Nu-Alprazt, Xanax *Benzodiazepine* *Antianxiety agent* Pregnancy Risk Category: D Controlled Substance Schedule: IV	*Anxiety* — **Adults:** initially, 0.25 to 0.5 mg P.O. t.i.d., to maximum of 4 mg q.d. in divided doses. For elderly or debilitated patients or those with advanced liver disease, initially, 0.25 mg P.O. b.i.d. or t.i.d., to maximum of 4 mg q.d. in divided doses. *Panic disorders* — **Adults:** 0.5 mg P.O. t.i.d., increased q 3 to 4 days ≤ 1 mg. Maximum 10 mg q.d. in divided doses.	▪ Not to be used for everyday stress or for more than 4 mo. ▪ Warn not to withdraw abruptly after long-term use; withdrawal symptoms may occur. Abuse or addiction possible. ▪ In repeated or prolonged therapy, monitor liver, renal, and hematopoietic studies periodically as ordered.
alprostadil Caverject *Prostaglandin* *Corrective agent for impotence* Pregnancy Risk Category: NR	*Erectile dysfunction due to vasculogenic, psychogenic, or mixed etiology* — **Adults:** dosages highly individualized, with initial dose of 2.5 mcg intracavernously. If partial response occurs, give second dose of 2.5 mcg; then increase in increments of 5 to 10 mcg until suitable erection. If no response to initial dose, may increase second dose to 7.5 mcg within 1 hr; then increase in increments of 5 to 10 mcg until suitable erection. *Erectile dysfunction of neurologic etiology* — **Adults:** dosage individualized, with initial dose of 1.25 mcg intracavernously. If partial response occurs, give second dose of 1.25 mcg, followed by increments of 1.25 mcg, to dose of 5 mcg, and then in incre-	▪ Regular follow-up care with thorough exam of penis strongly recommended to detect penile fibrosis. ▪ Erection should occur 5 to 20 min after administration and should last preferably ≤ 1 hr. Erection lasting > 6 hr requires immediate medical intervention. With initial dosing, patient must stay in doctor's office until complete detumescence. ▪ Should not be used > 3 times/wk. Interval of at least 24 hr required between uses. ▪ Monitor for adverse reactions, such as penile redness, swelling, tenderness, curvature, unusual pain, nodules, or priapism. ▪ Bleeding at injection site may increase risk of transmitting blood-borne disease to sexual partner.

ments of 5 mcg until suitable erection. If no initial response, may give next higher dose within 1 hr.

alprostadil
Prostin VR Pediatric
Prostaglandin
Ductus arteriosus patency adjunct
Pregnancy Risk Category: NR

Palliative therapy for temporary maintenance of patency of ductus arteriosus until surgery — **Infants:** 0.05 to 0.1 mcg/kg/min I.V. infusion. When response achieved, reduce rate to lowest dosage that will maintain response; maximum 0.4 mcg/kg/min. Or, give through umbilical artery catheter placed at ductal opening.

- Not for use in neonatal respiratory distress syndrome.
- Don't use diluents with benzyl alcohol.
- If apnea and bradycardia occur, stop infusion immediately.
- In restricted pulmonary blood flow, monitor blood oxygenation. In restricted systemic blood flow, monitor systemic BP and blood pH.

alteplase (tissue plasminogen activator, recombinant; t-PA)
Activase‡, Activase
Enzyme
Thrombolytic enzyme
Pregnancy Risk Category: C

Lysis of thrombi obstructing coronary arteries in acute MI — **Adults:** 100 mg I.V. infusion over 3 hr as follows: 60 mg in 1st hr, of which 6 to 10 mg given as bolus over 1st 1 to 2 min. Then 20 mg/hr infusion for 2 hr. Smaller adults (< 65 kg [143 lb]) should receive 1.25 mg/kg in similar fashion (60% in 1st hr, 10% as bolus; then 20% of total dose per hr for 2 hr).
Management of acute massive pulmonary embolism — **Adults:** 100 mg I.V. infusion over 2 hr. Begin heparin at end of infusion when PTT or thrombin time returns to twice normal or less. Don't exceed 100-mg dose.
Acute ischemic stroke — **Adults:** 0.9 mg/kg I.V. infusion over 1 hr with 10% of total

- Must be initiated as soon as possible after symptom onset when used to recanalize occluded coronary arteries.
- *I.V. use:* Check manufacturer's labeling for specific reconstitution information.
- Monitor vital signs and neurologic status carefully. Keep patient on strict bed rest.
- Have antiarrhythmics readily available, and carefully monitor ECG.
- Avoid invasive procedures. Carefully monitor for signs of internal bleeding, and frequently check all puncture sites.
- If uncontrollable bleeding occurs, stop infusion and concomitant heparin), apply pressure to site if possible, and notify doctor.

(continued)

11

‡Canadian, †Australian

DRUG / CLASS / CATEGORY	INDICATIONS / DOSAGES	KEY NURSING CONSIDERATIONS
alteplase (continued)	dose given as initial I.V. bolus over 1 min. Maximum 90 mg total. *Note:* Give within 3 hr after symptoms occur and only when intracranial bleeding has been ruled out.	
aluminum carbonate Basaljel *Inorganic aluminum salt* Antacid/hypophosphatemic Pregnancy Risk Category: B	*Antacid* — **Adults:** 5 to 10 ml of oral suspension P.O. q 2 hr, p.r.n.; or 1 to 2 tablets or capsules P.O. q 2 hr, p.r.n. Maximum 24 capsules, tablets, or tsp/24 hr. *To prevent urinary phosphate stones* — **Adults:** 15 to 30 ml oral suspension in water or juice P.O. 1 hr after meals and h.s.; or 2 to 6 tablets or capsules 1 hr after meals and h.s.	• When giving drug through NG tube, ensure correct tube placement and patency; after instilling, flush tube with water. • Monitor long-term, high-dose use in patients on restricted sodium intake. • Watch for hypophosphatemia symptoms with prolonged use.
aluminum hydroxide AlternaGEL, Alu-Cap, Amphojel, Dialume, Nephrox *Aluminum salt* Antacid/hypophosphatemic agent/adsorbent Pregnancy Risk Category: C	*Antacid* — **Adults:** 500 to 1,500 mg P.O. (5 to 30 ml of most suspension products) three to six times a day between meals and h.s.; or, 300-mg or 600-mg tablets (chewed before swallowing) taken with milk or water five to six times daily after meals and h.s.	• When giving drug through NG tube, ensure correct tube placement and patency; after instilling, flush tube with water. • Monitor long-term, high-dose use in patients on restricted sodium intake. • Watch for hypophosphatemia symptoms with prolonged use.

amantadine hydrochloride

Symadine, Symmetrel

Synthetic cyclic primary amine

Antiviral/antiparkinsonian

Pregnancy Risk Category: C

Prophylaxis or symptomatic treatment of influenza type A virus, respiratory tract illnesses — **Adults ≤ 65 yr with normal renal function and children > 9 yr weighing > 45 kg (99 lb):** 200 mg P.O. q.d. in single dose or divided b.i.d. **Children 1 to 9 yr or < 45 kg:** 4.4 to 8.8 mg/kg P.O. q.d. as single dose or divided b.i.d., up to 150 mg q.d. **Adults > 65 yr with normal renal function:** 100 mg P.O. q.d. Start treatment within 24 to 48 hr after symptoms appear and continue for 24 to 48 hr after they disappear. Start as soon as possible after initial exposure.

Parkinson's disease — **Adults:** 100 mg P.O. b.i.d. In patients receiving other antiparkinsonians or those who are seriously ill, 100 mg P.O. q.d. for 1 wk; then 100 mg P.O. b.i.d. May increase to 400 mg/day.

Adjust-a-dose: Patients with renal dysfunction should have maintenance dose based on creatinine clearance.

- Elderly patients are more susceptible to adverse neurologic effects.
- If insomnia occurs, advise taking drug several hr before bedtime.
- Use cautiously in elderly patients and in those with seizure disorders, heart failure, peripheral edema, hepatic illness, mental illness, eczematoid rash, renal impairment, orthostatic hypotension, or cardiovascular disease.
- If patient is also taking anticholinergic, dosage of anticholinergic may be reduced before start of amantadine therapy.
- Don't discontinue abruptly in patients with Parkinson's disease.
- If orthostatic hypotension occurs, instruct patient to stand or change position slowly.
- Observe for adverse reactions, especially dizziness, depression, anxiety, nausea, and urine retention.

amifostine

Ethyol

Organic thiophosphate

Cytoprotective agent

Pregnancy Risk Category: C

Reduction of cumulative renal toxicity associated with repeated cisplatin administration in patients with advanced ovarian cancer or non-small-cell lung cancer — **Adults:** 910 mg/m² q.d. as 15-min I.V. infusion, starting 30 min before chemotherapy. If hypotension occurs and BP doesn't return to normal within 5 min after treatment stops, use dose of 740 mg/m² for subsequent cycles.

- Should stop antihypertensive therapy 24 hr before amifostine administration.
- Patient should be adequately hydrated before administration. Keep supine during infusion. Monitor I&O.
- Monitor BP q 5 min during infusion.
- Don't infuse drug for > 15 min. Longer infusion has been associated with higher incidence of adverse reactions.

13

DRUG / CLASS / CATEGORY	INDICATIONS / DOSAGES	KEY NURSING CONSIDERATIONS
amikacin sulfate Amikin *Aminoglycoside* *Antibiotic* Pregnancy Risk Category: D	*Serious infections caused by sensitive strains of susceptible organisms* — **Adults and children:** 15 mg/kg/day divided q 8 to 12 hr by I.M. or I.V. infusion. **Neonates:** loading dose of 10 mg/kg I.V.: then 7.5 mg/kg q 12 hr. *Uncomplicated UTI* — **Adults:** 250 mg I.M. or I.V. b.i.d. **Adjust-a-dose:** Adults with renal dysfunction, intially 7.5 mg/kg I.V. or I.M. Subsequent doses and frequency based on blood levels and renal function studies.	▪ Obtain specimen for culture and sensitivity tests before 1st dose. ▪ Evaluate weight, hearing, and renal function before and during therapy. ▪ Peak levels > 35 mcg/ml and trough levels > 10 mcg/ml may indicate toxicity. ▪ Give I.V. infusions in 100 to 200 ml D₅W or 0.9% NaCl solution over 30 to 60 min.
amiloride hydrochloride Kalurit‡, Midamor *Potassium-sparing diuretic* *Diuretic/antihypertensive* Pregnancy Risk Category: B	*Hypertension; edema associated with heart failure, usually in patients also taking thiazide or other potassium-wasting diuretics* — **Adults:** initial dose 5 mg P.O. q.d. Increase to 10 mg q.d. if necessary. Maximum 20 mg daily.	▪ To prevent nausea, administer with meals. ▪ Monitor serum potassium. Alert doctor immediately if level is > 5.5 mEq/L, and expect to discontinue.
amino acid infusions Aminosyn, Aminosyn II in Dextrose, Aminosyn II with Electrolytes in Dextrose, Aminosyn-HBC, Aminosyn-	*TPN in patients who can't or won't eat* — **Adults:** 1 to 1.5 g/kg I.V. q.d. **Children < 10 kg (22 lb):** 2 to 4 g/kg I.V. q.d. **Children > 10 kg:** 2 to 2.5 g/kg I.V. q.d. for first 10 kg; then 1 to 1.25 g/kg I.V. q.d for each kg over 10 kg.	▪ Obtain baseline serum electrolytes, glucose, BUN, calcium, and phosphorus levels before therapy, as ordered. Monitor periodically throughout therapy. ▪ Limit peripheral infusions to 2.5% amino acids and dextrose 10%. Check infusion

RF, FreAmine III, Hepat-Amine, Travasol with Electrolytes
Protein substrates
Parenteral nutritional thera-py/caloric agent
Pregnancy Risk Category: C

Nutritional support in cirrhosis, hepatitis, and hepatic encephalopathy — **Adults:** 80 to 120 g of amino acids I.V. q.d. (hepatic failure form).
Nutritional support in high metabolic stress — **Adults:** 1.5 g/kg I.V. q.d. (high metabolic stress form).
Nutritional support in renal failure — **Adults:** 0.3 to 0.5 g/kg I.V. q.d. (maximum 26 g q.d.). Dialysis patients may require 1 to 1.2 g/kg q.d.

site frequently. Change peripheral sites routinely. If subclavian catheter is used, administer solution into midsuperior vena cava.

- Assess body temperature q 4 hr. If chills, fever, or other signs of sepsis occur, re-place I.V. tubing and bottle and send to lab for culture.

- Administer cautiously to diabetics and to patients with cardiac insufficiency.

---

aminocaproic acid
Amicar
Carboxylic acid derivative
Fibrinolysis inhibitor
Pregnancy Risk Category: C

Excessive bleeding resulting from hyperfib-rinolysis — **Adults:** initially, 5 g P.O. or slow I.V. infusion; then 1 to 1.25 g hourly until bleeding controlled. Maximum 30 g daily.

- *I.V. use:* Dilute solution with sterile water for injection, 0.9% NaCl for injection, D_5W, or Ringer's injection. Infuse slowly. Don't give by direct or intermittent injection.

- Monitor coagulation studies, as ordered, and HR and BP. Notify doctor immediately of any change.

---

aminoglutethimide
Cytadren
Antiadrenal hormone
Antineoplastic
Pregnancy Risk Category: D

Suppression of adrenal function in Cush-ing's syndrome and adrenal cancer — **Adults:** 250 mg q 6 hr. May increase dosage in increments of 250 mg q.d. q 1 to 2 wk, to maximum 2 g daily.

- Monitor BP frequently; monitor CBC and thyroid function tests periodically, as or-dered.

- May cause adrenal hypofunction, especially in stressful circumstances. Patients may need mineralocorticoid and glucocorticoid replacement. Monitor such patients carefully.

DRUG / CLASS / CATEGORY

aminophylline (theophylline ethylenediamine)
Phyllocontin, Truphylline
Xanthine derivative
Bronchodilator
Pregnancy Risk Category: C

INDICATIONS / DOSAGES

Symptomatic relief of acute broncho-spasm — **Patients not taking theophylline:** loading dose 6 mg/kg (equivalent to 4.7 mg/kg anhydrous theophylline) I.V.; then maintenance dose infusion. **Adults (nonsmokers) not taking theophylline:** 0.7 mg/kg/hr I.V. for 12 hr; then 0.5 mg/kg/hr. **Otherwise healthy adult smokers not taking theophylline:** 1 mg/kg/hr I.V. for 12 hr; then 0.8 mg/kg/hr. **Children 9 to 16 yr not taking theophylline:** 1 mg/kg/hr I.V. for 12 hr; then 0.8 mg/kg/hr. **Children 6 mo to 9 yr not taking theophylline:** 1.2 mg/kg/hr for 12 hr; then 1 mg/kg/hr.
Patients taking theophylline: Determine time, amount, route, and form of last dose. Infusions of 0.63 mg/kg (0.5 mg/kg anhydrous theophylline) increase plasma drug level by 1 mcg/ml. If no signs of toxicity, 3.1 mg/kg (2.5 mg/kg anhydrous theophylline).
Chronic bronchial asthma — **Adults and children:** 16 mg/kg or 400 mg (whichever less) P.O. q.d. in divided doses q 6 to 8 hr (for rapidly absorbed forms). May increase by 25% q 2 to 3 days. Or, 12 mg/kg or 400 mg (whichever less) P.O. q.d. in divided doses q 8 to 12 hr (for extended-release forms). May increase by 2 to 3 mg/kg q.d. q 3 days.

KEY NURSING CONSIDERATIONS

- Before loading dose, ensure that patient hasn't had recent theophylline therapy.
- Relieve GI symptoms by giving oral drug with full glass of water at meals (although food in stomach delays absorption).
- *I.V. use:* I.V. administration can cause burning; dilute with compatible I.V. solution and inject no faster than 25 mg/min.
- Monitor serum theophylline. Desirable levels is 10 to 20 mcg/ml; toxicity reported at > 20 mcg/ml.
- Inform elderly patient that dizziness is common adverse effect.
- Caution patient not to switch brands.
- Instruct patient to check with doctor or pharmacist before taking with other drugs.
- Rectal dosage same as recommended oral dosage.

amiodarone hydrochloride
Aratac, Cordarone, Cordarone X‡
Benzofuran derivative
Antiarrhythmic
Pregnancy Risk Category: D

Recurrent ventricular fibrillation and recurrent hemodynamically unstable ventricular tachycardia refractory to other antiarrhythmics — **Adults:** loading dose 800 to 1,600 mg P.O. q.d. for 1 to 3 wk until initial response; then 600 to 800 mg/day P.O. for 1 mo and maintenance of 200 to 600 mg/day P.O. q.d. Or, loading dose 150 mg I.V. over 10 min (15 mg/min); then 360 mg I.V. over next 6 hr (1 mg/min); then 540 mg I.V. over next 18 hr (0.5 mg/min). After 1st 24 hr, continue maintenance infusion of 720 mg/24 hr (0.5 mg/min).

- Obtain baseline thyroid and liver function tests.
- Continuously monitor cardiac status of patient receiving drug I.V.
- High incidence of adverse reactions limits use.
- Monitor carefully for pulmonary toxicity, which can be fatal. Incidence increases with doses > 400 mg/day.
- Methylcellulose ophthalmic solution recommended during therapy to minimize corneal microdeposits.

amitriptyline hydrochloride
Apo-Amitriptyline†, Elavil
TCA
Antidepressant
Pregnancy Risk Category: NR

Depression — **Adults:** initially, 50 to 100 mg P.O. h.s., increased to 150 mg q.d.; maximum 300 mg q.d., if needed. Maintenance: 50 to 100 mg/day P.O. or 20 to 30 mg I.M. q.i.d. **Elderly patients and adolescents:** 10 mg P.O. t.i.d. and 20 mg h.s. q.d.

- Parenteral form for I.M. use only.
- Has strong anticholinergic effects and is one of most sedating tricyclic antidepressants.
- If signs of psychosis occur or worsen, expect to reduce dosage.
- Don't withdraw abruptly.

amlodipine besylate
Norvasc
Dihydropyridine calcium channel blocker
Antianginal/antihypertensive
Pregnancy Risk Category: C

Chronic stable angina; vasospastic angina — **Adults:** initially, 5 to 10 mg P.O. q.d. *Hypertension —* **Adults:** initially, 2.5 to 5 mg P.O. q.d. **Elderly:** 2.5 mg P.O. q.d. With small or frail patients, those receiving other antihypertensives, or those with hepatic insufficiency, begin at 2.5 mg q.d. Adjust according to response. Maximum 10 mg/day. Adjust over 7 to 14 days.

- Monitor carefully for increased frequency, duration, or severity of angina or acute MI.
- Monitor BP frequently when therapy begins.
- Notify doctor if patient has signs of heart failure (shortness of breath, swelling of hands and feet).

DRUG / CLASS / CATEGORY	INDICATIONS / DOSAGES	KEY NURSING CONSIDERATIONS
amoxapine Asendin *Dibenzoxazepine* *TCA* Pregnancy Risk Category: C	*Depression —* **Adults:** 50 mg P.O. b.i.d. or t.i.d., increased to 100 mg b.i.d or t.i.d by end of 1st wk if tolerated. Make increases > 300 mg q.d. only if this dose ineffective during trial of at least 2 wk. Maximum recommended for outpatients, 400 mg q.d. When effective dose established, entire dose (≤ 300 mg) may be given h.s. **Elderly:** 25 mg b.i.d or t.i.d. If tolerated by end of 1st wk, increase to 50 mg b.i.d. or t.i.d. Carefully increase up to 300 mg q.d.	• Use with extreme caution in patients with history of seizure disorders. • Full effect may take 4 wk or more. • If signs of psychosis occur or worsen, expect to reduce dosage. • Monitor for tardive dyskinesia, especially in elderly women. • Drug has been linked to neuroleptic malignant syndrome.
amoxicillin/clavulanate potassium (amoxycillin/clavulanate potassium) Augmentin, Clavulin† *Aminopenicillin and beta-lactamase inhibitor* *Antibiotic* Pregnancy Risk Category: B	*Lower respiratory infections, otitis media, sinusitis, skin and skin-structure infections, and UTIs caused by susceptible strains of gram-positive and gram-negative organisms —* **Adults and children ≥ 40 kg (88 lb):** 250 to 500 mg (based on amoxicillin component) P.O. q 8 hr. **Children < 40 kg:** 20 to 40 mg/kg (based on amoxicillin component) P.O. daily in divided doses q 8 hr.	• Assess history of drug allergies. • Obtain specimen for culture and sensitivity tests before first dose. • Know that two 250-mg tablets are not equivalent to one 500-mg tablet. • Give at least 1 hr before bacteriostatic antibiotics. • Advise to take with food. • Instruct to call doctor if rash occurs.
amoxicillin trihydrate (amoxycillin trihydrate) Amoxil, Cilamox‡, Larotid, Polymox, Trimox, Wymox	*Systemic infections, acute and chronic UTIs caused by susceptible strains of gram-positive and gram-negative organisms —* **Adults and children ≥ 20 kg (44 lb):** 250 to 500 mg P.O. q 8 hr. **Children < 20 kg:** 20	• Assess history of allergic reactions to penicillin. (However, negative history doesn't preclude future reactions.) • Obtain specimen for culture and sensitivity tests before first dose.

Aminopenicillin
Antibiotic
Pregnancy Risk Category: NR

mg/kg P.O. q.d. in divided doses q 8 hr; in severe infection, 40 mg/kg P.O. in divided doses q 8 hr or 500 mg to 1 g/m² P.O. in divided doses q 8 hr.

Uncomplicated gonorrhea — **Adults and children > 45 kg (99 lb):** 3 g P.O. with 1 g probenecid as single dose. Don't give to children < 2 yr.

Endocarditis prophylaxis for dental procedures — **Adults:** 2 g P.O. as single dose 1 hr before procedure. **Children > 2 yr:** 50 mg/kg P.O. as single dose 1 hr before procedure.

- With prolonged therapy, observe for fungal or bacterial superinfection, especially in elderly, debilitated, or immunosuppressed patients.
- Give at least 1 hr before bacteriostatic antibiotics.
- Advise patient taking oral suspension form that drug can be stored at room temperature for up to 2 wk, but is preferable to store in refrigerator.

---

amphotericin B
Amphocin, Amphotericin B for Injection, Fungilin Oral‡, Fungizone Intravenous
Polyene macrolide
Antifungal
Pregnancy Risk Category: B

Systemic fungal infections; meningitis — **Adults:** test dose of 1 mg in 20 ml D₅W infused I.V. over 20 to 30 min may be recommended. If tolerated, start as 0.25 to 0.3 mg/kg/day by slow I.V. infusion (0.1 mg/ml) over 2 to 6 hr. Increase dosage gradually to maximum of 1 mg/kg q.d. If stopped for ≥ 1 wk, resume drug with initial dose and increase gradually.

GI tract infections caused by Candida albicans — **Adults:** 100 mg P.O. q.i.d. for 2 wk.

Oral and perioral candidal infections — **Adults:** 1 lozenge q.i.d. for 7 to 14 days. Lozenge should dissolve slowly.

- For severe reactions, discontinue and notify doctor.
- *I.V. use:* Monitor pulse, respiratory rate, temperature, and BP for at least 4 hr with initial test dose.
- Monitor vital signs q 30 min; fever, shaking chills, and hypotension may appear 1 to 2 hr after I.V. infusion starts and should subside within 4 hr of stopping drug.
- Report change in urine appearance or volume. Monitor BUN and creatinine q wk.
- Use infusion pump and in-line filter with mean pore diameter > 1 micron.

DRUG/CLASS/CATEGORY	INDICATIONS/DOSAGES	KEY NURSING CONSIDERATIONS
amphotericin B cholesteryl sulfate complex Amphotec *Polyene macrolide* *Antifungal* Pregnancy Risk Category: B	*Invasive aspergillosis in patients in whom renal impairment or unacceptable toxicity precludes use of amphotericin B deoxycholate or in those with invasive aspergillosis in whom prior amphotericin B deoxycholate therapy has failed —* **Adults and children:** 3 to 4 mg/kg/day I.V. Dilute in D₅W and administer by continuous infusion at 1 mg/kg/hr. Perform a test dose before beginning new course of treatment; infuse a small amount of drug (10 ml of final preparation containing 1.6 to 8.3 mg of drug) over 15 to 30 min and monitor for next 30 min. Can shorten infusion time to 2 hr or lengthen infusion time based on patient tolerance.	▪ Monitor I&O; report changes in urine appearance or volume. ▪ Monitor renal and hepatic function tests, serum electrolytes, CBC, and PT. ▪ *I.V. use:* Reconstitute with sterile water for injection only and dilute in D₅W. Drug is incompatible with saline, electrolyte solutions, and bacteriostatic agents. ▪ Pretreating with antihistamines and corticosteroids or reducing rate of infusion (or both) may reduce the acute infusion-related reactions. ▪ Monitor vital signs every 30 min during initial therapy. Acute infusion-related reactions usually occur 1 to 3 hr after starting I.V. infusion.
ampicillin sodium/sulbactam sodium Unasyn *Aminopenicillin/beta-lactamase inhibitor combination* *Antibiotic* Pregnancy Risk Category: B	*Intra-abdominal, gynecologic, and skin-structure infections caused by susceptible strains —* **Adults and children ≥ 40 kg (88 lb):** dosage expressed as total drug (each 1.5-g vial contains 1 g ampicillin sodium and 0.5 g sulbactam sodium) — 1.5 to 3 g I.M. or I.V. q 6 hr. Maximum daily dose 4 g sulbactam and 8 g ampicillin (12 g of combined drugs). **Children ≥ 1 yr and ≥ 40 kg:** 300 mg/kg/day I.V. divided equally q 6 hr.	▪ Assess history of allergic reactions to penicillin. (However, negative history doesn't preclude future reactions.) ▪ Obtain specimen for culture and sensitivity tests before first dose. ▪ *I.V. use:* Give I.V. over 10 to 15 min, or dilute in 50 to 100 ml of compatible diluent and infuse over 15 to 30 min. If permitted, give intermittently. Change site every 48 hr.

- For I.M. injection, reconstitute with sterile water for injection or 0.5% or 2% lidocaine.

Adjust-a-dose: Dose adjustment necessary in patients with renal insufficiency.

amprenavir
Agenerase
*HIV protease inhibitor/
sulfonamide*
Antiretroviral
Pregnancy Risk Category: C

Treatment of HIV-1 infection in combination with other antiretroviral agents — **Adults and children 13 to 16 yr weighing > 50 kg (110 lb):** 1,200 mg P.O. b.i.d. **Children 4 to 12 yr or 13 to 16 yr and weighing < 50 kg:** *Capsules:* 20 mg/kg P.O. b.i.d. or 15 mg/kg P.O. t.i.d. (to a maximum daily dose of 2,400 mg). *Oral solution:* 22.5 mg/kg P.O. (1.5 ml/kg) b.i.d. or 17 mg/kg P.O. (1.1 ml/kg) t.i.d. (to a maximum daily dose of 2,800 mg).

Adjust-a-dose: Use with caution in patients with moderate or severe hepatic impairment. In those with Child-Pugh score of 5 to 8, reduce capsule dose to 450 mg b.i.d. In those with a Child-Pugh score of 9 to 12, reduce capsule dose to 300 mg b.i.d.

- Don't give with astemizole, bepridil, cisapride, dihydroergotamine, midazolam, rifampin, sildenafil, triazolam, or vitamin E. Obtain a drug history.
- Always use in combination with other antiretroviral agents.
- Know that capsules and oral solution are not interchangeable on a mg per mg basis.
- Use cautiously in patients with sulfonamide allergy.
- Instruct patients receiving hormonal contraceptives to use alternative contraceptives during therapy.
- Know that high fat meals may decrease absorption of drug.

amrinone lactate
Inocor
Bipyridine derivative
Inotropic/vasodilator
Pregnancy Risk Category: C

Short-term management of heart failure — **Adults:** initially, 0.75 mg/kg I.V. bolus over 2 to 3 min. Then start maintenance infusion of 5 to 10 mcg/kg/min. May give additional bolus of 0.75 mg/kg 30 min after therapy starts. Don't exceed 10 mg/kg total daily dose. Dosage depends on clinical response.

- Primarily given to patients unresponsive to cardiac glycosides, diuretics, and vasodilators.
- Don't dilute with solution containing dextrose. Can be injected into free-flowing dextrose infusions through Y-connector or directly into tubing.
- Monitor BP and HR throughout infusion.
- Drug contains bisulfites; use with caution in sulfite-sensitive patients.

21

DRUG/CLASS/ CATEGORY	INDICATIONS/ DOSAGES	KEY NURSING CONSIDERATIONS
anagrelide hydrochloride Agrylin *Platelet-reducing agent* *Anticoagulant* Pregnancy Risk Category: C	*Treatment of patients with essential thrombocythemia to reduce elevated platelet count and risk of thrombosis and to ameliorate associated symptoms* — **Adults:** 0.5 mg P.O. q.i.d. or 1 mg P.O. b.i.d. for at least 1 wk; then lowest effective dose required to maintain platelet count below 600,000/mm³ and, ideally, to normal range. Do not increase dosage by more than 0.5 mg/day in any 1 wk; do not exceed 10 mg/day or 2.5 mg in single dose.	■ Use cautiously in patients with cardiovascular disease or serum creatinine over 2 mg/dl and in those with liver function tests exceeding 1.5 times the upper normal limits. ■ Use cautiously in breast-feeding women. ■ During first 2 wk of treatment, monitor blood counts and liver and renal function tests. ■ Monitor patient for bleeding, bruising, and cardiac symptoms. ■ Give drug 1 hr before or 2 hr after meals.
anastrozole Arimidex *Nonsteroidal aromatase inhibitor* *Antineoplastic* Pregnancy Risk Category: D	*Treatment of advanced breast cancer in postmenopausal women with disease progression after tamoxifen therapy* — **Adults:** 1 mg P.O. q.d.	■ Use cautiously in breast-feeding women. ■ Give under supervision of qualified doctor experienced in use of anticancer drugs.
antihemophilic factor (AHF) Hemofil M, Humate-P, Hyate:C, Koate-HP, Koate-HS *Blood derivative* *Antihemophilic* Pregnancy Risk Category: C	*Spontaneous hemorrhage in patients with hemophilia A (factor VIII deficiency)* — **Adults and children:** calculate dosage using this formula: AHF required (IU) = body weight (kg) × desired factor VIII increase (% of normal) ×0.5.	■ Monitor coagulation studies and vital signs before and regularly during therapy. Monitor for hemolysis if patient has blood type A, B, or AB. ■ Change in urine color to orange or red hue may signify hemolytic reaction. ■ Refrigerate concentrate until ready to use. Warm concentrate and diluent bottle to

To prevent spontaneous hemorrhage, desired level of factor VIII is 5% of normal; for mild hemorrhage, 30% of normal; for moderate hemorrhage and minor surgery, 30% to 50% of normal; for severe hemorrhage, 80% to 100% of normal.

Treatment of bleeding in patients with hemophilia A — **Adults and children:** for minor hemorrhage into muscle and joints, 8 to 10 IU/kg I.V. (or calculated dose to raise plasma factor VIII levels to 20% to 40% of normal) q 8 to 12 hr for 1 to 3 days, p.r.n.

For overt bleeding, initial dose of 15 to 25 IU/kg I.V., followed by 8 to 15 IU/kg q 8 to 12 hr for 3 to 4 days. To treat massive bleeding or hemorrhage involving major organs, initial dose of 40 to 50 IU/kg I.V., followed by 20 to 25 IU/kg I.V. q 8 to 12 hr.

Prevention of bleeding in hemophilic patients requiring surgery — **Adults:** 25 to 30 IU/kg I.V. 1 hr before surgery, followed by half of initial dose 5 hr later. Dosage adjusted to achieve level of AHF 80% to 100% of normal during surgery and maintained at 30% to 60% of normal for 10 to 14 days postoperatively.

room temperature before reconstituting. To mix drug, gently roll vial between hands.

- **I.V. use:** Use plastic syringe; drug may interact with glass syringe and bind to surface.
- Use reconstituted solution within 3 hr. Store away from heat and don't refrigerate. Don't shake or mix with other I.V. solutions. Filter solution before administration.
- Don't give S.C. or I.M.
- Some patients develop inhibitors to factor VIII, resulting in decreased drug response.
- Monitor for allergic reactions.
- Risk of hepatitis must be weighed against risks involved if patient doesn't receive drug.
- Because of manufacturing process, risk of HIV transmission is extremely low.

DRUG / CLASS / CATEGORY

antithrombin III, human (AT-III, heparin cofactor I)
ATnativ, Thrombate III
Glycoprotein
Anticoagulant/antithrombotic
Pregnancy Risk Category: C

INDICATIONS / DOSAGES

Thromboembolism associated with hereditary AT-III deficiency — **Adults and children:** initial dose individualized to quantity required to increase AT-III activity to 120% of normal activity as determined 30 min after administration. Usual dose 50 to 100 IU/min I.V., not to exceed 100 IU/min. Dose calculated based on anticipated 1% increase in plasma AT-III activity produced by 1 IU/kg of body weight using the formula:

Dose required (IU) = (desired activity [%] − baseline activity [%]) × weight (kg) ÷ 1.4

Maintenance dose individualized to quantity required to increase AT-III activity to 80% of normal activity, and given at 24-hr intervals. To calculate subsequent doses, multiply desired AT-III activity (as percentage of normal) minus baseline AT-III activity (as percentage of normal) by body weight (in kg). Divide by actual increase in AT-III activity (as percentage) produced by 1 IU/kg as determined 30 min after initial dose given. Treatment usually continues for 2 to 8 days but may be prolonged in pregnancy or when used with surgery or immobilization.

KEY NURSING CONSIDERATIONS

- **I.V. use:** Reconstitute using 10 ml of sterile water (provided). 0.9% NaCl solution, or D₅W. Don't shake vial. Dilute further in same diluent solution if desired.
- Obtain AT-III activity levels b.i.d. until dosage requirement stabilizes, then q.d. immediately before dose. Functional assays preferred.
- Monitor for dyspnea and increased BP, which may occur with too-rapid administration rate.
- Heparin binds to AT-III lysine binding sites, resulting in increased heparin efficacy.
- 1 IU equivalent to quantity of endogenous AT-III present in 1 ml normal human plasma.
- Prepared from pooled plasma from human donors; carries minimal risk of transmission of viruses, including hepatitis and HIV.
- Risk of neonatal thromboembolism (sometimes fatal) in children of parents with hereditary AT-III deficiency. Obtain AT-III levels immediately after birth.

apraclonidine hydrochloride
Iopidine
Alpha-adrenergic agonist
Ocular hypotensive agent
Pregnancy Risk Category: C

Prevention or control of elevated IOP before and after ocular laser surgery — **Adults:** 1 drop of 1% solution instilled 1 hr before initiation of laser surgery on anterior segment; then 1 drop immediately after surgery.
Short-term adjunct therapy in patients who require additional IOP reduction — **Adults:** 1 or 2 drops of 0.5% solution instilled into affected eye t.i.d.

- Allow 5 min to elapse between each drop.
- Closely monitor patients who tend to develop exaggerated IOP decreases after drug therapy.
- Observe closely for vasovagal attack during laser surgery.
- Closely monitor patients with severe systemic disease, including hypertension.

aprotinin
Trasylol
Naturally occurring protease inhibitor
Systemic hemostatic agent
Pregnancy Risk Category: B

To reduce blood loss or need for transfusion in patients undergoing CABG — **Adults:** 10,000 U (1 ml) test dose ≥ 10 min before loading dose. If no allergic reaction, anesthesia may be induced while loading dose of 2 million U is given slowly over 20 to 30 min. When loading dose is complete, sternotomy may be performed. Before bypass is initiated, cardiopulmonary bypass circuit is primed with 2 million U of drug by replacing aliquot of priming fluid with drug. Continuous infusion at 500,000 U/hr is given until patient leaves operating room. This is *regimen A*. Or, *regimen B* may be used: give half dosage of *regimen A* (except for test dose).

- Be prepared to administer test dose. Test dose particularly important in patients with history of allergies or who have previously received drug. In such patients, pretreat with antihistamine, as ordered.
- Monitor closely for hypersensitivity reaction. Patient may experience anaphylaxis even if no symptoms occurred with test dose. If hypersensitivity symptoms occur, stop infusion immediately, notify doctor, and provide supportive treatment.
- Administer through central line. Don't mix with other drugs.
- Monitor for signs of nephrotoxicity.

25

†Canadian. ‡Australian

DRUG/CLASS/ CATEGORY	INDICATIONS/ DOSAGES	KEY NURSING CONSIDERATIONS
ardeparin sodium Normiflo Injection *Low-molecular-weight heparin* *Anticoagulant* Pregnancy Risk Category: C	*Prevention of deep vein thrombosis that may lead to pulmonary embolism following knee replacement surgery* — **Adults:** 50 anti-Xa U/kg S.C. q 12 hr for 14 days or until patient is ambulatory, whichever is shorter. Give initial dose in evening of day of surgery or following morning.	• Use cautiously in patients at increased risk for hemorrhage. • Administer drug with deep S.C. injection. Don't rub injection site. • Know that ardeparin cannot be used interchangeably (unit for unit) with heparin sodium or other low-molecular-weight heparins. • Bleeding is the principal sign of drug overdose. • Routinely monitor CBC, platelet counts, urinalysis, and occult blood in stools. Monitoring of coagulation parameters not required.
asparaginase (L-asparaginase) Elspar, Kidrolase† *Enzyme* *Antineoplastic* Pregnancy Risk Category: C	*Acute lymphocytic leukemia (in combination with other drugs)* — **Adults and children:** 1,000 IU/kg I.V. q.d. for 10 days, injected over 30 min; or 6,000 IU/m² I.M. at intervals specified in protocol. *Sole induction agent for acute lymphocytic leukemia* — **Adults:** 200 IU/kg I.V. q.d. for 28 days.	• Risk of hypersensitivity increases with repeated doses. Intradermal skin test should be done. • Monitor CBC, bleeding studies, glucose, and serum amylase levels. • If drug contacts skin, flush with copious amounts of water for ≥ 15 min. • *I.V. use:* Administer through side arm of infusion of normal saline or D₅W. • Limit I.M. injection to 2 ml.

aspirin (acetylsalicylic acid)

A.S.A., Ascriptin, Bayer
Timed-Release, Bufferin,
Ecotrin
Salicylate
Nonnarcotic analgesic/
antipyretic/anti-inflammatory/antiplatelet
Pregnancy Risk Category: C
(D in third trimester)

*Rheumatoid arthritis; other inflammatory
conditions* — **Adults:** initially, 2.4 to 3.6 g
P.O. q.d. in divided doses. Maintenance: 3.2
to 6 g P.O. q.d. in divided doses.
Mild pain or fever — **Adults and children
> 11 yr:** 325 to 650 mg P.O. or P.R. q 4 hr,
p.r.n. **Children 2 to 11 yr :** 10 to 15 mg/kg
P.O. or P.R. q 4 hr up to 60 to 80 mg/kg/day.
Reduction of MI risk in patients with previous MI or unstable angina — **Adults:** 160 to
325 mg P.O. q.d.
MI prophylaxis — **Adults:** 160 to 325 mg
P.O. q.d.

- Don't give to children or teenagers with
chickenpox or flulike illness; use cautiously
at all times.
- Give on scheduled basis for inflammatory
conditions, rheumatic fever, and thrombosis.
- Monitor blood drug levels. Tinnitus may
occur at 30 mg/100 ml and above.
- During prolonged therapy, periodically assess Hct, Hgb, PT, and renal function.
- Instruct to discontinue aspirin 5 to 7 days
before elective surgery.

atenolol

Apo-Atenolol†, Noten‡,
Nu-Atenol†, Tenormin
Beta blocker
Antihypertensive/antianginal
Pregnancy Risk Category: D

Hypertension — **Adults:** initially, 50 mg P.O.
q.d. as single dose, increased to 100 mg
once daily after 7 to 14 days. Dosages > 100
mg unlikely to bring further benefit.
Angina pectoris — **Adults:** 50 mg P.O. once
daily, increased to 100 mg q.d. after 7 days
for optimal effect. Maximum 200 mg q.d.
To reduce CV mortality and risk of reinfarction in acute MI — **Adults:** 5 mg I.V., repeat
10 min later. After additional 10 min, 50 mg
P.O.; then 50 mg P.O. in 12 hr. Then, 100 mg
P.O. q.d. (or 50 mg b.i.d.) for ≥ 7 days.
Adjust-a-dose: Patients with creatinine
clearance < 35 ml/min require dosage adjustment.

- If apical pulse < 60, withhold drug and call
doctor.
- *I.V. use:* Give by slow I.V. injection, not
exceeding 1 mg/min.
- Monitor BP.
- Caution not to increase dosage without
consulting doctor. High dosages may lead
to arrhythmias.
- Instruct to take on empty stomach at least
2 hr after meals and avoid eating for at
least 1 hr after taking.
- Withdraw gradually over 2 wk.

DRUG/CLASS/CATEGORY	INDICATIONS/DOSAGES	KEY NURSING CONSIDERATIONS
atorvastatin calcium Lipitor *Hydroxymethylglutaryl-coenzyme A reductase inhibitor* *Antilipemic* Pregnancy Risk Category: X	*Adjunct to diet in primary hypercholesterolemia and mixed dyslipidemia* — **Adults:** 10 mg P.O. q.d.; increase as needed to maximum of 80 mg q.d. Dosage based on blood lipid levels drawn 2 to 4 wk after therapy starts. *Alone or as adjunct to lipid-lowering treatments in homozygous familial hypercholesterolemia* — **Adults:** 10 to 80 mg P.O. q.d.	▪ Initiate only after diet and other nonpharmacologic treatments prove ineffective. ▪ Obtain periodic liver function tests and lipid levels before initiating drug, 6 and 12 wk after initiation or after dosage increase, and periodically thereafter. ▪ Watch for signs of myositis.
atovaquone Mepron *Ubiquinone analogue* *Antiprotozoal* Pregnancy Risk Category: C	*Acute, mild to moderate Pneumocystis carinii pneumonia in patients who can't tolerate co-trimoxazole* — **Adults:** 750 mg P.O. b.i.d. with food for 21 days.	▪ Risk of concurrent pulmonary infections; monitor patient closely during therapy. ▪ Instruct to take with meals.
atropine sulfate (systemic) *Anticholinergic/belladonna alkaloid* *Antiarrhythmic/vagolytic* Pregnancy Risk Category: C	*Symptomatic bradycardia, bradyarrhythmia* — **Adults:** usually 0.5 to 1 mg I.V. push; repeat q 3 to 5 min to maximum of 2 mg as needed. **Children:** 0.01 mg/kg I.V.; may repeat q 4 to 6 hr; maximum of 0.4 mg or 0.3 mg/m². *Preoperatively to diminish secretions and block cardiac vagal reflexes* — **Adults and children ≥ 20 kg (44 lb):** 0.4 to 0.6 mg I.M. or S.C. 30 to 60 min before anesthesia. **Children < 20 kg:** 0.01 mg/kg I.M. or S.C. (maximum 0.4 mg) 30 to 60 min before anesthesia.	▪ May administer via ET tube. Dose is 2 to 2½ times I.V. dose diluted with 10 ml 0.9% NaCl solution or sterile water. ▪ *I.V. use:* Administer by direct I.V. into large vein or I.V. tubing over at least 1 min. ▪ Monitor for paradoxical initial bradycardia (usually disappears within 2 min). ▪ Monitor I&O. Watch for urine retention and urinary hesitancy. ▪ Doses < 0.5 mg can cause bradycardia.

atropine sulfate (ophthalmic)

Atropisol, Atropt†, BufOpto Atropine, Isopto Atropine

Anticholinergic/belladonna alkaloid

Cycloplegic/mydriatic

Pregnancy Risk Category: C

Acute iritis; uveitis — **Adults:** 1 to 2 drops instilled into eyes up to t.i.d., or small strip of ointment applied to conjunctival sac up to t.i.d. **Children:** 1 to 2 drops of 0.5% solution instilled into eyes up to t.i.d., or 0.3 to 0.5 cm of ointment applied to conjunctival sac up to t.i.d.

Cycloplegic refraction — **Adults:** 1 to 2 drops of 1% solution instilled 1 hr before refraction. **Children:** 1 to 2 drops of 0.5% solution instilled in each eye b.i.d. for 1 to 3 days before eye exam and 1 hr before refraction.

- Not for internal use; signs of poisoning are disorientation and confusion. Antidote is physostigmine salicylate.
- Watch for signs of glaucoma: increased IOP (ocular pain, headache, progressive blurring of vision).
- Apply light finger pressure on lacrimal sac for 1 min after instillation.
- Excessive use in children and in certain susceptible patients may produce symptoms of atropine poisoning.

---

attapulgite

Children's Kaopectate, Diasorb, Donnagel, Fowler's†, Rheaban Maximum Strength

Hydrated magnesium aluminum silicate

Antidiarrheal

Pregnancy Risk Category: NR

Acute, nonspecific diarrhea — **Adults and adolescents:** 1.2 to 1.5 g (up to 3 g of Diasorb) P.O. after each loose bowel movement, up to 9 g/24 hr. **Children 6 to 12 yr:** 600 mg (suspension) or 750 mg (tablets) P.O. after each loose bowel movement, up to 4.2 g (suspension) or 4.5 g (tablets)/24 hr. **Children 3 to 6 yr:** 300 mg P.O. after each loose bowel movement, up to 2.1 g/24 hr.

- Don't give if diarrhea accompanied by fever or by blood or mucus in stool.
- Instruct to take after each loose bowel movement until diarrhea controlled.
- Advise to notify doctor if diarrhea not controlled within 48 hr or if fever develops.
- Instruct to chew tablets well before swallowing or to shake liquid well before measuring dose.

---

auranofin

Ridaura

Gold salt

Antarthritic

Pregnancy Risk Category: C

Rheumatoid arthritis — **Adults:** 6 mg P.O. q.d., either as 3 mg b.i.d. or 6 mg q.d. After 6 mo, may increase to 9 mg daily.

- Stop drug if monthly platelet count < 100,000/mm³, if Hgb drops suddenly, if granulocytes < 1,500/mm³, or if patient develops leukopenia or eosinophilia.
- Monitor urinalysis for proteinuria or hematuria.

DRUG / CLASS / CATEGORY	INDICATIONS / DOSAGES	KEY NURSING CONSIDERATIONS
aurothioglucose Gold-50‡, Solganal **gold sodium thiomalate** Myochrysine *Gold salt* *Antarthritic* Pregnancy Risk Category: C	*Rheumatoid arthritis* **aurothioglucose — Adults:** 10 mg I.M.; then 25 mg for second and third doses at weekly intervals. Then, 50 mg q wk until 800 mg to 1 g given. If improvement occurs without toxicity, 25 to 50 mg q 3 to 4 wk indefinitely. **Children 6 to 12 yr:** 25% of usual adult dosage. Don't exceed 25 mg/dose. **gold sodium thiomalate — Adults:** 10 mg I.M.; then 25 mg in 1 wk. Then, 25 to 50 mg q wk to total dose of 1 g. If improvement occurs without toxicity, 25 to 50 mg q 2 wk for 2 to 20 wk; then, 25 to 50 mg q 3 to 4 wk as maintenance therapy. If relapse occurs, resume injections q wk. **Children:** 10 mg I.M.; then 1 mg/kg I.M. q wk. Follow adult intervals of doses.	▪ Watch for anaphylactoid reaction for 30 min after administration. ▪ Keep dimercaprol on hand to treat acute toxicity. ▪ Give I.M. as ordered, preferably intra-gluteally. Drug is pale yellow; don't use if it darkens. ▪ Immerse aurothioglucose vial in warm wa-ter; shake vigorously before injecting. ▪ When injecting gold sodium thiomalate, have patient lie down for 10 to 20 min to minimize hypotension. ▪ Analyze urine for protein and sediment changes before each injection. Monitor CBC, platelet count, and liver function tests.
azathioprine Imuran, Thioprine‡ *Purine antagonist* *Immunosuppressive* Pregnancy Risk Category: D	*Immunosuppression in kidney transplanta-tion* — **Adults and children:** initially, 3 to 5 mg/kg P.O. or I.V. daily, usually starting on day of transplantation. Maintain at 1 to 3 mg/kg daily (dosage varies considerably ac-cording to patient response).	▪ Administer after meals. ▪ Monitor Hgb and WBC and platelet counts at least q mo, as ordered, more often at beginning of treatment. ▪ Watch for early signs of hepatotoxicity and for increased alkaline phosphatase, biliru-bin, AST, and ALT levels.

- **I.V. use:** Reconstitute 100-mg vial with 10 ml sterile water for injection. May give by direct I.V. injection or further dilute in 0.9% NaCl for injection or D$_5$W, and infuse over 30 to 60 min. Use only for patients unable to tolerate oral medications.

Severe, refractory rheumatoid arthritis — **Adults:** initially, 1 mg/kg P.O. as single dose or divided into 2 doses. If response not satisfactory after 6 to 8 wk, may increase by 0.5 mg/kg daily (to maximum of 2.5 mg/kg daily) at 4-wk intervals.

---

azithromycin
Zithromax
Azalide macrolide
Antibiotic
Pregnancy Risk Category: B

Acute bacterial exacerbations of COPD; mild community-acquired pneumonia; second-line therapy of pharyngitis or tonsillitis caused by susceptible organisms — **Adults and adolescents ≥ 16 yr:** 500 mg P.O. as single dose on day 1; then 250 mg daily on days 2 through 5. Total dose 1.5 g.
Otitis media; community acquired pneumonia — **Children ≥ 6 mo:** 10 mg/kg P.O. (up to 500 mg) as a single dose; then 5 mg/kg (up to 250 mg) on days 2 to 5.
Nongonococcal urethritis or cervicitis caused by C. trachomatis — **Adults and adolescents ≥ 16 yr:** 1 g P.O. as single dose.
Prevention of disseminated MAC disease in advanced HIV infection — **Adults:** 1,200 mg P.O. q wk, as indicated.

- Obtain specimen for culture and sensitivity tests before first dose.
- Give capsules and multidose suspension 1 hr before or 2 hr after meals; don't give with antacids. Tablets and single-dose packets for oral suspension can be taken with or without food.
- Reduce GI distress by taking with food or milk.
- Caution to avoid alcohol and activities requiring alertness until CNS effects known.
- Suspension doesn't require refrigeration.
- Monitor blood counts (including platelets) during long-term therapy. Watch for signs of blood dyscrasias.
- Monitor for superinfection.

DRUG/CLASS/ CATEGORY	INDICATIONS/ DOSAGES	KEY NURSING CONSIDERATIONS
aztreonam Azactam Monobactam Antibiotic Pregnancy Risk Category: B	*UTIs, lower respiratory tract infections, septicemia, skin and skin-structure infections, intra-abdominal infections, surgical infections, and gynecologic infections caused by susceptible strains of gram-negative aerobic organisms; respiratory infections caused by* H. influenzae — **Adults:** 500 mg to 2 g I.V. or I.M. q 8 to 12 hr. For severe systemic or life-threatening infections, may give 2 g q 6 to 8 hr, up to 8 g daily. **Children 9 mo to 15 yr:** 30 mg/kg I.V. q 6 to 8 hr, up to 120 mg/kg/day. **Adjust-a-dose:** Patients with impaired renal function and alcoholic cirrhosis require reduced dose.	• Obtain culture and sensitivity tests before first dose. • **I.V. use:** Inject bolus dose slowly (over 3 to 5 min) directly into vein or I.V. tubing. Give infusions over 20 min to 1 hr. • Administer I.M. deep into large muscle mass. Give doses > 1 g I.V. • Don't give I.M. injection to pediatric patients.
bacitracin (ophthalmic) AK-Tracin Polypeptide antibiotic Ophthalmic antibiotic Pregnancy Risk Category: NR	*Surface bacterial infections involving conjunctiva and cornea* — **Adults and children:** small amount of ointment applied into conjunctival sac q.d. or p.r.n. until favorable response seen.	• Clean eye area of excessive exudate before application. • Ophthalmic ointment may be stored at room temperature. • Don't touch tip of tube to eye.
bacitracin (topical) Baciguent, Bacitin† Polypeptide antibiotic	*Topical infections; abrasions; cuts; minor burns or wounds* — **Adults and children:** clean area and apply thin film q.d. to t.i.d., depending on severity of condition. Don't	• Anticipate alternative treatment for burns covering > 20% of body surface. • Prolonged use may result in overgrowth of nonsusceptible organisms.

Topical antibiotic
Pregnancy Risk Category: C

■ May cover drug with sterile bandage.

use for > 1 wk.

■ Obtain culture and sensitivity tests before first dose.
■ Assess baseline renal function studies before and during therapy; monitor urine output.
■ Maintain urine pH > 6.0.

bacitracin (systemic)
Baciguent, Baci-IM, Bacitin†
Polypeptide antibiotic
Systemic antibiotic
Pregnancy Risk Category: C

Pneumonia or empyema caused by suscep-tible staphylococci — **Infants > 2.5 kg (5.5 lb):** 1,000 U/kg I.M. daily, divided q 8 to 12 hr. **Infants < 2.5 kg:** 900 U/kg daily, divided q 8 to 12 hr.

■ With test dose, markedly decreased severi-ty or frequency of spasms or reduced mus-cle tone should appear within 4 to 8 hr.
■ After test dose, give maintenance dose by implantable infusion pump. Most patients need 300 to 800 mcg daily.
■ Don't give orally to treat muscle spasm caused by rheumatic disorders, cerebral palsy, Parkinson's disease, or CVA; effica-cy not established.
■ Watch for sensitivity reactions, such as skin eruptions and respiratory distress.
■ Observe for increased risk of seizures in patients with seizure disorder.
■ Amount of relief determines whether dosage can be reduced.
■ Don't withdraw abruptly after long-term use unless required by severe adverse re-actions; doing so may trigger hallucina-tions or rebound spasticity.

baclofen
Clofen‡, Lioresal, Lioresal Intrathecal
Chlorphenyl derivative
Skeletal muscle relaxant
Pregnancy Risk Category: C

Spasticity in multiple sclerosis, spinal cord injury — **Adults:** 5 mg P.O. t.i.d. for 3 days, then 10 mg t.i.d. for 3 days, 15 mg t.i.d. for 3 days, 20 mg t.i.d. for 3 days. Increase p.r.n. to maximum of 80 mg daily.
Management of severe spasticity in patients who can't tolerate or don't respond to oral therapy — **Adults:** *Test dose:* 1 ml of 50-mcg/ml dilution into intrathecal space by bar-botage over ≥ 1 min. If poor response, give second test dose (75 mcg/1.5 ml) 24 hr after first. If poor response, give test dose (100 mcg/2 ml) 24 hr later. Patients unresponsive to final test dose shouldn't have implantable pump. Initial maintenance dose titrated based on test-dose response. Effective dose doubled and given over 24 hr. If test-dose efficacy maintained for ≥ 12 hr, don't double dose. After 1st 24 hr, increase dose slowly, p.r.n. and as tolerated, by 10% to 30% q.d.

DRUG / CLASS / CATEGORY	INDICATIONS / DOSAGES	KEY NURSING CONSIDERATIONS
basiliximab Simulect *Recombinant chimeric human monoclonal antibody* *Immunosuppressant* Pregnancy Risk Category: B	*Prophylaxis of acute organ rejection in patients receiving renal transplantation when used as part of an immunosuppressive regimen that includes cyclosporine and corticosteroids* — Used only under the supervision of a doctor qualified and experienced in immunosuppression therapy and management of organ transplantation. **Adults:** 20 mg I.V. given within 2 hr before transplant surgery, and 20 mg I.V. given 4 days after transplantation. **Children 2 to 15 yr:** 12 mg/m² (up to 20 mg) I.V. given within 2 hr before transplant surgery, and 12 mg/m² (up to 20 mg) I.V. given 4 days after transplantation.	■ Reconstitute with 5 ml sterile water for injection. Shake gently to dissolve. Dilute to volume of 50 ml with 0.9% NaCl or dextrose 5% for infusion. When mixing, gently invert bag to avoid foaming. Don't shake. Infuse over 20 to 30 min via central or peripheral vein. Don't add or infuse other drugs through same I.V. line. Use solution immediately. ■ Use with caution in elderly patients. ■ Anaphylactoid reactions may occur. ■ Monitor for electrolyte imbalances and acidosis during therapy. ■ Monitor I&O, vital signs, Hgb, and Hct.
becaplermin Regranex Gel *Recombinant human platelet-derived growth factor* *Wound repair enhancer* Pregnancy Risk Category: C	*Treatment of lower extremity diabetic neuropathic ulcers that extend into or beyond subcutaneous tissue and have adequate blood supply* — **Adults:** apply daily in ¹⁄₁₆″ even thickness to entire surface of wound. If tube size is 2 g, length of gel to apply by taking wound length (inches) × wound width × 1.3, or wound length (cm) × wound width ÷ 2. If tube size is 7.5 or 15 g, find length of gel to apply by taking wound length (inches) × wound width ×	■ Used as an adjunct to good ulcer care practices (initial sharp debridement, infection control, pressure relief). ■ Measure ulcer's greatest length and width. Squeeze calculated length of gel onto clean measuring surface, such as waxed paper. Use cotton swab or other applicator to transfer and spread drug over entire ulcer area. Place saline-moistened dressing over site and leave in place for 12 hr. Then re-

move dressing and rinse away residual gel with 0.9% NaCl or water; apply fresh, moist dressing without becaplermin for rest of day. Recalculate dose at least each wk.
- Monitor for application site reactions.

0.6, or wound length (cm) × wound width ÷ 4.

---

beclomethasone dipropionate (oral inhalant) Becloforte Inhaler‡, Beclovent, Vanceril *Glucocorticoid* *Anti-inflammatory/anti-asthmatic* Pregnancy Risk Category: C	*Steroid-dependent asthma* — **Adults and children ≥ 12 yr:** 2 inhalations t.i.d. or q.i.d. or 4 inhalations b.i.d. up to 20 inhalations (840 mcg) q.d. **Children 6 to 12 yr:** 1 to 2 inhalations t.i.d. or q.i.d. or 2 to 4 inhalations b.i.d., up to 10 inhalations (420 mcg) q.d. *Note:* Above doses for adults and children based on regular strength formulation (42 mcg/metered spray).	- Taper oral therapy slowly. Acute adrenal insufficiency and death have occurred in asthmatics who changed abruptly from oral corticosteroids to beclomethasone. - Spacer device may ensure proper dose and decrease local (oral) adverse effects. - Rinse mouth with water after each use.
beclomethasone dipropionate (nasal) Beconase AQ Nasal Spray, Beconase Nasal Inhaler, Vancenase AQ Double Strength, Vancenase AQ Nasal Spray, Vancenase Nasal Inhaler *Glucocorticoid* *Anti-inflammatory* Pregnancy Risk Category: C	*Relief of symptoms of seasonal or perennial rhinitis; prevention of recurrence of nasal polyps after surgical removal* — **Adults and children > 12 yr:** usual dosage 1 or 2 sprays in each nostril b.i.d, t.i.d., or q.i.d. **Children 6 to 12 yr:** 1 spray in each nostril t.i.d. *Double strength form* — **Adults and children > 6 yr:** 1 or 2 sprays in each nostril once daily.	- Observe for fungal infections. - Not effective for acute rhinitis exacerbations. Decongestants or antihistamines may be needed. - Don't use longer than 3 wk if no improvement noted.

DRUG/CLASS/ CATEGORY	INDICATIONS/ DOSAGES	KEY NURSING CONSIDERATIONS
benazepril hydrochloride Lotensin *ACE inhibitor* *Antihypertensive* Pregnancy Risk Category: C (D in second and third trimesters)	*Hypertension* — **Adults:** in patients not receiving diuretics, 10 mg P.O. q.d. initially. Most patients receive 20 to 40 mg q.d. in 1 or 2 doses; patient receiving diuretic, 5 mg P.O. q.d. **Adjust-a-dose:** For patients with creatinine clearance < 30 ml/min, give 5 mg P.O. q.d. Dose may be adjusted up to 40 mg/day.	• Measure BP 2 to 6 hr after dose and just before next dose. Monitor for hypotension. • Assess renal and hepatic function before and during therapy. Monitor serum potassium levels. • Safety and efficacy of doses over 80 mg have not been established.
benzonatate Tessalon *Local anesthetic (ester)* *Nonnarcotic antitussive* Pregnancy Risk Category: C	*Symptomatic relief of cough* — **Adults and children > 10 yr:** 100 mg P.O. t.i.d.; up to 600 mg daily may be needed.	• Don't give when cough is valuable diagnostic sign or is beneficial. • Don't crush capsules. • Monitor cough type and frequency. • Use with percussion and chest vibration.
benztropine mesylate Apo-Benztropine†, Cogentin, PMS-Benztropine† *Anticholinergic* *Antiparkinsonian* Pregnancy Risk Category: C	*Drug-induced extrapyramidal disorders (except tardive dyskinesia)* — **Adults:** 1 to 4 mg P.O. or I.M. q.d. or b.i.d. *Acute dystonic reaction* — **Adults:** 1 to 2 mg I.V. or I.M.; then 1 to 2 mg P.O. b.i.d. *Parkinsonism* — **Adults:** 0.5 to 6 mg P.O. or I.M. daily. Initial dose 0.5 mg to 1 mg, increased by 0.5 mg q 5 to 6 days. Adjust dosage to meet individual requirements.	• Give initial dose h.s. • Never discontinue abruptly. • Monitor vital signs carefully. Watch for adverse reactions, especially in elderly or debilitated patients. • May aggravate tardive dyskinesia. • Watch for intermittent constipation and abdominal distention and pain; may indicate onset of paralytic ileus.

bepridil hydrochloride
Bepadin†, Vascor
Calcium channel blocker
Antianginal
Pregnancy Risk Category: C

Chronic stable angina in patients who can't tolerate or don't respond to other agents — **Adults:** initially, 200 mg P.O. daily. After 10 days, increase dosage based on response. Maintenance dosage in most patients 300 mg/day. Maximum 400 mg daily.

- Use cautiously in left bundle-branch block, sinus bradycardia, impaired renal or hepatic function, or heart failure.
- Can cause severe ventricular arrhythmias.
- Don't adjust dosage more often than every 10 to 14 days.

beractant (natural lung surfactant)
Survanta
Bovine lung extract
Lung surfactant
Pregnancy Risk Category: NR

Prevention of respiratory distress syndrome (RDS) in premature neonates weighing 1,250 g or less at birth or having symptoms of surfactant deficiency — **Neonates:** 4 ml/kg intratracheally; give each dose in 4 quarter-doses; in between, use handheld resuscitation bag at rate of 60 breaths/min and sufficient oxygen to prevent cyanosis. Give within 15 min of birth, if possible. Repeat in 6 hr if respiratory distress continues. Give no more than 4 doses in 48 hr.

Rescue treatment of RDS in premature neonates — **Neonates:** 4 ml/kg intratracheally; before giving, increase ventilator rate to 60 with inspiratory time of 0.5 sec and FiO_2 of 1. Give each dose in 4 quarter-doses; in between, continue ventilation for 30 sec or until RDS stable. Give dose as soon as RDS confirmed. Repeat in 6 hr if distress continues. Give no more than 4 doses in 48 hr.

- Continuous monitoring of ECG and Sao_2 essential; frequent arterial BP monitoring and frequent ABG sampling highly desirable.
- Accurate weight determination essential to proper dosage measurements.
- Can rapidly affect oxygenation and lung compliance. May need to adjust peak ventilator inspiratory pressures if chest expansion improves markedly after administration. Notify doctor and adjust immediately as directed.
- Homogeneous drug distribution important.

37

DRUG/CLASS/CATEGORY	INDICATIONS/DOSAGES	KEY NURSING CONSIDERATIONS
betamethasone Betnesol†, Celestone **betamethasone acetate and betamethasone sodium phosphate** Celestone Soluspan **betamethasone sodium phosphate** Celestone Phosphate *Glucocorticoid* Anti-inflammatory Pregnancy Risk Category: C	*Conditions with severe inflammation; conditions requiring immunosuppression —* **Adults:** 0.6 to 7.2 mg P.O. q.d.; or 0.5 to 9 mg I.M., I.V., or into joint or soft tissue q.d. Betamethasone sodium phosphate-acetate suspension 6 to 12 mg injected into large joints or 1.5 to 6 mg injected into smaller joints. May give both injections q 1 to 2 wk, p.r.n. *Note:* Betamethasone sodium phosphate and betamethasone acetate suspension combination product should *not* be given I.V.	• Don't use for alternate-day therapy. • Obtain baseline weight before starting therapy and weigh daily; report sudden gain. • For better results and less toxicity, give once-daily dose in morning. • To reduce GI irritation, give with milk or food. • Monitor blood glucose and serum potassium regularly, as ordered. Diabetics may require insulin dosage adjustments.
betamethasone dipropionate Alphatrex, Diprolene, Diprolene AF, Diprosone, Maxivate **betamethasone valerate** Betatrex, Beta-Val, Betnovate†‡, Valisone *Topical glucocorticoid* Anti-inflammatory Pregnancy Risk Category: C	*Inflammation associated with corticosteroid-responsive dermatoses —* **Adults and children:** clean area; apply cream, ointment, lotion, or aerosol spray sparingly. Give dipropionate q.d. or b.i.d.; valerate q.d. to q.i.d. Maximum dosage 45 g/wk for Diprolene cream, 50 ml/wk for Diprolene lotion.	• Gently wash skin before applying. Rub in gently, leaving thin coat. When treating hairy sites, part hair and apply directly to lesions. For patients with eczematous dermatitis, hold dressing in place with gauze, elastic bandage, stocking, or stockinette. • Don't apply near eyes or mucous membranes or in ear canal. • Notify doctor and remove occlusive dressing if fever, infection, striae, or atrophy occurs. • Don't discontinue abruptly.

betaxolol hydro-chloride (oral) Kerlone *Beta blocker* *Antihypertensive* Pregnancy Risk Category: C	*Hypertension (used alone or with other an-tihypertensives)* — **Adults:** initially, 10 mg P.O. q.d.; if necessary, 20 mg P.O. q.d. if de-sired response not achieved in 7 to 14 days.	• May mask tachycardia associated with hy-perthyroidism. In suspected thyrotoxico-sis, withdraw gradually, as ordered. • Abrupt discontinuation may trigger angina pectoris in unrecognized CAD. • Monitor BP closely.
betaxolol hydro-chloride (oph-thalmic) Betoptic, Betoptic S, Kerlone *Beta blocker* *Antiglaucoma agent* Pregnancy Risk Category: C	*Chronic open-angle glaucoma and ocular hypertension* — **Adults:** 1 or 2 drops of 0.5% solution or 0.25% suspension b.i.d.	• Wash hands before and after instilling. Ap-ply light finger pressure on lacrimal sac for 1 min after instillation. Don't touch dropper tip to eye or surrounding tissue. Shake suspension well before instilling. • Some patients may need several weeks of treatment to stabilize IOP-lowering re-sponse. Determine IOP after 4 wk.
bethanechol chloride Duvoid, Myotonachol, Urabeth, Urecholine, Urocarb Tablets‡ *Cholinergic agonist* *Urinary tract and GI tract stimulant* Pregnancy Risk Category: C	*Acute postoperative and postpartum nonobstructive urine retention; neurogenic atony of urinary bladder with urine reten-tion* — **Adults:** 10 to 50 mg P.O. t.i.d. to q.i.d. Or 2.5 to 5 mg S.C. Never give I.M. or I.V. For urine retention, may require 50 to 100 mg P.O. per dose. Use such doses with extreme caution. *Test dose:* 2.5 mg S.C., re-peated at 15- to 30-min intervals to total of 4 doses to determine minimal effective dose; then use minimal effective dose q 6 to 8 hr. All doses adjusted individually.	• Never give I.M. or I.V. • Give on empty stomach; otherwise, may cause nausea and vomiting. • Monitor vital signs frequently, especially respirations. Always have atropine injec-tion available. • Watch for toxicity. Edrophonium ineffec-tive against muscle relaxation caused by bethanechol. • Inform patient that drug usually effective within 30 to 90 min after oral dose and 5 to 15 min after S.C. dose.

DRUG / CLASS / CATEGORY	INDICATIONS / DOSAGES	KEY NURSING CONSIDERATIONS
biperiden hydrochloride Akineton **biperiden lactate** Akineton Lactate *Anticholinergic* *Antiparkinsonian* Pregnancy Risk Category: C	*Drug-induced extrapyramidal disorders —* **Adults:** 2 mg P.O. q.d., b.i.d., or t.i.d., depending on severity. Usual dosage 2 mg daily, or 2 mg I.M. or I.V. q ½ hr; not to exceed 4 doses or 8 mg daily. *Parkinsonism —* **Adults:** 2 mg P.O. t.i.d. or q.i.d. Dosage individualized and adjusted to maximum of 16 mg/24 hr.	• ***I.V. use:*** Administer very slowly. Keep patient supine. • Monitor vital signs carefully. • Instruct to take oral form with or after meals. • Warn to avoid activities that require alertness until CNS effects known. • Advise to report signs of urinary hesitancy or urine retention.
bisacodyl Bisac-Evac, Bisacodyl Uni-serts, Carter's Little Pills, Dacodyl, Deficol, Dulcagen, Dulcolax, Durolax‡, Fleet Bisacodyl, Fleet Bisacodyl Prep, Fleet Laxative, Theralax *Diphenylmethane derivative* *Stimulant laxative* Pregnancy Risk Category: B	*Chronic constipation; preparation for delivery, surgery, or rectal or bowel examination —* **Adults and children > 12 yr:** 10 to 15 mg P.O. in evening or before breakfast. May give up to 30 mg P.O. or 10 mg P.R. for evacuation before examination or surgery. **Children 6 to 12 yr:** 5 mg P.O. or P.R. h.s. or before breakfast. Oral form not recommended if unable to swallow tablet whole.	• Soft, formed stools usually produced 15 to 60 min after P.R. administration. • For constipation, determine if patient has adequate fluid intake, exercise, and diet. • Avoid embedding suppositories in fecal material; may delay drug onset. • Don't crush tablets; they must be swallowed whole. • Don't give within 1 hr of milk or antacid. • Discourage excessive use.
bismuth subsalicylate Bismatrol, Pepto-Bismol, Pink Bismuth *Adsorbent* *Antidiarrheal* Pregnancy Risk Category: C	*Mild, nonspecific diarrhea —* **Adults:** 30 ml or 2 tablets P.O. q ½ to 1 hr, to maximum of 8 doses for ≤ 2 days. **Children 3 to 6 yr:** 5 ml or ⅓ tablet P.O. **Children 6 to 9 yr:** 10 ml or ⅔ tablet P.O. **Children 9 to 12 yr:** 15 ml or 1 tablet P.O. *Note:* Give children's doses q ½ to 1 hr, to maximum of 8 doses for ≤ 2 days.	• Use cautiously in patients taking aspirin. • Don't use in children with chickenpox or flu. • Know that suspension should be shaken well before use. • Tell patient that drug may darken stools. • Avoid use before GI radiologic procedures.

bisoprolol fumarate
Zebeta
Beta blocker
Antihypertensive
Pregnancy Risk Category: C

Hypertension (drug used alone or in combination) — **Adults:** 5 mg P.O. q.d. If response inadequate, increase to 10 to 20 mg P.O. q.d. Maximum dose 20 mg q.d.
Adjust-a-dose: In patients with hepatic insufficiency or creatinine clearance < 40 ml/min, start dose at 2.5 mg daily.

- Use cautiously in bronchospastic disease, diabetes, PVD, or thyroid disease and in history of heart failure.
- Monitor BP frequently.
- May mask hypoglycemia signs.

bleomycin sulfate
Blenoxane
Antibiotic/antineoplastic (cell cycle–phase specific, G_2 and M phase)
Antineoplastic
Pregnancy Risk Category: D

Squamous cell carcinoma; lymphosarcoma; reticulum cell carcinoma; testicular carcinoma — **Adults:** 10 to 20 U/m² I.V., I.M., or S.C. once or twice weekly to total of 300 to 400 U.
Hodgkin's disease — **Adults:** 10 to 20 U/m² I.V., I.M., or S.C. once or twice/wk. After 50% response, maintenance dosage is 1 U I.M. or I.V. q.d. or 5 U I.M. or I.V./wk.
Treatment of malignant pleural effusion; prevention of recurrent pleural effusions — **Adults:** 60 U in 50 to 100 ml 0.9% NaCl solution as single-dose bolus intrapleural injection.

- Dosage and indications may vary.
- Obtain pulmonary function tests as ordered. Pulmonary toxic effects may increase in patients receiving radiation therapy.
- Watch for hypersensitivity reactions. May need to give test dose. Monitor for fever, which may be treated with antipyretics.
- Reconstitute per manufacturer's labeling. Administer I.V. infusion over 10 min.

bretylium tosylate
Bretylate†, Bretylol
Adrenergic blocker
Antiarrhythmic
Pregnancy Risk Category: C

Ventricular fibrillation or hemodynamically unstable ventricular tachycardia unresponsive to other antiarrhythmics — **Adults:** 5 mg/kg I.V. push over 1 min. If necessary, increase dose to 10 mg/kg and repeat q 15 to 30 min until 30 mg/kg given. For continuous suppression, diluted solution given at 1 to 2

- To prevent nausea and vomiting, follow dosage directions carefully.
- Keep patient supine until tolerance to hypotension develops.
- Monitor patient closely for transient hypertension and arrhythmias.

(continued)

†Canadian ‡Australian

41

DRUG / CLASS / CATEGORY	INDICATIONS / DOSAGES	KEY NURSING CONSIDERATIONS
bretylium tosylate *(continued)*	mg/min continuously or 5 to 10 mg/kg diluted and given over more than 8 min q 6 hr.	- Monitor BP and HR continuously. - Observe susceptible patients for increased angina.
bromocriptine mesylate Parlodel *Dopamine receptor agonist Semisynthetic ergot alkaloid/dopaminergic agonist/antiparkinsonian/inhibitor of prolactin release/inhibitor of growth hormone release* Pregnancy Risk Category: B	*Amenorrhea and galactorrhea associated with hyperprolactinemia; female infertility* — **Adults:** 1.25 to 2.5 mg P.O. q.d., increased by 2.5 mg q.d. at 3- to 7-day intervals until response achieved. Therapeutic dosage range 2.5 to 15 mg/day. Doses > 100 mg q.d. not studied. *Parkinson's disease* — **Adults:** 1.25 mg P.O. b.i.d. with meals. Increase dose q 14 to 28 days, up to 100 mg daily, p.r.n. *Acromegaly* — **Adults:** 1.25 to 2.5 mg P.O. with snack h.s. for 3 days. Additional 1.25 to 2.5 mg may be added q 3 to 7 days until benefit obtained. Maximum 100 mg/day.	- Monitor for adverse reactions. Incidence of such reactions high, especially at start of therapy; however, most are mild to moderate, with nausea being most common. - For Parkinson's disease, usually given in conjunction with levodopa or carbidopa-levodopa. - Give with meals. - May lead to early postpartum conception. Test for pregnancy every 4 wk or whenever menses missed after menses resume.
brompheniramine maleate Bromphen, Chlorphed, Codimal-A, Dimetane, Veltane *Alkylamine antihistamine Antihistamine (H₁-receptor antagonist)*	*Rhinitis; allergy symptoms* — **Adults:** 4 to 8 mg P.O. t.i.d. or q.i.d.; or 8 to 12 mg extended-release P.O. b.i.d. or t.i.d. Maximum P.O. dose 24 mg/day. Or, 5 to 20 mg P.O. q 6 to 12 hr I.M., I.V., or S.C. Maximum parenteral dose 40 mg/day. **Children 6 to 12 yr:** 2 to 4 mg P.O. t.i.d. or q.i.d.; or 8 to 12 mg extended-release P.O. q 12 hr; or 0.5 mg/kg I.M.,	- **I.V. use:** Can give injectable form containing 10 mg/ml diluted or undiluted very slowly I.V. - Don't give 100 mg/ml injection I.V. - Monitor blood count during long-term therapy, as ordered; observe for blood dyscrasias.

Pregnancy Risk Category: C	I.V., or S.C. q.d. in divided doses t.i.d. or q.i.d. **Children < 6 yr:** 0.5 mg/kg P.O., I.M., I.V., or S.C. q.d. in divided doses t.i.d. or q.i.d.	▪ Children < 12 yr should use only as directed by doctor.
budesonide (nasal) Rhinocort *Glucocorticoid* *Anti-inflammatory* Pregnancy Risk Category: C	*Symptoms of seasonal or perennial allergic rhinitis —* **Adults and children ≥ 6 yr:** 2 sprays in each nostril in morning and evening, or 4 sprays in each nostril in morning. Maintenance dose should be fewest number of sprays needed to control symptoms.	▪ Shake well prior to use. ▪ Instruct to avoid exposure to chickenpox or measles. ▪ Don't break or incinerate canister or store in extreme heat.
budesonide (oral inhalant) Pulmicort Turbuhaler *Glucocorticoid* *Anti-inflammatory* Pregnancy Risk Category: C	*Prophylactic therapy in maintenance treatment of asthma —* **Adults previously on bronchodilators alone:** initially, inhaled dose of 200 to 400 mcg b.i.d., to maximum of 400 mcg b.i.d. **Adults previously on inhaled corticosteroids:** initially, inhaled dose of 200 to 400 mcg b.i.d., to maximum of 800 mcg b.i.d. **Adults previously on oral corticosteroids:** initially, inhaled dose of 400 to 800 mcg b.i.d., to maximum of 800 mcg b.i.d. **Children > 6 yr previously on bronchodilators alone or inhaled corticosteroids:** initially, inhaled dose of 200 mcg b.i.d., to maximum of 400 mcg b.i.d. **Children > 6 yr previously on oral corticosteroids:** highest recommended dose is 400 mcg b.i.d. *Note:* In all patients, use lowest effective dose after stabilization of asthma occurs.	▪ Use cautiously, if at all, in patients with active or quiescent TB of the respiratory tract; untreated systemic fungal, bacterial, viral, or parasitic infections; or ocular herpes. ▪ Use caution when transferring from systemic steroid to budesonide; gradually decrease steroid dose to prevent adrenal insufficiency. ▪ If bronchospasm occurs after giving drug, stop therapy and treat with bronchodilator. ▪ Improved lung function may occur within 24 hr of initiating treatment, although maximum benefit may not occur for ≥ 1 to 2 wk. ▪ Watch for *Candida* infections of mouth or pharynx. ▪ Corticosteroid use may increase risk of developing serious or fatal infections in patients exposed to viral illnesses, such as chickenpox or measles.

†Canadian ‡Australian

DRUG/CLASS/ CATEGORY	INDICATIONS/ DOSAGES	KEY NURSING CONSIDERATIONS
bumetanide Bumex, Burinex‡ *Loop diuretic* *Diuretic* Pregnancy Risk Category: C	*Edema in heart failure or hepatic or renal disease —* **Adults:** 0.5 to 2 mg P.O. q.d. as single dose. If diuretic response inadequate, may give 2nd or 3rd dose at 4- to 5-hr intervals. Maximum 10 mg/day. May be given I.V. if P.O. not feasible. Usual initial dose 0.5 to 1 mg, given I.V. or I.M. If response inadequate, may give 2nd or 3rd dose at 2- to 3-hr intervals. Maximum 10 mg/day.	▪ *I.V. use:* Give direct I.V. doses over 1 to 2 min. For intermittent infusion, give diluted at ordered rate. ▪ Intermittent dosage is safest and most effective way to control edema. ▪ Monitor I&O, weight, BP, pulse, oxygen, and serum electrolyte, BUN, creatinine, glucose, and uric acid levels. ▪ Watch for signs of hypokalemia.
bupropion hydrochloride (antidepressant) Wellbutrin *Aminoketone* *Antidepressant* Pregnancy Risk Category: B	*Depression —* **Adults:** initially, 100 mg P.O. b.i.d., increased after 3 days to 100 mg P.O. t.i.d. if needed. If no response after several weeks of therapy, increase to 150 mg t.i.d. No single dose should exceed 150 mg.	▪ May cause agitation, insomnia, or anxiety. ▪ To minimize risk of seizure, don't exceed 450 mg/day, and give daily dosage in 3 to 4 equally divided doses. ▪ Closely monitor patients with history of bipolar disorders.
bupropion hydrochloride (nicotine replacement) Zyban *Norepinephrine, serotonin, and dopamine inhibitor* *Nicotine replacement/antidepressant*	*Aid to smoking cessation treatment —* **Adults:** 150 mg P.O. daily for 3 days; increased to maximum of 300 mg P.O. daily given in 2 divided doses at least 8 hr apart. Tapering dose is not required.	▪ To reduce seizure risk, don't exceed daily dose of 300 mg. Divide dose (150 mg b.i.d.) so that no single dose exceeds 150 mg. ▪ Stop therapy if patient has not made progress by wk 7 of therapy. ▪ Start therapy while patient is still smoking; about 1 wk is required to achieve steady-state plasma drug levels.

Pregnancy Risk Category: B

buspirone hydrochloride BuSpar Azaspirodecanedione derivative *Antianxiety agent* Pregnancy Risk Category: B	*Anxiety disorders; short-term relief of anxiety* — **Adults:** initially, 5 mg P.O. t.i.d., increased at 3-day intervals in 5-mg increments. Usual maintenance dosage 20 to 30 mg daily in divided doses. Don't exceed 60 mg daily.	▪ Monitor closely for adverse CNS reactions. ▪ Less sedating than other antianxiety agents. ▪ Has shown no potential for abuse. ▪ Before initiating in patient also receiving benzodiazepines, warn against stopping benzodiazepines abruptly; withdrawal reaction may occur.
busulfan Myleran Alkylating agent (cell cycle–phase nonspecific) *Antineoplastic* Pregnancy Risk Category: D	*Palliative treatment of chronic myelocytic leukemia* — **Adults:** 4 to 8 mg P.O. q.d., up to 12 mg P.O. q.d., until WBC ≤ 15,000/mm³; drug stopped until WBC ≥ 50,000/mm³, and then resumed as before; or 4 to 8 mg P.O. q.d. until WBC ≤ 10,000 to 20,000/mm³; then daily dose reduced as needed to maintain WBC at this level (usually 1 to 3 mg q.d.). **Children:** 0.06 to 0.12 mg/kg/day or 1.8 to 4.6 mg/m²/day P.O.; dosage adjusted to maintain WBC count at 20,000/mm³, but never < 10,000/mm³.	▪ To prevent bleeding, avoid all I.M. injections when platelet count < 100,000/mm³. ▪ Administer drug at same time each day. ▪ Monitor patient response (increased appetite and sense of well-being, decreased total WBC count, reduced spleen size), which usually begins within 1 to 2 wk. ▪ Monitor serum uric acid. To prevent hyperuricemia, allopurinol may be ordered. Keep patient adequately hydrated. ▪ Anticipate possible blood transfusion. ▪ Toxicity can accompany therapeutic effects.
butoconazole nitrate Femstat 3 Synthetic imidazole derivative *Topical fungistat* Pregnancy Risk Category: C	*Vulvovaginal mycotic infections caused by Candida species* — **Adults:** for nonpregnant patient, 1 applicatorful intravaginally h.s. for 3 days. If needed, treat for another 3 days. For pregnant patient during second or third trimester, 1 applicatorful intravaginally h.s. for 6 days.	▪ Confirm diagnosis by smears or cultures, as ordered. ▪ May be used with oral contraceptives and antibiotic therapy.

45

†Canadian ‡Australian

DRUG/CLASS/ CATEGORY	INDICATIONS/ DOSAGES	KEY NURSING CONSIDERATIONS
butorphanol tartrate Stadol, Stadol NS *Narcotic agonist-antagonist/ opioid partial agonist* *Analgesic/adjunct to anesthesia* Pregnancy Risk Category: C	*Moderate to severe pain* — **Adults:** 1 to 4 mg I.M. q 3 to 4 hr, p.r.n. or around the clock; or 0.5 to 2 mg I.V. q 3 to 4 hr, p.r.n. or around the clock. Not to exceed 4 mg per dose. Or, 1 mg by nasal spray q 3 to 4 hr (1 spray in one nostril); repeated in 60 to 90 min if pain relief inadequate. *Preoperative anesthesia or preanesthesia* — **Adults:** 2 mg I.M. 60 to 90 min before surgery.	• Periodically monitor postoperative vital signs and bladder function. • Respiratory depression apparently doesn't increase with larger dose. • Psychological and physical addiction may occur.
calcifediol Calderol *Vitamin D analogue* *Antihypocalcemic* Pregnancy Risk Category: C	*Metabolic bone disease and hypocalcemia associated with chronic renal failure* — **Adults:** initially, 300 to 350 mcg P.O. weekly. Dosage may be increased at 4-wk intervals.	• Monitor serum calcium level; during adjustment, at least weekly. • If hypercalcemia occurs, discontinue calcifediol and notify doctor.
calcipotriene Dovonex *Synthetic vitamin D₃ analogue* *Topical antipsoriatic* Pregnancy Risk Category: C	*Moderate plaque psoriasis* — **Adults:** Apply thin layer to affected area b.i.d. Rub in gently and completely.	• Use cautiously in elderly patients; they may have more severe adverse skin reactions. • Advise to apply thin layer of ointment to avoid transient elevations of serum calcium. • Advise not to use drug on face, in eyes, orally, or vaginally.

calcitonin (human)
Cibacalcin

calcitonin (salmon)
Calcimar, Miacalcin, Miacalcin Nasal Spray, Osteocalcin, Salmonine

Thyroid hormone
Hypocalcemic
Pregnancy Risk Category: C

Paget's disease of bone (osteitis deformans) — **Adults:** 100 IU of calcitonin (salmon) q.d. S.C. or I.M.: maintenance dose is 50 to 100 IU q.d. or q.o.d. Or, calcitonin (human) 0.5 mg three or three times weekly or 0.25 mg q.d., up to 0.5 mg b.i.d.
Hypercalcemia — **Adults:** 4 IU/kg of calcitonin (salmon) q12 hr I.M. If poor response after 1 or 2 days, increase to 8 IU/kg I.M. q 12 hr. If response remains poor after 2 more days, increase to maximum 8 IU/kg I.M. q 6 hr.
Postmenopausal osteoporosis — **Adults:** 100 IU of calcitonin (salmon) q.d. I.M. or S.C. Or, 200 IU (1 activation) of calcitonin (salmon) q.d. intranasally, alternating nostrils q.d.

- Skin test usually done before therapy.
- Systemic allergic reactions possible. Keep epinephrine handy.
- Administer at bedtime.
- Use reconstituted solution within 2 hr.
- Observe for signs of hypocalcemic tetany.
- Monitor serum calcium, alkaline phosphatase, and 24-hr urine hydroxyproline levels closely.
- Store calcitonin (human) at room temperature; refrigerate calcitonin (salmon).
- Facial flushing and warmth may occur within min of injection and usually last about 1 hr.

calcitriol (1,25-dihydroxycholecalciferol)
Calcijex, Delta D, Rocaltrol

Vitamin D analogue
Antihypocalcemic
Pregnancy Risk Category: A (D if given in doses above RDA)

Hypocalcemia in patients undergoing chronic dialysis — **Adults:** 0.25 mcg P.O. q.d. Increased by 0.25 mcg q.d. q 4 to 8 wk. Maintenance is 0.25 mcg q.o.d., up to 1.25 mcg q.d.
Hypoparathyroidism and pseudohypoparathyroidism — **Adults and children > 6 yr:** 0.25 mcg P.O. q.d. May be increased at 2- to 4-wk intervals. Maintenance, 0.25 to 2 mcg q.d.
Hypoparathyroidism — **Children 1 to 6 yr:** 0.25 to 0.75 mcg P.O. q.d.

- Monitor serum calcium level. Discontinue drug if hypercalcemia occurs, and notify doctor.
- Protect from heat and light.
- Tell patient to immediately report weakness, nausea, vomiting, dry mouth, constipation, muscle or bone pain, or metallic taste.
- Drug not to be taken by anyone without a prescription for it.

47

DRUG/CLASS/ CATEGORY	INDICATIONS/ DOSAGES	KEY NURSING CONSIDERATIONS
calcium acetate Phos-Ex, Phos-Lo **calcium chloride** Calciject **calcium citrate** Citracal **calcium glubionate** Neo-Calglucon **calcium gluceptate** **calcium gluconate** **calcium lactate** **calcium phosphate, tribasic** Posture *Calcium supplement* *Therapeutic agent for electrolyte balance/cardiotonic* Pregnancy Risk Category: C	*Hypocalcemic emergency* — **Adults:** 7 to 14 mEq calcium I.V. (as 10% gluconate solution, 2% to 10% chloride solution, or 22% gluceptate solution). **Children:** 1 to 7 mEq calcium I.V. **Infants:** up to 1 mEq calcium I.V. *Hypocalcemic tetany* — **Adults:** 4.5 to 16 mEq calcium I.V. Repeat until controlled. **Children:** 0.5 to 0.7 mEq/kg calcium I.V. 3 to 4 times/day until controlled. **Neonates:** 2.4 mEq/kg I.V. q.d. in divided doses. *Adjunctive treatment of cardiac arrest* — **Adults:** 0.027 to 0.054 mEq/kg calcium chloride I.V., 4.5 to 6.3 mEq calcium gluceptate I.V., or 2.3 to 3.7 mEq calcium gluconate I.V. **Children:** 0.27 mEq/kg calcium chloride I.V. May repeat in 10 min; check serum calcium before administering further doses. *During exchange transfusions* — **Adults:** 1.35 mEq I.V. concurrently with each 100 ml citrated blood. **Neonates:** 0.45 mEq I.V. after each 100 ml citrated blood. *Hyperphosphatemia* — **Adults:** 1,334 to 2,000 mg P.O. acetate t.i.d. with meals. Dialysis patients need 3 to 4 tablets with meals.	• Use all calcium products with extreme caution in patients with sarcoidosis and renal or cardiac disease, and in digitalized patients. • *I.V. use (direct injection):* Give slowly through small needle into large vein or I.V. line with free-flowing, compatible solution at maximum 1 ml/min (1.5 mEq/min) for chloride, 1.5 to 5 ml/min for gluceptate, and 2 ml/min for gluceptate. Don't use scalp veins. *(Intermittent infusion):* Infuse diluted solution through I.V. line with compatible solution at maximum rate of 200 mg/min for gluceptate and gluconate. • Give chloride and gluceptate I.V. only. Use in-line filter. • Drug will precipitate if given I.V. with alkaline drugs. • Monitor ECG when giving calcium I.V. Stop for complaints of discomfort, and notify doctor. Following I.V. injection, patient should remain recumbent for 15 min. • Ensure that doctor specifies form of calcium to be used. • Monitor blood calcium levels frequently. • Severe necrosis and tissue sloughing can occur after extravasation.

calcium carbonate
Alka-Mints, CalCarb-HD,
Calcarb 600, Calci-Chew,
Chooz, Os-Cal 500, Rolaids
Calcium Rich, Tums
Calcium supplement
Therapeutic agent for elec-
trolyte balance
Pregnancy Risk Category: NR

Antacid — **Adults:** 350 mg to 1.5 g P.O. or 2 pieces of chewing gum 1 hr after meals and h.s., p.r.n.
Dietary supplement — **Adults:** 500 mg to 2 g P.O. b.i.d. to q.i.d.

- Watch for nausea, vomiting, headache, mental confusion, and anorexia.
- Monitor serum calcium level.
- Record amount and consistency of stools.
- Tell patient to shake suspension and take with small amount of water.

calcium polycarbophil
Equalactin, Fiberall, Fiber-
Con, Fiber-Lax, FiberNorm
Hydrophilic agent
Bulk laxative/antidiarrheal
Pregnancy Risk Category: NR

Constipation; diarrhea associated with irrita-
ble bowel syndrome; acute nonspecific diar-
rhea — **Adults:** 1 g P.O. q.i.d., p.r.n. Maximum 6 g in 24-hr period. **Children 2 to 6 yr:**
as directed by doctor. 500 mg P.O. b.i.d., p.r.n.
Maximum 1.5 g in 24-hr period. **Children 6 to
12 yr:** 500 mg P.O. q.d. to t.i.d., p.r.n. Maximum 3 g in 24-hr period.

- Before giving for constipation, determine if patient has adequate fluid intake, exercise, and diet.
- If given for diarrhea, dose may be repeat-ed q 30 min.
- If given as laxative, tell patient to drink 8 oz water with each dose.
- Rectal bleeding or failure to respond to therapy may indicate need for surgery.

candesartan cilexetil
Atacand
Selective angiotensin II
receptor antagonist
Antihypertensive
Pregnancy Risk Category: C
(first trimester); D (second
and third trimesters)

Treatment of hypertension (alone or in com-
bination with other antihypertensive
agents) — **Adults:** initially, 16 mg P.O. once
daily when used as monotherapy; usual
dosage range is 8 to 32 mg P.O. q.d. as a
single dose or divided b.i.d.

- Use cautiously in patients (such as those with heart failure) whose renal function depends on the renin-angiotensin-aldosterone system because of potential for oliguria and progressive azotemia with acute renal failure or death.
- Use cautiously in patients who are vol-ume- or salt-depleted because of potential
(continued)

49

†Canadian ‡Australian

DRUG/CLASS/ CATEGORY	INDICATIONS/ DOSAGES	KEY NURSING CONSIDERATIONS
candesartan cilexetil *(continued)*		for symptomatic hypotension. Start therapy with a lower dosage range, as ordered, and monitor blood pressure carefully. • Know that drug can cause fetal and neonatal morbidity and death when administered to pregnant women. These problems haven't been detected when exposure has been limited to first trimester. If pregnancy is suspected, notify doctor because drug should be discontinued. • If hypotension occurs after dose, place patient in the supine position and give an I.V. infusion of 0.9% NaCl solution, as ordered. • Monitor therapeutic response and occurrence of adverse reactions carefully in the elderly and in patients with renal disease.
capecitabine Xeloda *Thymidylate inhibitor Antineoplastic* Pregnancy Risk Category: D	*Treatment of patients with metastatic breast cancer resistant to both paclitaxel and an anthracycline-containing chemotherapy regimen or resistant to paclitaxel and for whom further anthracycline therapy isn't indicated*— **Adults:** 2,500 mg/m² P.O. q.d. in 2 divided doses (about 12 hr apart) after meals for 2 wk, followed by 1-wk rest period; given as 3-wk cycles.	• Use cautiously in patients with history of CAD, mild-to-moderate hepatic dysfunction caused by liver metastases, hyperbilirubinemia, or renal insufficiency, and in the elderly. • Know that patients age 80 and older may experience greater incidence of GI adverse effects. • If severe diarrhea occurs, notify doctor. If patient becomes dehydrated, give fluid

Adjust-a-dose: National Cancer Institute of Canada (NCIC) Common Toxicity Criteria: NCIC grade 2: first appearance, interrupt treatment until resolved to grade 0 to 1, then restart at 100% of starting dose for next cycle; second appearance, interrupt treatment until resolved to grade 0 to 1 and use 75% of starting dose for next cycle; third appearance, interrupt treatment until resolved to grade 0 to 1 and use 50% of starting dose for next cycle; fourth appearance, discontinue treatment permanently.

NCIC grade 3: first appearance, interrupt treatment until resolved to grade 0 to 1 and use 75% of starting dose for next cycle; second appearance, interrupt treatment until resolved to grade 0 to 1 and use 50% of starting dose for next cycle; third appearance, discontinue treatment permanently.

NCIC grade 4: first appearance, discontinue treatment permanently or interrupt treatment until resolved to grade 0 to 1 and use 50% of starting dose for next cycle.

Note: Toxicity criteria relate to degrees of severity of diarrhea, nausea, vomiting, stomatitis, and hand-and-foot syndrome. Refer to capecitabine package insert for specific toxicity definitions.

and electrolyte replacement, as ordered. Drug may need to be immediately interrupted until diarrhea resolves or decreases in intensity.

- Adjust drug therapy immediately if patient exhibits symptoms of hand-and-foot syndrome (numbness, paresthesia, tingling, painless or painful swelling, erythema, desquamation, blistering and severe pain of hands or feet), hyperbilirubinemia, or severe nausea.

- Know that hyperbilirubinemia may require stopping drug.

- Monitor patient carefully for toxicity. Toxicity may be managed by symptomatic treatment, dose interruptions, and dosage adjustments.

51

DRUG / CLASS / CATEGORY	INDICATIONS / DOSAGES	KEY NURSING CONSIDERATIONS
capsaicin Axsain, Zostrix, Zostrix-HP 0.075% *Naturally occurring chemical derived from plants of the Solanaceae family* *Topical analgesic* Pregnancy Risk Category: NR	*Temporary relief of pain after herpes zoster infections; neuralgias; pain associated with osteoarthritis or rheumatoid arthritis* — **Adults and children > 2 yr:** apply to affected areas no more than q.i.d.	• For external use only. • Warn patient to avoid getting drug in eyes or on broken skin. • Advise patient not to bandage area tightly after application. • Wash hands thoroughly after use.
captopril Apo-Capto†, Capoten, Novo-Captopril† *ACE inhibitor* *Antihypertensive/adjunctive treatment of heart failure* Pregnancy Risk Category: C (D in second and third trimesters)	*Hypertension* — **Adults:** initially, 25 mg P.O. b.i.d. or t.i.d. If BP not controlled in 1 to 2 wk, increase to 50 mg b.i.d. or t.i.d. If BP not controlled after another 1 to 2 wk, expect to add diuretic. If further BP reduction needed, may increase dosage to 150 mg t.i.d. while continuing diuretic. Maximum 450 mg q.d. *Heart failure; to reduce risk of death and to slow development of heart failure after MI* — **Adults:** initially, 6.25 to 12.5 mg P.O. t.i.d. Gradually increase to 50 mg t.i.d., p.r.n. Maximum 450 mg q.d.	• Monitor BP and HR frequently. • Elderly patients may be more sensitive to hypotensive effects. • In impaired renal function or collagen vascular disease, monitor WBC and differential before treatment starts and every 2 wk for first 3 mo of therapy. • Give capsule 1 hr before meals because food in GI tract may reduce absorption. • Inform patient that dizziness may occur during first few days of therapy.
carbachol (intraocular) Miostat **carbachol (topical)** Isopto Carbachol	*To produce pupillary miosis during ocular surgery* — **Adults:** before or after securing sutures, doctor gently instills 0.5 ml (intraocular form) into anterior chamber.	• In case of toxicity, give atropine parenterally. • Patients with dark eyes may require stronger solutions or more frequent instillation.

Cholinergic agonist
Miotic
Pregnancy Risk Category: C

Open-angle glaucoma — **Adults:** 1 to 2 drops instilled (topical form) q 4 to 8 hr.

- Warn patient to avoid hazardous activities until temporary blurring subsides.

carbamazepine

Apo-Carbamazepine†, Epitol, Novo-Carbamaz†, Tegretol

Iminostilbene derivative; chemically related to TCAs

Anticonvulsant/analgesic

Pregnancy Risk Category: C

Generalized tonic-clonic and complex partial seizures; mixed seizure patterns — **Adults and children > 12 yr:** 200 mg P.O. b.i.d. (tablets) or 1 tsp (suspension) P.O. q.i.d. Increase at weekly intervals by 200 mg P.O. q.d., in divided doses at 6- to 8-hr intervals. Adjust to minimum effective level. Maximum 1 g/day in ages 12 to 15 or 1.2 g/day in patients > age 15. **Children 6 to 12 yr:** 100 mg P.O. b.i.d. or ½ tsp of suspension P.O. q.i.d. Increase weekly by 100 mg P.O. q.d. Maximum 1 g/day. **Children < 6 yr:** 10 to 20 mg/kg/day P.O. b.i.d. or t.i.d. (tablets) or q.i.d. (suspension). Maximum 35 mg/kg/day.

- Therapeutic blood level is 4 to 12 mcg/ml.
- Observe for appetite changes.
- Monitor urinalysis, BUN, liver function tests, CBC, platelet and reticulocyte counts, and serum iron level.
- Institute seizure precautions.
- When giving by NG tube, mix with equal volume water, 0.9% NaCl solution, or D₅W. Then flush with 100 ml diluent.
- Tell patient not to discontinue drug suddenly and to notify doctor immediately if adverse reactions occur.

carbamide peroxide

Debrox

Urea hydrogen peroxide

Ceruminolytic/topical antiseptic

Pregnancy Risk Category: NR

Impacted cerumen — **Adults and children:** 5 to 10 drops into ear canal b.i.d. for up to 4 days. Allow to remain in ear canal for 15 to 30 min; remove with warm water.

- Use in children < 12 years only under a doctor's direction.
- Tell patient to flush ear gently with warm water, using a rubber bulb syringe.
- Tell patient to call doctor if redness, pain, or swelling persists.

†Canadian ‡Australian

DRUG/CLASS/CATEGORY	INDICATIONS/DOSAGES	KEY NURSING CONSIDERATIONS
carbidopa-levodopa Sinemet, Sinemet CR *Decarboxylase inhibitor-dopamine precursor* *Antiparkinsonian* Pregnancy Risk Category: C	*Idiopathic Parkinson's disease; postencephalitic parkinsonism; symptomatic parkinsonism resulting from carbon monoxide or manganese intoxication* — **Adults:** 1 tablet 25 mg carbidopa/100 mg levodopa P.O. t.i.d.; then increase by 1 tablet q.d. or q.o.d., p.r.n. to maximum 8 tablets q.d. 25 mg carbidopa/250 mg levodopa or 10 mg carbidopa/100 mg levodopa tablet substituted as required to obtain maximum response. Optimum dosage determined by individual titration. Patients treated with conventional tablets may receive extended-release tablets; dosage calculated on current levodopa intake. Initially, extended-release tablet dosage should amount to 10% more levodopa per day, increased as needed and tolerated to 30% more per day. Give in divided doses at intervals of 4 to 8 hr.	▪ Muscle twitching and blepharospasm may be early signs of overdose. ▪ Discontinue levodopa at least 8 hr before starting carbidopa-levodopa. ▪ Therapeutic and adverse reactions more rapid with carbidopa-levodopa than levodopa alone. Monitor vital signs, especially while adjusting dosage. ▪ Tell patient not to crush or chew sustained-release tablets; however, they can be broken in half. ▪ With long-term therapy, patient should be tested regularly for diabetes and acromegaly and have periodic tests of liver, renal, and hematopoietic function.
carboplatin Paraplatin, Paraplatin-AQ† *Alkylating agent* *Antineoplastic* Pregnancy Risk Category: D	*Palliative treatment of ovarian cancer* — **Adults:** 360 mg/m² I.V. on day 1 q 4 weeks; doses not repeated until platelet count > 100,000/mm³ and neutrophil count > 2,000/mm³. Subsequent doses based on blood counts. ***Adjust-a-dose:*** Adjust dosage in renal failure and for creatinine clearance < 60 ml/min.	▪ Check serum electrolyte, creatinine, BUN, CBC, and creatinine clearance before first infusion and each course of treatment. ▪ I.V. form associated with mutagenic, teratogenic, and carcinogenic risks for personnel. Have emergency drugs available when administering drug.

- Do not use needles or I.V. administration sets containing aluminum to administer drug.
- Monitor vital signs during infusion.

Drug not recommended for patients with creatinine clearance ≤ 15 ml/min.

carisoprodol
Sodol, Soma
Carbamate derivative
Skeletal muscle relaxant
Pregnancy Risk Category: NR

As adjunct in acute, painful musculoskeletal conditions — **Adults:** 350 mg P.O. t.i.d. and h.s.

- Watch for idiosyncratic reactions (weakness, ataxia, visual and speech difficulties, fever, skin eruptions, and mental changes) after first to fourth dose and for severe reactions (including bronchospasm, hypotension, and anaphylactic shock).
- Record amount of relief to help determine whether dosage can be reduced.
- Don't stop drug abruptly.

---

carmustine (BCNU)
BiCNU
Alkylating agent
Antineoplastic
Pregnancy Risk Category: D

Brain tumors; Hodgkin's disease; malignant lymphoma; multiple myeloma — **Adults:** 75 to 100 mg/m^2 I.V. by slow infusion q.d. for 2 days; repeated q 6 wk if platelet count is > 100,000/mm^3 and WBC count is > 4,000/mm^3. Dosage reduced by 30% when WBC count is 2,000 to 3,000/mm^3 and platelet count is 2,000 to 3,000/mm^3 and platelet count falls. Or, 150 to 200 mg/m^2 I.V. by slow infusion as single dose, repeated q 6 weeks.
Adjust-a-dose: Reduced dosage required when WBC count < 4,000/mm^3.

- Parenteral form associated with carcinogenic, mutagenic, and teratogenic risks for personnel.
- Dilute solution with 27 ml sterile water for injection. Resultant solution contains 3.3 mg of carmustine/ml when further diluted in 0.9% NaCl solution or D$_5$W for I.V. infusion. Give at least 250 ml over 1 to 2 hr.
- Monitor CBC, uric acid, and liver, renal, and pulmonary function tests periodically.

DRUG / CLASS / CATEGORY	INDICATIONS / DOSAGES	KEY NURSING CONSIDERATIONS
carteolol hydrochloride (oral) Cartrol *Beta blocker* *Antihypertensive* Pregnancy Risk Category: C	*Hypertension* — **Adults:** initially, 2.5 mg P.O. as single daily dose; increase gradually to 5 or 10 mg as single daily dose, as needed. Doses > 10 mg q.d. don't produce greater response (may actually decrease response). **Adjust-a-dose:** In patients with creatinine clearance from 20 to 60 ml/min, dosage interval is 48 hr. In those with creatinine clearance < 20 ml/min, interval is 72 hr.	• Monitor BP frequently. • May inhibit glycogenolysis and hypoglycemia signs and symptoms. • May mask tachycardia associated with hyperthyroidism. • Patients with unrecognized CAD may experience angina pectoris on withdrawal.
carteolol hydrochloride (ophthalmic) Ocupress Ophthalmic Solution, 1% *Beta blocker* *Antihypertensive* Pregnancy Risk Category: C	*Chronic open-angle glaucoma; intraocular hypertension* — **Adults:** 1 drop b.i.d. in conjunctival sac of affected eye.	• Discontinue drug at first sign of cardiac failure and notify doctor. • If signs of serious adverse reactions or hypersensitivity occur, tell patient to discontinue drug and notify doctor immediately.
carvedilol Coreg *Beta blocker* *Vasodilator/antihypertensive* Pregnancy Risk Category: C	*Hypertension* — **Adults:** dosage highly individualized. Initially, 6.25 mg P.O. b.i.d. Obtain a standing BP 1 hr after initial dose. If tolerated, continue dosage for 7 to 14 days. May increase to 12.5 mg P.O. b.i.d. for 7 to 14 days, following BP monitoring protocol noted above. Maximum dose 25 mg P.O. b.i.d., as tolerated.	• Be aware that prior to starting drug, dosages of digoxin, diuretics, or ACE inhibitors should be stabilized. • Use cautiously in hypertensive patients with left-sided heart failure, perioperative patients who receive anesthetics that depress myocardial function, diabetic patients receiving insulin or oral antidiabetic agents,

and in those subject to spontaneous hypoglycemia. Also use with caution in patients with thyroid disease, pheochromocytoma, Prinzmetal's or variant angina, bronchospastic disease, or PVD, and in breast-feeding women.

- Patients on beta-blocker therapy with history of severe anaphylactic reaction to several allergens may be more reactive to repeated challenge. They may be unresponsive to dosages of epinephrine typically used to treat allergic reactions.
- If patient needs to be taken off drug, discontinue gradually over 1 to 2 wk.
- Monitor patient with heart failure for worsened condition, renal dysfunction, or fluid retention; diuretics may need to be increased.
- Observe patient for dizziness or light-headedness for 1 hr after administration of each new dose.

Heart failure — **Adults:** dosage highly individualized. Initially, 3.125 mg P.O. b.i.d. for 2 weeks; if tolerated, can increase to 6.25 mg P.O. b.i.d. Dosage may be doubled q 2 wk, as tolerated. Maximum for patients < 85 kg (187 lb) 25 mg P.O. b.i.d.; for those > 85 kg, 50 mg P.O. b.i.d. **Children:** Safety and efficacy in patients < 18 years have not been established.

Adjust-a-dose: If patient experiences bradycardia with pulse rate < 55 beats/min, use reduced dose.

- Before giving for constipation, determine if fluid intake, exercise, and diet are adequate.
- Give with full glass of water.
- Monitor serum electrolytes.

---

cascara sagrada
Anthraquinone glycoside
mixture
Laxative
Pregnancy Risk Category: C

Acute constipation; preparation for bowel or rectal exam — **Adults and children ≥ 12 yr:** one 325-mg tablet P.O. q.d. h.s. **Children < 2 yr:** one-quarter adult dosage. **Children 2 to 12 yr:** one-half adult dosage.

DRUG / CLASS / CATEGORY	INDICATIONS / DOSAGES	KEY NURSING CONSIDERATIONS
cefaclor Ceclor *Second-generation cephalosporin Antibiotic* Pregnancy Risk Category: B	*Respiratory, urinary tract, skin, or soft-tissue infections and otitis media caused by susceptible organisms —* **Adults:** 250 to 500 mg P.O. q 8 hr. For pharyngitis or otitis media, may give daily dose in 2 equally divided doses q 12 hr. **Children:** 20 mg/kg q.d. P.O. in divided doses q 8 hr. For pharyngitis or otitis media, may give daily dose in 2 equally divided doses q 12 hr. In more serious infections, 40 mg/kg q.d. recommended, not to exceed 1 g q.d.	▪ Obtain specimen for culture and sensitivity tests before first dose. ▪ With large doses or prolonged therapy, monitor for superinfection, especially in high-risk patients. ▪ Store reconstituted suspension in refrigerator for up to 14 days. Shake well before using. ▪ Tell patient to call doctor if rash occurs.
cefadroxil monohydrate Duricef, Ultracef *First-generation cephalosporin Antibiotic* Pregnancy Risk Category: B	*UTIs, skin and soft-tissue infections, and pharyngitis or tonsillitis caused by susceptible organisms —* **Adults:** 1 to 2 g P.O. q.d., depending on infection type. Usually given q.d. or b.i.d. **Children:** 30 mg/kg P.O. q.d. in 2 divided doses q 12 hr. **Adjust-a-dose:** In patients with creatinine clearance < 50 ml/min, reduce dosage.	▪ Obtain specimen for culture and sensitivity tests before first dose. ▪ With large doses or prolonged therapy, monitor for superinfection, especially in high-risk patients. ▪ Instruct patient to take with food or milk. ▪ Advise patient to call doctor if rash occurs.
cefazolin sodium Ancef, Kefzol, Zolicef *First-generation cephalosporin Antibiotic* Pregnancy Risk Category: B	*Prophylaxis in contaminated surgery —* **Adults:** 1 g I.M. or I.V. 30 to 60 min before surgery; then 0.5 to 1 g I.M. or I.V. q 6 to 8 hr for 24 hr. In operations > 2 hr, may give another 0.5 to 1 g I.M. intraoperatively.	▪ Obtain specimen for culture and sensitivity tests before first dose. ▪ **I.V. use:** Reconstitute with diluent: 2 ml to 500-mg vial; 2.5 ml to 1-g vial. Shake until dissolved. Resultant concentration: 225 mg/ml or 330 mg/ml, respectively.

Where infection would be devastating, prophylaxis may continue for 3 to 5 days. *Respiratory; biliary; GU; skin; soft-tissue; bone and joint infections; septicemia; endocarditis caused by susceptible organisms* — **Adults:** 250 mg I.M. or I.V. q 8 hr to 1.5 g P.O. q 6 hr. Maximum 12 g/day in life-threatening situations. **Infants > 1 mo:** 25 to 50 mg/kg or 1.25 g/m² q.d. I.M. or I.V. in three or four divided doses. May increase to 100 mg/kg/day.

Adjust-a-dose: If creatinine clearance 11 to 34 ml/min, give 50% usual dose q 12 hr; if creatinine clearance < 10 ml/min, give 50% usual dose q 18 to 24 hr.

- For direct injection, dilute Ancef with 5 ml or Kefzol with 10 ml of sterile water for injection. Inject into large vein or tubing of free-flowing I.V. solution over 3 to 5 min. For intermittent infusion, add reconstituted drug to 50 to 100 ml of compatible solution or use a premixed solution.
- With large doses or prolonged therapy, monitor for superinfection.

cefdinir
Omnicef
*Broad-spectrum
cephalosporin
Antibiotic*
Pregnancy Risk Category: B

Treatment of mild to moderate infections caused by susceptible strains of microorganisms for conditions of community-acquired pneumonia; acute exacerbations of chronic bronchitis; acute maxillary sinusitis; acute bacterial otitis media; uncomplicated skin and skin-structure infections — **Adults and children ≥ 13 yr:** 300 mg P.O. q 12 hr or 600 mg P.O. q 24 hr for 10 days. (Use q-12-hr doses for pneumonia and skin infections.) **Children 6 mo to 12 yr:** 7 mg/kg P.O. q 12 hr or 14 mg/kg P.O. q 24 hr for 10 days, up to maximum of 600 mg q.d. (Use q-12-hr doses for skin infections.)

- Use cautiously in patients with known hypersensitivity to penicillin, because of possible cross-sensitivity with other beta-lactam antibiotics, and in those with history of colitis and renal insufficiency.
- Prolonged drug treatment may result in possible emergence and overgrowth of resistant organisms. Monitor for symptoms of superinfection.
- Pseudomembranous colitis has been reported with cefdinir and should be considered in patients with diarrhea subsequent

(continued)

†Canadian ‡Australian

DRUG/CLASS/ CATEGORY	INDICATIONS/ DOSAGES	KEY NURSING CONSIDERATIONS
cefdinir *(continued)*	*Treatment of pharyngitis and tonsillitis —* **Adults and children ≥ 13 yr:** 300 mg P.O. q 12 hr for 5 to 10 days or 600 mg P.O. q 24 hr for 10 days. **Children 6 mo to 12 yr:** 7 mg/kg P.O. q 12 hr for 5 to 10 days or 14 mg/kg P.O. q 24 hr for 10 days. *Adjust-a-dose:* If creatinine clearance < 30 ml/min, reduce dosage to 300 mg P.O. once daily for adults and 7 mg/kg (up to 300 mg) P.O. once daily for children. In patients receiving chronic hemodialysis, 300 mg or 7 mg/kg P.O. at end of each dialysis session and subsequently q.o.d.	to antibiotic therapy or in those with history of colitis. ▪ Tell diabetic patients that each tsp of suspension contains 2.86 g of sucrose. ▪ Antacids, iron supplements, and multivitamins containing iron reduce rate of absorption and bioavailability; administer these types of preparations 2 hr before or after cefdinir. ▪ Know that cephalosporins may induce a positive Coombs' test.
cefepime hydrochloride Maxipime *Semisynthetic cephalosporin* *Antibiotic* Pregnancy Risk Category: B	*Mild to moderate UTI caused by susceptible organisms —* **Adults and children ≥ 12 yr:** 0.5 to 1 g I.M. (I.M. used only for infections caused by *E. coli*) or I.V. infused over 30 min q 12 hr for 7 to 10 days. *Severe UTI —* **Adults and children ≥ 12 yr:** 2 g I.V. infused over 30 min q 12 hr for 10 days. *Moderate to severe pneumonia —* **Adults and children ≥ 12 yr:** 1 to 2 g I.V. infused over 30 min q 12 hr for 10 days. *Adjust-a-dose:* Reduce dose in patients with renal failure.	▪ Obtain specimens for culture and sensitivity tests before first dose, if appropriate. ▪ *I.V. use:* Give resulting solution over about 30 min. ▪ Monitor PT, as ordered. Give exogenous vitamin K, as ordered. ▪ Monitor for superinfection. ▪ Instruct patient to report adverse reactions promptly.

cefmetazole sodium (cefmetazone)
Zefazone
Second-generation cephalosporin
Antibiotic
Pregnancy Risk Category: B

Lower respiratory tract, intra-abdominal, skin, and skin-structure infections caused by susceptible organisms — **Adults:** 2 g I.V. q 6 to 12 hr for 5 to 14 days.
UTIs caused by E. coli — **Adults:** 2 g I.V. q 12 hr.
Adjust-a-dose: Patients with renal failure may receive reduced dose, longer dosing interval, or both.

- Obtain specimen for culture and sensitivity tests before first dose.
- Monitor for superinfection.
- Monitor PT in patients at risk from renal or hepatic impairment, malnutrition, or prolonged therapy.
- Tell patient to report adverse reactions promptly.

cefonicid sodium
Monocid
Second-generation cephalosporin
Antibiotic
Pregnancy Risk Category: B

Perioperative prophylaxis in contaminated surgery — **Adults:** 1 g I.M. or I.V. 30 to 60 min before surgery; then 1 g I.M. or I.V. q.d. for 2 days after surgery. If used for prophylaxis in cesarean section, 1 g I.M. or I.V. after umbilical cord is clamped.
Serious infections of lower respiratory and urinary tracts; skin and skin-structure infections; septicemia; bone and joint infections; preoperative prophylaxis — **Adults:** usual dose 1 g I.V. or I.M. q 24 hr; in life-threatening infections, 2 g q 24 hr.
Adjust-a-dose: Patients with creatinine clearance < 80 ml/min require dosage adjustment.

- Obtain specimen for culture and sensitivity tests before first dose.
- With large doses or prolonged therapy, monitor for superinfection.
- When giving 2-g I.M. doses q.d., divide dose equally and inject deeply into large muscle mass, such as gluteus maximus or lateral aspect of thigh.

DRUG / CLASS / CATEGORY	INDICATIONS / DOSAGES	KEY NURSING CONSIDERATIONS
cefoperazone sodium Cefobid *Third-generation cephalosporin* *Antibiotic* Pregnancy Risk Category: B	*Serious respiratory tract infections; intra-abdominal, gynecologic, and skin infections; bacteremia; septicemia caused by susceptible organisms* — **Adults:** usual dose 1 to 2 g q 12 hr I.M. or I.V. In severe infections or infections caused by less sensitive organisms, total daily dose or frequency may increase to 16 g/day in certain situations. *Adjust-a-dose:* In patients with hepatic and biliary obstruction, total daily dose shouldn't exceed 4 g/day.	• Obtain specimen for culture and sensitivity tests before first dose. • Give doses of 4 g/day cautiously in hepatic disease or biliary obstruction. • With large doses or prolonged therapy, monitor for superinfection. • Monitor PT regularly. Vitamin K promptly reverses bleeding. • For I.M. use, inject deeply into large muscle mass.
cefotaxime sodium Claforan *Third-generation cephalosporin* *Antibiotic* Pregnancy Risk Category: B	*Perioperative prophylaxis in contaminated surgery* — **Adults:** 1 g I.M. or I.V. 30 to 60 min before surgery. For cesarean section, 1 g I.M. or I.V. as soon as umbilical cord clamped; then 1 g I.M. or I.V. 6 and 12 hr later. *Serious infections of lower respiratory and urinary tracts, CNS, skin, bone, and joints; gynecologic and intra-abdominal infections; bacteremia; septicemia caused by susceptible organisms* — **Adults:** usual dose 1 g I.V. or I.M. q 6 to 8 hr. Up to 12 g q.d. can be given in life-threatening infections.	• Obtain specimen for culture and sensitivity tests before first dose. • *I.V. use:* Inject into large vein or into tubing of free-flowing I.V. solution over 3 to 5 min. For infusion, infuse over 20 to 30 min. • For I.M. use, inject deeply into large muscle mass, such as gluteus maximus or lateral aspect of thigh. • With large doses or prolonged therapy, monitor for superinfection. • Advise patient to report adverse reactions promptly.

Children ≥ 50 kg (110 lb): usual adult dose, but don't exceed 12 g q.d. **Children 1 mo to 12 yr weighing < 50 kg:** 50 to 180 mg/kg/day I.M. or I.V. in 4 to 6 divided doses.
Neonates to 1 wk: 50 mg/kg I.V. q 12 hr.
Neonates 1 to 4 wk: 50 mg/kg I.V. q 8 hr.
Adjust-a-dose: If creatinine clearance < 20 ml/min, give ½ usual dose at usual interval.

cefotetan disodium Cefotan *Second-generation cephalosporin/cephamycin Antibiotic* Pregnancy Risk Category: B	*Serious UTI and lower respiratory tract infections and gynecologic, skin and skin-structure, intra-abdominal, and bone and joint infections caused by susceptible organisms* — **Adults:** 1 to 2 g I.V. or I.M. q 12 hr for 5 to 10 days. Up to 6 g q.d. in life-threatening infections. *Perioperative prophylaxis* — **Adults:** 1 to 2 g I.V. given once 30 to 60 min before surgery. In cesarean section, give dose as soon as umbilical cord clamped. *Adjust-a-dose:* If creatinine clearance 10 to 30 ml/min, give usual dose q 24 hr. If < 10 ml/min, give usual dose q 48 hr.	▪ Obtain specimen for culture and sensitivity tests before first dose. ▪ *I.V. use:* Reconstitute with sterile water for injection. Then drug may be mixed with 50 to 100 ml D_5W or 0.9% NaCl solution. ▪ With large doses or prolonged therapy, monitor for superinfection.
cefoxitin sodium Mefoxin *Second-generation cephalosporin/cephamycin Antibiotic*	*Serious infections of respiratory and GU tracts; skin, soft-tissue, bone, and joint infections; bloodstream and intra-abdominal infections caused by susceptible organisms; perioperative prophylaxis* — **Adults:** 1 to 2 g q 6 to 8 hr in uncomplicated infec-	▪ Obtain specimen for culture and sensitivity tests before first dose. ▪ *I.V. use:* For direct injection, inject into large vein or into tubing of free-flowing

(continued)

DRUG/CLASS/ CATEGORY	INDICATIONS/ DOSAGES	KEY NURSING CONSIDERATIONS
cefoxitin sodium *(continued)* Pregnancy Risk Category: B	tions. Up to 12 g q.d. in life-threatening infections. **Children > 3 mo:** 80 to 160 mg/kg q.d. in 4 to 6 equally divided doses. Maximum 12 g q.d. *Prophylactic use in surgery* — **Adults:** 2 g I.M. or I.V. 30 to 60 min before surgery; then 2 g I.M. or I.V. q 6 hr for 24 hr (72 hr after prosthetic arthroplasty). **Children ≥ 3 mo:** 30 to 40 mg/kg I.M. or I.V. 30 to 60 min before surgery; then 30 to 40 mg/kg q 6 hr for 24 hr (72 hr after prosthetic arthroplasty). *Adjust-a-dose:* If creatinine clearance < 50 ml/min, dosage reduction required.	• I.V. solution over 3 to 5 min. For intermittent infusion, add reconstituted drug to 50 or 100 ml D_5W, $D_{10}W$, or 0.9% NaCl injection. Interrupt flow of primary I.V. solution during infusion. • Assess I.V. site frequently. I.V. use linked to thrombophlebitis. • For I.M. use, reconstitute I.M. injection with 0.5% or 1% lidocaine hydrochloride (without epinephrine) to minimize pain. Inject deeply into large muscle mass. • With large doses or prolonged therapy, monitor for superinfection.
cefpodoxime proxetil Vantin *Second-generation cephalosporin Antibiotic* Pregnancy Risk Category: B	*Acute, community-acquired pneumonia caused by susceptible organisms* — **Adults and children ≥ 13 yr:** 200 mg P.O. q 12 hr for 14 days. *Acute bacterial exacerbation of chronic bronchitis caused by susceptible organisms* — **Adults and children ≥ 13 yr:** 200 mg P.O. q 12 hr for 10 days. *Uncomplicated UTI due to E. coli, K. pneumoniae, P. mirabilis, or S. saprophyticus* — **Adults:** 100 mg P.O. q 12 hr for 7 days. *Adjust-a-dose:* If creatinine clearance < 30 ml/min, increase dose interval to q 24 hr.	• Obtain specimen for culture and sensitivity tests before first dose. • Keep oral suspension refrigerated. Shake well before measuring dose. • Give tablets with food to enhance absorption. • Monitor for superinfection. • May cause false-positive urine glucose results with copper sulfate tests (Clinitest). Glucose enzymatic tests (Diastix) not affected.

cefprozil
Cefzil
Second-generation cephalosporin
Antibiotic
Pregnancy Risk Category: B

Pharyngitis or tonsillitis caused by S. pyogenes — **Adults and children ≥ 13 yr:** 500 mg P.O. q.d. for at least 10 days.
Otitis media caused by S. pneumoniae, H. influenzae, *or* M. (Branhamella) catarrhalis — **Infants and children 6 mo to 12 yr:** 15 mg/kg P.O. q 12 hr for 10 days.
Acute sinusitis caused by susceptible organisms — **Adults and children ≥ 13 yr:** 250 to 500 mg P.O. q 12 hr for 10 days. **Children 6 mo to 12 yr:** 7.5 to 15 mg/kg P.O. q 12 hr for 10 days.
Adjust-a-dose: If creatinine clearance < 30 ml/min, give 50% of usual dose.

- Obtain specimen for culture and sensitivity tests before first dose.
- Removed by hemodialysis; give after hemodialysis treatment is completed.
- Monitor for superinfection.
- Tell patient to shake suspension well before measuring dose.
- Instruct patient to notify doctor if rash develops.

---

ceftazidime
Ceptaz, Fortaz, Tazicef, Tazidime
Third-generation cephalosporin
Antibiotic
Pregnancy Risk Category: B

Serious infections of lower respiratory and urinary tracts; gynecologic, intra-abdominal, CNS, and skin infections; bacteremia; septicemia — **Adults and children ≥ 12 yr:** 1 g I.V. or I.M. q 8 to 12 hr; up to 6 g q.d. in life-threatening infections. **Children 1 mo to 12 yr:** 25 to 50 mg/kg I.V. q 8 hr (sodium carbonate formulation). **Neonates 0 to 4 wk:** 30 mg/kg I.V. q 12 hr (sodium carbonate formulation).
Adjust-a-dose: Patients with creatinine clearance < 50 ml/min require dosage adjustment.

- Obtain specimen for culture and sensitivity tests before first dose.
- *I.V. use:* Read and follow instructions for reconstitution carefully.
- Removed by hemodialysis; give supplemental dose after each dialysis period, as ordered.
- For I.M. use, inject deeply into large muscle mass.
- With large doses or prolonged therapy, monitor for superinfection.

DRUG/CLASS/CATEGORY	INDICATIONS/DOSAGES	KEY NURSING CONSIDERATIONS
ceftibuten Cedax *Second-generation cephalosporin* *Antibiotic* Pregnancy Risk Category: B	*Acute bacterial exacerbation of chronic bronchitis due to susceptible organisms* — **Adults and children ≥ age 12:** 400 mg P.O. q.d. for 10 days. *Pharyngitis and tonsillitis due to S. pyogenes; acute bacterial otitis media due to H. influenzae, M. catarrhalis, or S. pyogenes* — **Adults and children ≥ age 12:** 400 mg P.O. q.d. for 10 days. **Children < age 12:** 9 mg/kg P.O. q.d. for 10 days. **Children > 45 kg:** maximum 400 mg P.O. q.d. for 10 days. *Adjust-a-dose:* Patients with renal impairment and those undergoing hemodialysis require dosage adjustment.	▪ Obtain specimen for culture and sensitivity tests before giving first dose. ▪ Discontinue if allergic reaction suspected. Emergency treatment may be required. ▪ Consider possibility of pseudomembranous colitis in patients who develop diarrhea secondary to therapy. Obtain specimens for *C. difficile,* as ordered. ▪ Monitor patient for superinfection.
ceftizoxime sodium Cefizox *Third-generation cephalosporin* *Antibiotic* Pregnancy Risk Category: B	*Serious infections of lower respiratory and urinary tracts; gynecologic, intra-abdominal, bone, joint, and skin infections; bacteremia; septicemia; meningitis caused by susceptible microorganisms* — **Adults:** usual dose 1 to 2 g I.V. or I.M. q 8 to 12 hr. In life-threatening infections, up to 2 g I.V. q 4 hr. **Children > 6 mo:** 33 to 50 mg/kg I.V. q 6 to 8 hr. Serious infections: up to 200 mg/kg/day in divided doses. Don't exceed 12 g/day.	▪ Obtain specimen for culture and sensitivity tests before first dose. ▪ *I.V. use:* To reconstitute powder, add 5 ml sterile water to 500-mg vial, 10 ml to 1-g vial, or 20 ml to 2-g vial. Reconstitute piggyback vials with 50 to 100 ml 0.9% NaCl solution or D_5W. Shake well. ▪ For I.M. use, inject deeply into large muscle mass. Divide larger doses (2 g) and inject at two separate sites. ▪ Monitor for superinfection.

ceftriaxone sodium
Rocephin
Third-generation cephalosporin
Antibiotic
Pregnancy Risk Category: B

Most infections caused by susceptible organisms — **Adults:** 1 to 2 g I.M. or I.V. q.d. or b.i.d. depending on severity of infection. *Serious infections of lower respiratory and urinary tracts; gynecologic, bone, joint, intra-abdominal, and skin infections; bacteremia; septicemia; Lyme disease caused by susceptible organisms* — **Adults and children > 12 yr:** 1 to 2 g I.M. or I.V. q.d. or in equally divided doses b.i.d. Maximum 4 g/day. **Children ≤ 12 yr:** 50 to 75 mg/kg I.M. or I.V., not to exceed 2 g/day, in divided doses q 12 hr.

Meningitis — **Adults and children:** initially, 100 mg/kg I.M. or I.V. (not to exceed 4 g); thereafter, 100 mg/kg I.M. or I.V., once daily or in divided doses q 12 hr, not to exceed 4 g, for 7 to 14 days.

- Obtain specimen for culture and sensitivity tests before first dose.
- For I.M. use, inject deeply into large muscle mass.
- Monitor for superinfection.
- Commonly used in home antibiotic programs for outpatient treatment of serious infections such as osteomyelitis.

cefuroxime axetil
Ceftin
cefuroxime sodium
Kefurox, Zinacef
Second-generation cephalosporin
Antibiotic
Pregnancy Risk Category: B

Injectable form used for serious infections and for perioperative prophylaxis. Oral form used for otitis media, pharyngitis, tonsillitis, infections of urinary and lower respiratory tracts, and skin and skin-structure infections due to susceptible organisms — **Adults and children ≥ 12 yr:** usual dosage of cefuroxime sodium: 750 mg to 1.5 g I.M. or I.V. q 8 hr for 5 to 10 days. For life-threatening infections and less susceptible organisms, 1.5 g I.M. or I.V. q 6 hr; for bacterial menin-

- Obtain specimen for culture and sensitivity tests before first dose.
- *I.V. use:* For direct injection, inject into large vein or into tubing of free-flowing I.V. solution over 3 to 5 min.
- For I.M. doses, inject deeply into large muscle mass.
- Food enhances absorption of cefuroxime axetil.

(continued)

67

†Canadian ‡Australian

DRUG/CLASS/ CATEGORY	INDICATIONS/ DOSAGES	KEY NURSING CONSIDERATIONS
cefuroxime axetil *(continued)*	gitis, up to 3 g I.V. q 8 hr. Or, 250 to 500 mg of cefuroxime axetil P.O. q 12 hr. **Children and infants > 3 mo:** 50 to 100 mg/kg/day of cefuroxime sodium I.M. or I.V. in divided doses q 6 to 8 hr. Higher doses used for meningitis. Or, 125 mg of cefuroxime axetil P.O. q 12 hr; for bacterial meningitis, 200 to 240 mg/kg I.V. in divided doses q 6 to 8 hr. *Otitis media* — **Children < 2 yr:** 125 mg P.O. q 12 hr. **Children ≥ 2 yr:** 250 mg P.O. q 12 hr. *Early Lyme disease caused by B. burgdorferi* — **Adults and children ≥ 13 yr:** 500 mg P.O. b.i.d. for 20 days. ***Adjust-a-dose:*** For parenteral administration, patients with creatinine clearance < 20 ml/min require dosage adjustment.	▪ With large doses or prolonged therapy, monitor for superinfection, especially in high-risk patients. ▪ Advise patient to report pain at I.V. site. ▪ Tell patient to report adverse reactions promptly.
celecoxib Celebrex *COX-2 inhibitor* *NSAID* Pregnancy Risk Category: C	*Relief of signs and symptoms of osteoarthritis* — **Adults:** 200 mg P.O. q.d. as a single dose or divided equally b.i.d. *Relief of signs and symptoms of rheumatoid arthritis* — **Adults:** 100 to 200 mg P.O. b.i.d. ***Adjust-a-dose:*** In patients < 50 kg (110 lb), start at lowest recommended dosage. In patients with moderate hepatic impairment	▪ Patients with history of ulcers or GI bleeding are at higher risk for GI bleeding while taking NSAIDs. Other risk factors for GI bleeding include treatment with corticosteroids or anticoagulants, longer duration of NSAID treatment, smoking, alcoholism, older age, and poor overall health. ▪ Monitor for signs and symptoms of overt and occult bleeding.

Drug	Indications & Dosages	Nursing Considerations

(Child-Pugh Class II), start therapy with reduced dosage.

- Know that NSAIDs can cause fluid retention. Also, closely monitor patients who have hypertension, edema, or heart failure.
- Know that NSAIDs may be hepatotoxic. Monitor for such signs and symptoms as nausea, fatigue, lethargy, and jaundice.
- Aluminum and magnesium antacids may decrease the effect of celecoxib and should be administered at least 1 hr apart.

---

cephalexin hydrochloride
Keftab

cephalexin monohydrate
Apo-Cephalex†, Biocef, Cefanex, Keflex
First-generation cephalosporin
Antibiotic
Pregnancy Risk Category: B

Respiratory and GI tract, skin, soft-tissue, bone, and joint infections and otitis media caused by E. coli and other coliform bacteria, group A beta-hemolytic streptococci, Klebsiella, P. mirabilis, S. pneumoniae, and staphylococci — **Adults:** 250 mg to 1 g P.O. q 6 hr. **Children:** 6 to 12 mg/kg P.O. q 6 hr (monohydrate only). Maximum 25 mg/kg q 6 hr.

- Ask about previous allergic reactions to cephalosporins or penicillin before giving first dose.
- Obtain specimen for culture and sensitivity tests before first dose.
- With large doses or prolonged therapy, monitor for superinfection.
- Group A beta-hemolytic streptococcal infections should be treated for ≥ 10 days.

---

cephradine
Velosef
First-generation cephalosporin
Antibiotic
Pregnancy Risk Category: B

Serious infections of respiratory, GI, or GU tract; skin and soft-tissue infections; bone and joint infections; septicemia; endocarditis; otitis media caused by susceptible organisms; perioperative prophylaxis — **Adults:** 250 to 500 mg P.O. q 6 hr. **Children > 9 mo:** 25 to 50 mg/kg P.O. q.d. in divided doses.

- Obtain specimen for culture and sensitivity tests before first dose.
- Group A beta-hemolytic streptococcal infections should be treated for ≥ 10 days.
- With large doses or prolonged therapy, monitor for superinfection, especially in high-risk patients.
- Tell patient to take with food or milk.

(continued)

69

†Canadian ‡Australian

DRUG/CLASS/CATEGORY	INDICATIONS/DOSAGES	KEY NURSING CONSIDERATIONS
cephradine *(continued)*	*Otitis media —* **Children:** 75 to 100 mg/kg P.O. q.d. Don't exceed 4 g q.d. Any patient, regardless of age and weight, may receive doses up to 1 g q.i.d. for severe or chronic infections.	• Instruct patient to shake oral suspension well before measuring dose. • Advise patient to report rash immediately.
cerivastatin sodium Baycol *Hydroxymethylglutaryl coenzyme A (HMG CoA) reductase inhibitor* *Cholesterol reducer* Pregnancy Risk Category: X	*Adjunct to diet, to reduce total and LDL cholesterol levels in patients with primary hypercholesterolemia or mixed dyslipidemia when diet and other nonpharmacologic measures have been inadequate —* **Adults:** 0.3 mg P.O. q.d. in evening. **Children:** safety and efficacy in children have not been established. ***Adjust-a-dose:*** In patients with moderate or severe renal dysfunction (creatinine clearance ≤ 60 ml/min), starting dose is 0.2 mg P.O. q.d.	• Use cautiously in patients with history of liver disease or heavy alcohol use. • Know that drug should be given to women of childbearing age only if conception is highly unlikely and they have been warned of potential risks to fetus. • Know that therapy with lipid-lowering drugs should be started after appropriate diet, exercise, and weight-reduction programs have been unsuccessful in controlling cholesterol levels. • Perform liver function tests before starting treatment, at 6 and 12 wk after initiating therapy, and periodically thereafter. • Withhold drug temporarily in patients experiencing an acute or serious condition predisposing them to renal failure secondary to rhabdomyolysis. Rare cases of rhabdomyolysis have been reported with other HMG CoA reductase inhibitors.

cetirizine hydrochloride
Zyrtec
Selective H₁-receptor antagonist
Antihistamine
Pregnancy Risk Category: B

Seasonal allergic rhinitis; perennial allergic rhinitis; chronic urticaria — **Adults and children ≥ 12 yr:** 5 or 10 mg P.O. q.d. depending on symptom severity; 5 mg P.O. q.d. in renal or hepatic impairment. **Children 6 to 11 yr:** 5 or 10 mg (1 or 2 tsp) P.O. q.d. depending on symptom severity.
Adjust-a-dose: In renally impaired patients with creatinine clearance of 11 to 31 ml/min, those on dialysis (creatinine clearance < 7 ml/min), or those with hepatic impairment, give 5 mg P.O. q.d.

- Not recommended for breast-feeding patients.
- Warn patient to avoid hazardous activities until CNS effects known.
- Advise patient to avoid alcohol and other CNS depressants.

chloral hydrate
Aquachloral Suppretes, Noctec, Novo-Chlorhydrate†
General CNS depressant
Sedative-hypnotic
Pregnancy Risk Category: C
Controlled Substance
Schedule: IV

Sedation — **Adults:** 250 mg P.O. or P.R. t.i.d. after meals. **Children:** 8.3 mg/kg or 250 mg/m² P.O. or P.R. t.i.d. Maximum daily dose 500 mg t.i.d.
Insomnia — **Adults:** 500 mg to 1 g P.O. or P.R. 15 to 30 min before bedtime. **Children:** 50 mg/kg or 1.5 g/m² P.O. or P.R. 15 to 30 min before bedtime. Maximum single dose 1 g.
Preoperative — **Adults:** 500 mg to 1 g P.O. or P.R. 30 min before surgery.
Premedication for EEG — **Children:** 20 to 25 mg/kg P.O. or P.R.

- Note two strengths of oral liquid form.
- Double-check dose, especially when giving to children. Fatal overdoses have occurred.
- To minimize unpleasant taste and stomach irritation, dilute or give with liquid. Should be taken after meals.
- Take steps to prevent hoarding or self-overdosing by depressed, suicidal, or drug-dependent patients or those with history of drug abuse.
- Don't administer for 48 hr before fluorometric test, as ordered.
- Monitor BUN as ordered. Large dosage may raise BUN.

†Canadian ‡Australian

DRUG / CLASS / CATEGORY	INDICATIONS / DOSAGES	KEY NURSING CONSIDERATIONS
chlorambucil Leukeran *Alkylating agent* *Antineoplastic* Pregnancy Risk Category: D	*Chronic lymphocytic leukemia; malignant lymphomas, including lymphosarcoma, giant follicular lymphoma, and Hodgkin's disease* — **Adults:** 0.1 to 0.2 mg/kg P.O. q.d. for 3 to 6 wk; then adjusted for maintenance (usually 4 to 10 mg q.d.).	▪ Monitor CBC and serum uric acid level. ▪ If WBC count < 2,000/mm³ or granulocyte count < 1,000/mm³, follow institutional policy for infection control in immuno-compromised patients. ▪ Avoid I.M. injections when platelet count < 100,000/mm³.
chloramphenicol (ophthalmic) AK-Chlor, Chloromycetin Ophthalmic, Chloroptic, Chloroptic S.O.P., Ophthochlor Ophthalmic *Dichloroacetic acid derivative* *Antibiotic* Pregnancy Risk Category: C	*Surface bacterial infection involving conjunctiva or cornea* — **Adults and children:** 1 or 2 drops of solution in eye q 3 to 6 hr or more often, if necessary. Or, small amount of ointment to lower conjunctival sac q 3 to 6 hr or more often, if necessary. Continued for at least 48 hr after eye appears normal.	▪ If chloramphenicol drops are given q hr and then the dosage is tapered, follow order closely to ensure adequate anterior chamber levels. ▪ Teach patient how to instill drops or apply ointment. ▪ Instruct patient to apply light finger pressure on lacrimal sac for 1 min after drops are instilled.
chloramphenicol (otic) Chloromycetin Otic *Dichloroacetic acid derivative* *Antibiotic* Pregnancy Risk Category: C	*External ear canal infection* — **Adults and children:** 2 to 3 drops into ear canal t.i.d.	▪ Watch for signs of superinfection or sore throat (early sign of toxicity). ▪ Reculture persistent drainage.

chlordiazepoxide
Libritabs
chlordiazepoxide hydrochloride
Librium, Novo-Poxide†
Benzodiazepine
Antianxiety agent/anticonvulsant/sedative-hypnotic
Pregnancy Risk Category: D
Controlled Substance
Schedule: IV

Mild to moderate anxiety — **Adults:** 5 to 10 mg P.O. t.i.d. or q.i.d. **Children > 6 yr:** 5 mg P.O. b.i.d. to q.i.d. Maximum 10 mg P.O. b.i.d. or t.i.d.
Severe anxiety — **Adults:** 20 to 25 mg P.O. t.i.d. or q.i.d. **Elderly:** 5 mg P.O. b.i.d. to q.i.d.
Withdrawal symptoms of acute alcoholism — **Adults:** 50 to 100 mg P.O., I.M., or I.V.; repeat in 2 to 4 hr, p.r.n. Maximum 300 mg q.d.
Note: Parenteral form not recommended in children < 12 yr.
Adjust-a-dose: In debilitated patients, give 5 mg P.O. b.i.d. to q.i.d.

- *I.V. use:* Use 5 ml 0.9% NaCl solution or sterile water for injection as diluent; don't give packaged diluent. Administer over 1 min.
- When giving I.V., be sure equipment for emergency airway management is available. Monitor respirations every 5 to 15 min and before each repeated I.V. dose.
- Injectable form comes in two types of ampules. Read directions carefully.
- Don't withdraw abruptly.

chloroquine hydrochloride
Aralen HCl, Chlorquin‡
chloroquine phosphate
Aralen Phosphate, Chloroquin‡
4-Aminoquinoline
Antimalarial/amebicide/antiinflammatory
Pregnancy Risk Category: C

Acute malarial attacks — **Adults:** 1 g (600 mg base) P.O.: then 500 mg (300 mg base) at 6, 24, and 48 hr. Or, 160 to 200 mg (base) I.M. initially; repeat in 6 hr, p.r.n. Switch to P.O. as soon as possible. **Children:** 10 mg (base)/kg P.O.: then 5 mg (base)/kg at 6, 24, and 48 hr (maximum < adult dose). Or 5 mg (base)/kg I.M. initially; repeated in 6 hr, p.r.n. Switch to P.O. as soon as possible.
Malaria prophylaxis — **Adults and children:** 5 mg (base)/kg P.O. (maximum 300 mg) weekly (begun 2 wk before exposure and continued for 4 to 6 wk after). If treatment begins after exposure, initial dose doubled in 2 divided doses P.O. q 6 hr.

- Monitor for possible overdose, which can quickly lead to toxic symptoms. Children are extremely susceptible to toxicity.
- Baseline and periodic ophthalmic and audiometric exams needed.
- Monitor CBC and liver function studies.
- Advise patient to take immediately before or after meals on same day each wk.
- Tell patient to report adverse reactions promptly.
- Instruct patient to avoid exposure to sunlight.

73

DRUG / CLASS / CATEGORY	INDICATIONS / DOSAGES	KEY NURSING CONSIDERATIONS
chlorpheniramine maleate Aller-Chlor L, Chlor-Trimeton, Teldrin *Propylamine-derivative antihistamine* *Antihistamine (H_1-receptor antagonist)* Pregnancy Risk Category: B	*Rhinitis; allergy symptoms —* **Adults:** 4 mg P.O. q 4 to 6 hr, not to exceed 24 mg/day; or 8 to 12 mg timed-release capsule P.O. q 8 to 12 hr, not to exceed 24 mg q.d. Or, 5 to 20 mg I.M., I.V., or S.C. as single dose. Maximum 40 mg/24 hr. **Children 6 to 12 yr:** 2 mg P.O. q 4 to 6 hr, not to exceed 12 mg/day. Or, may give 8 mg timed-release capsule P.O. h.s. **Children 2 to 6 yr:** 1 mg P.O. q 4 to 6 hr, not to exceed 4 mg q.d.	▪ *I.V. use:* Available in 10-mg/ml ampules. Don't give 100 mg/ml strength I.V. Drug compatible with most I.V. solutions. Check with pharmacist before mixing with I.V. solutions to verify specific compatibilities. Give injection over 1 min. ▪ If symptoms occur during or after parenteral dose, discontinue drug.
chlorpromazine hydrochloride Chlorpromanyl-5†, Chlorpromanyl-20†, Chlorpromanyl-40†, Ormazine, Thorazine *Aliphatic phenothiazine* *Antipsychotic/antiemetic* Pregnancy Risk Category: C	*Psychosis —* **Adults:** 25 to 75 mg P.O. q.d. in 2 to 4 divided doses. Increase by 20 to 50 mg twice weekly until symptoms controlled. May need up to 800 mg q.d. Or, 25 to 50 mg I.M. q 1 to 4 hr, p.r.n. I.M. doses gradually increased over several days to maximum 400 mg q 4 to 6 hr. Switch to P.O. as soon as possible. **Children ≥ 6 mo:** 0.55 mg/kg P.O. q 4 to 6 hr or I.M. q 6 to 8 hr; or 1.1 mg/kg P.R. q 6 to 8 hr. Maximum I.M. dose in children < 5 yr or < 22.7 kg (50 lb): 40 mg. Maximum I.M. dose in children 5 to 12 yr or 22.7 to 45.5 kg (100 lb): 75 mg. *Nausea and vomiting —* **Adults:** 10 to 25 mg P.O. q 4 to 6 hr, p.r.n.; or 50 to 100 mg P.R. q 6 to 8 hr, p.r.n.; or 25 to 50 mg I.M. q 3 to 4	▪ Obtain baseline BP before starting therapy and monitor BP regularly. Watch for orthostatic hypotension, especially with parenteral use. Monitor BP before and after I.M. administration; keep patient supine 1 hr afterward and instruct to get up slowly. ▪ Monitor for tardive dyskinesia, which may follow prolonged use (up to mo or yr later) and may disappear spontaneously or persist for life despite drug discontinuation. ▪ Watch for signs of neuroleptic malignant syndrome. ▪ Know that acute dystonic reactions may be treated with diphenhydramine.

	hr, p.r.n. **Children ≥ 6 mo:** 0.55 mg/kg q 4 to 6 hr, or I.M. q 6 to 8 hr; or 1.1 mg/kg P.R. q 6 to 8 hr. Maximum I.M. dose in children < 5 yr or < 22.7 kg: 40 mg. Maximum I.M. dose in children 5 to 12 yr or 22.7 to 45.5 kg: 75 mg.	
chlorthalidone Apo-Chlorthalidone†, Hygroton, Novo-Thalidone†, Uridon† *Thiazide-like diuretic* *Diuretic/antihypertensive* *Pregnancy Risk Category: D*	*Edema* — **Adults:** initially, 50 to 100 mg P.O. q.d., or up to 200 mg P.O. on alternate days. **Children:** 2 mg/kg or 60 mg/m² P.O. three times weekly. *Hypertension* — **Adults:** 12.5 to 50 mg P.O. q.d.	▪ To prevent nocturia, give in morning. ▪ Monitor I&O, weight, BP, electrolytes, glucose, creatinine, BUN, and uric acid. ▪ Watch for signs of hypokalemia. ▪ Don't confuse various brands.
cholestyramine Prevalite, Questran, Questran Light *Anion exchange resin* *Antilipemic/bile acid* *sequestrant* *Pregnancy Risk Category: B*	*Primary hyperlipidemia or pruritus caused by partial bile obstruction; adjunct for reduction of elevated serum cholesterol in primary hypercholesterolemia* — **Adults:** 4 g q.d. or b.i.d. Maintenance: 8 to 16 g q.d. divided into 2 doses. Maximum 24 g q.d.	▪ Monitor serum cholesterol and triglyceride levels regularly. ▪ If patient also receiving cardiac glycoside, monitor serum cardiac glycoside levels. ▪ Don't give in dry form. ▪ Monitor bowel habits. Encourage diet high in fiber and fluids.
choline magnesium trisalicylate (choline salicylate and magnesium salicylate) Tricosal, Trilisate *Salicylate*	*Rheumatoid arthritis (RA) and other inflammatory conditions* — **Adults:** initially, 1.5 to 2.5 g P.O. q.d. as single dose or in 2 or 3 divided doses. Adjust dosage according to response. Maintenance: 1 to 4.5 g q.d. *Juvenile RA* — **Children:** 60 to 110 mg/kg/ day P.O. in divided doses (q 6 to 8 hr).	▪ Monitor Hgb levels and PT in long-term or high-dose therapy. ▪ Monitor serum salicylate in long-term therapy. In arthritis, therapeutic level is 10 to 30 mg/100 ml.

(continued)

†Canadian ‡Australian

DRUG / CLASS / CATEGORY	INDICATIONS / DOSAGES	KEY NURSING CONSIDERATIONS
choline magnesium trisalicylate *(continued)* *Nonnarcotic analgesic/antipyretic/anti-inflammatory* Pregnancy Risk Category: C	*Mild to moderate pain and fever* — **Adults:** 2 to 3 g P.O. q.d. in divided doses q 4 to 6 hr. **Children ≤37 kg (81.5 lb):** 25 mg/kg P.O. b.i.d. **Children >37 kg:** 2,250 mg/day.	
cidofovir Vistide *Nucleotide analogue* *Antiviral* Pregnancy Risk Category: C	*CMV retinitis in patients with AIDS* — **Adults:** initially, 5 mg/kg I.V. infused over 1 hr once weekly for 2 consecutive wk; then maintenance dose of 5 mg/kg I.V. infused over 1 hr once q 2 wk. Must give probenecid and prehydration with 0.9% NaCl solution I.V. concomitantly (may reduce potential for nephrotoxicity). *Adjust-a-dose:* In patients with renal failure, if serum creatinine increases 0.3 to 0.4 mg/dl above baseline, reduce dose to 3 mg/kg at same rate and frequency. If serum creatinine increases ≥ 0.5 mg/dl above baseline, discontinue drug.	• Give 1 L 0.9% NaCl solution, usually over 1 to 2 hr, immediately before each infusion. • Monitor eye exam results periodically. • To prepare for infusion, transfer dose to bag containing 100 ml 0.9% NaCl solution. • Mutagenic; prepare drug by following facility protocols. • If drug contacts skin, wash mucous membranes and flush thoroughly with water. • Don't administer by intraocular injection. • Monitor renal function.
cilostazol Pletal *Phosphodiesterase III inhibitor*	*Reduction of symptoms of intermittent claudication* — **Adults:** 100 mg P.O. b.i.d., taken at least 30 min before or 2 hr after breakfast and dinner. Decrease dose to 50 mg P.O. b.i.d. during administration with	• Give at least ½ hr before or 2 hr after breakfast and dinner. • Know that beneficial effect may not be observed for up to 12 wk after initiating therapy.

- Use cautiously in combination with other drugs metabolized by the cytochrome P-450 enzyme system. May need to initiate therapy at a lower dose in patients taking other drugs metabolized by the cytochrome P-450 enzyme system.
- Cytochrome P-4503A4 enzyme is inhibited by grapefruit juice and may result in increased cilostazol levels; tell patient to avoid grapefruit juice while taking drug.
- Know that several drugs that inhibit the enzyme phosphodiesterase have caused decreased survival compared to placebo in patients with class III-IV heart failure.

Platelet aggregation inhibitor/vasodilator
Pregnancy Risk Category: C

drugs that may interact to increase cilostazol serum levels.

---

cimetidine
Tagamet, Tagamet HB
H₂-receptor antagonist
Antiulcer agent
Pregnancy Risk Category: B

Duodenal ulcer (short-term treatment and maintenance) — **Adults and children ≥ 16 yr:** 800 mg P.O. h.s. Or, 400 mg P.O. b.i.d. or 300 mg q.i.d. with meals and h.s. Maintenance therapy: 400 mg h.s. Parenteral therapy: 300 mg diluted to 20 ml by I.V. push over at least 5 min q 6 hr; or 300 mg diluted in 50 ml D₅W or other compatible I.V. solution by I.V. infusion over 15 to 20 min q 6 hr; or 300 mg I.M. q 6 hr (no dilution necessary). Maximum 2,400 mg q.d., p.r.n. Or, 900 mg/day (37.5 mg/hr) I.V. diluted in 100 to 1,000 ml by continuous I.V. infusion.

- *I.V. use:* Dilute I.V. solutions with 0.9% NaCl solution, D₅W and D₁₀W (and combinations of these), lactated Ringer's solution, or 5% sodium bicarbonate injection. Don't dilute with sterile water for injection.
- Don't infuse I.V. too rapidly; bradycardia may occur. Some authorities recommend infusing over at least 30 min to reduce risk of adverse cardiac effects. Sometimes given as continuous I.V. infusion. Use infusion pump if given in total volume of 250 ml over ≤ 24 hr.
- Identify tablet strength when obtaining drug history.

(continued)

DRUG / CLASS / CATEGORY	INDICATIONS / DOSAGES	KEY NURSING CONSIDERATIONS
cimetidine *(continued)*	*Active benign gastric ulceration* — **Adults:** 800 mg P.O. h.s., or 300 mg P.O. q.i.d. (with meals and h.s.) for up to 6 wk. *Gastroesophageal reflux disease* — **Adults:** 800 mg P.O. b.i.d. or 400 mg q.i.d. before meals and h.s. for up to 12 wk.	• Schedule dose at end of hemodialysis treatment. • Up to 10-g overdose can occur without adverse reactions.
ciprofloxacin Cipro, Cipro I.V., Ciproxin‡ *Fluoroquinolone antibiotic* Antibiotic Pregnancy Risk Category: C	*Mild to moderate UTI caused by susceptible organisms* — **Adults:** 250 mg P.O. or 200 mg I.V. q 12 hr. *Severe or complicated UTI or mild to moderate bone, joint, skin, or skin-structure infections caused by susceptible organisms* — **Adults:** 500 mg P.O. or 400 mg I.V. q 12 hr. *Chronic bacterial prostatitis caused by E. coli or P. mirabilis* — **Adults:** 500 mg P.O. q 12 hr for 28 days. *Adjust-a-dose:* In patients with renal failure, if creatinine clearance < 50 ml/min, reduce dose or frequency.	• Obtain specimen for culture and sensitivity tests before first dose. • Give oral form 2 hr after meal or 2 hr before or after taking antacids, sucralfate, or products that contain iron. • *I.V. use:* Infuse slowly (over 1 hr) into large vein. • Preferable to give I.V. dose 2 hr after meal. • Don't give antacids, magnesium, aluminum, or iron products within 4 hr before or 2 hr after I.V. dose. • Instruct patient to avoid excessive artificial ultraviolet light and to stop drug and call doctor if phototoxicity occurs. • Encourage high fluid intake to avoid crystalluria.

ciprofloxacin hydrochloride
CILOXAN
Fluoroquinolone
Antibacterial agent
Pregnancy Risk Category: C

Corneal ulcers caused by susceptible organisms — **Adults and children > 12 yr:** 2 drops in affected eye q 15 min for first 6 hr; then 2 drops q 30 min for remainder of 1st day. On day 2, 2 drops q hr. On days 3 to 14, 2 drops q 4 hr.
Bacterial conjunctivitis caused by susceptible organisms — **Adults and children > 12 yr:** 1 or 2 drops in affected eye q 2 hr *while awake* for first 2 days. Then 1 or 2 drops q 4 hr *while awake* for next 5 days.

- Discontinue at first sign of hypersensitivity and notify doctor.
- Prolonged use may result in superinfection.
- Teach patient how to instill drops.
- Instruct patient to apply light finger pressure on lacrimal sac for 1 min after drops instilled.

---

cisapride
PROPULSID
Serotonin-4 receptor agonist
GI prokinetic agent
Pregnancy Risk Category: C

Symptoms of nocturnal heartburn caused by gastroesophageal reflux disease —
Adults: initially, 10 mg P.O. q.i.d. 15 min before meals and h.s. If response inadequate, increase to 20 mg q.i.d.

- Use cautiously in breast-feeding patient.
- Protect 20-mg tablets from light; protect all products from moisture.
- Remind patient to avoid alcohol and sedatives while taking drug.
- Monitor for drug interactions.

---

cisplatin (cis-platinum, CDDP)
PLATAMINE‡, PLATINOL, PLATINOL AQ
Alkylating agent
Antineoplastic
Pregnancy Risk Category: D

Adjunctive therapy in metastatic testicular cancer — **Adults:** 20 mg/m² I.V. q.d. for 5 days. Repeated q 3 wk for three cycles or longer.
Adjunctive therapy in metastatic ovarian cancer — **Adults:** 100 mg/m² I.V.; repeated q 4 wk. Or 75 to 100 mg/m² I.V. once q 4 wk in combination with cyclophosphamide.
Advanced bladder cancer — **Adults:** 50 to 70 mg/m² I.V. q 3 to 4 wk. Patients who have re-

- Monitor CBC, electrolyte levels, platelet count, and renal function studies.
- Hydrate patient with 0.9% NaCl solution before giving drug. Maintain urine output of ≥ 100 ml/hr for 4 hr before therapy and for 24 hr after therapy.
- Monitor for tinnitus.
- Have anaphylactic medications readily available during administration.

(continued)

DRUG/CLASS/CATEGORY	INDICATIONS/DOSAGES	KEY NURSING CONSIDERATIONS
cisplatin *(continued)*	ceived other antineoplastic agents or radiation therapy should receive 50 mg/m² q 4 wk.	- Parenteral form associated with carcinogenic, mutagenic, and teratogenic risks for personnel. - Do not use needles or I.V. administration sets that contain aluminum. - Administer antiemetics, as ordered.
citalopram hydrobromide Celexa *Selective serotonin reuptake inhibitor* *Antidepressant* Pregnancy Risk Category: C	*Depression* — **Adults:** initially, 20 mg P.O. once daily, increasing to 40 mg q.d. after no less than 1 wk. Maximum recommended dose 40 mg q.d. **Elderly:** 20 mg/day P.O. with titration to 40 mg/day only for nonresponding patients. ***Adjust-a-dose:*** For patients with hepatic impairment, give 20 mg/day P.O. with titration to 40 mg/day only for nonresponding patients.	- Use cautiously in patients with history of mania, seizures, suicidal ideation, or hepatic or renal impairment. - Safety and effectiveness have not been established in children. - Be aware that, although drug has not been shown to impair psychomotor performance, any psychoactive drug has the potential to impair judgment, thinking, or motor skills. - Be aware that possible suicide attempt is inherent in depression and may persist until significant remission occurs. Closely supervise high-risk patients at the start of drug therapy. Reduce risk of overdose by limiting amount of drug available per refill. - Know that at least 14 days should elapse between MAO inhibitor therapy and citalopram therapy.

cladribine (2-chlorodeoxy-adenosine, CdA)

Leustatin

Purine nucleoside analogue

Antineoplastic

Pregnancy Risk Category: D

Active hairy cell leukemia — **Adults:** 0.09 mg/kg q.d. by continuous I.V. infusion for 7 consecutive days.

- **I.V. use:** For 24-hr infusion, add calculated dose to 500-ml infusion bag of 0.9% NaCl for injection. Don't use dextrose solutions.
- Because of risk of hyperuricemia from tumor lysis, administer allopurinol, as ordered, during therapy.
- Monitor hematologic function closely.
- Fever is common during 1st mo of therapy.

clarithromycin

Biaxin

Macrolide

Antibiotic

Pregnancy Risk Category: C

Pharyngitis or tonsillitis caused by S. pyogenes — **Adults:** 250 mg P.O. q 12 hr for 10 days. **Children:** 15 mg/kg/day P.O. in divided doses q 12 hr for 10 days.

Acute maxillary sinusitis caused by S. pneumoniae, H. influenzae, or M. (Branhamella) catarrhalis — **Adults:** 500 mg P.O. q 12 hr for 14 days. **Children:** 15 mg/kg/day P.O. in divided doses q 12 hr for 10 days.

MAC disease in HIV infection — **Adults:** 500 mg P.O. q 12 hr, in combination with other antimycobacterial drugs, for life. **Children:** 7.5 mg/kg P.O. (maximum of 500 mg) q 12 hr, in combination with other antimycobacterial drugs, for life.

H. pylori infection — **Adults:** 500 mg P.O. q 8 hr for 14 days with omeprazole 40 mg P.O. each morning. Continue omeprazole (20 mg P.O. each morning) for total of 28 days.

- Obtain specimen for culture and sensitivity tests before first dose.
- May cause overgrowth of nonsusceptible bacteria or fungi. Monitor for superinfection.
- May take with or without food. Instruct patient not to refrigerate suspension.
- Advise patient to report persistent adverse reactions.
- Not recommended for patients with creatinine clearance < 25 ml/min.
- May administer without dosage adjustment in patients with hepatic impairment but normal renal function.

DRUG/CLASS/ CATEGORY	INDICATIONS/ DOSAGES	KEY NURSING CONSIDERATIONS
clemastine fumarate Tavist, Tavist-1 *Ethanolamine-derivative antihistamine* *Antihistamine (H_1-receptor antagonist)* Pregnancy Risk Category: B	*Rhinitis; allergy symptoms* — **Adults and children ≥12 yr:** 1.34 mg P.O. q 12 hr, or 2.68 mg P.O. q.d. to t.i.d., p.r.n. Maximum dose 8.04 mg/day. **Children 6 to 12 yr:** 0.67 to 1.34 mg (syrup only) P.O. b.i.d. Maximum dose 4.02 mg/day. *Urticaria; angioedema* — **Adults and children ≥12 yr:** 2.68 mg P.O. q.d. to t.i.d. Maximum dose 8.04 mg/day. **Children 6 to 12 yr:** 1.34 mg (syrup only) P.O. b.i.d. Maximum 4.02 mg/day.	• Monitor blood counts during long-term therapy, as ordered; observe for blood dyscrasias. • Instruct patient not to drink alcohol and to avoid activities that require alertness until CNS effects are known. • Tell patient to report tolerance to drug.
clindamycin hydrochloride Cleocin HCl, Dalacin C‡ **clindamycin palmitate hydrochloride** Cleocin Pediatric, Dalacin C **clindamycin phosphate** Cleocin Phosphate, Cleocin T, Dalacin C‡ *Lincomycin derivative* *Antibiotic* Pregnancy Risk Category: B	*Infections caused by sensitive aerobic and anaerobic organisms* — **Adults:** 150 to 450 mg P.O. q 6 hr; or, 300 to 600 mg I.M. or I.V. q 6, 8, or 12 hr. **Children >1 mo:** 8 to 20 mg/kg P.O. q.d. in divided doses q 6 to 8 hr; or, 20 to 40 mg/kg I.M. or I.V. q.d. in divided doses q 6 or 8 hr. *Endocarditis prophylaxis for dental procedures in patients allergic to penicillin* — **Adults:** initially, 600 mg P.O. 1 hr before procedure. **Children:** initially, 10 mg/kg P.O. 1 hr before procedure. *Pelvic inflammatory disease* — **Adults:** 900 mg I.V. q 8 hr in conjunction with gentamicin. Continue at least 48 hr after symptoms	• Obtain specimen for culture and sensitivity tests before first dose. • *I.V. use:* Check I.V. site daily for phlebitis and irritation. For infusion, dilute each 300 mg in 50 ml solution, and give no faster than 30 mg/min (over 10 to 60 min). Never give undiluted as bolus. • For I.M. use, inject deeply. Rotate sites. Doses > 600 mg per injection not recommended. • Observe for signs of superinfection. • Don't give opioid antidiarrheals to treat drug-induced diarrhea; may prolong and worsen diarrhea.

improve; then switch to oral clindamycin 450 mg five times daily for total course of 10 to 14 days.

Inflammatory acne vulgaris — **Adults and adolescents:** Apply to skin b.i.d., morning and evening.

Bacterial vaginosis — **Adults:** 1 applicatorful intravaginally h.s. for 7 consecutive days.

- Drug can cause excessive dryness.
- Tell patient to avoid too-frequent washing of area and to cover entire affected area but avoid contact with eyes, nose, mouth, and other mucous membranes.
- Warn patient not to smoke while applying topical solution.

---

clindamycin phosphate
Cleocin T Gel, Lotion, Solution; Cleocin Vaginal Cream
Lincomycin derivative
Antibiotic
Pregnancy Risk Category: B

---

clomipramine hydrochloride
Anafranil
TCA
Antiobsessional agent
Pregnancy Risk Category: C

Obsessive-compulsive disorder — **Adults:** initially, 25 mg P.O. q.d. with meals, gradually increased to 100 mg q.d. in divided doses during first 2 wk. Thereafter, increase to maximum 250 mg q.d. in divided doses with meals, p.r.n. After adjustment, total daily dose may be given h.s. **Children and adolescents:** initially, 25 mg P.O. q.d. with meals, gradually increased over first 2 wk to daily maximum 3 mg/kg or 100 mg P.O. in divided doses, whichever is smaller. Maximum daily dose 3 mg/kg or 200 mg, whichever is smaller; may be given h.s. after adjustment. Periodic reassessment and adjustment necessary.

- Gradually discontinue drug several days before surgery.
- Adverse anticholinergic effects can occur rapidly.
- Advise patient to use sunblock, wear protective clothing, and avoid prolonged exposure to strong sunlight.
- Don't withdraw abruptly.

DRUG/CLASS/CATEGORY	INDICATIONS/DOSAGES	KEY NURSING CONSIDERATIONS
clonazepam Klonopin *Benzodiazepine* *Anticonvulsant* Pregnancy Risk Category: C Controlled Substance Schedule: IV	*Lennox-Gastaut syndrome; atypical absence seizures; akinetic and myoclonic seizures* — **Adults:** initially, not to exceed 1.5 mg P.O. q.d. in 3 divided doses. May increase by 0.5 to 1 mg q 3 days until seizures controlled. If given in unequal doses, give largest dose h.s. Maximum recommended daily dose 20 mg. **Children ≤ 10 yr or 30 kg (66 lb):** initially, 0.01 to 0.03 mg/kg P.O. q.d. (not to exceed 0.05 mg/kg q.d.), in 2 or 3 divided doses. Increase by 0.25 to 0.5 mg q 3rd day to maximum maintenance dose: 0.1 to 0.2 mg/kg q.d., p.r.n.	• Never withdraw suddenly because seizures may worsen. Monitor for oversedation. Call doctor at once if adverse reactions develop. • Monitor blood drug levels. Therapeutic level is 20 to 80 ng/ml. • Withdrawal symptoms resemble those of barbiturates.
clonidine Catapres-TTS **clonidine hydrochloride** Catapres, Dixarit‡ *Centrally acting adrenergic agent* *Antihypertensive* Pregnancy Risk Category: C	*Essential and renal hypertension* — **Adults:** initially, 0.1 mg P.O. b.i.d.; then increase by 0.1 to 0.2 mg q.d. on weekly basis. Usual range 0.2 to 0.8 mg q.d. in divided doses. Infrequently, doses up to 2.4 mg q.d. used. Or, as transdermal patch applied to nonhairy area of intact skin on upper arm or torso q 7 days, starting with 0.1-mg system and titrated with another 0.1-mg or larger system.	• May give to lower BP rapidly in some hypertensive emergencies. • Monitor BP and pulse frequently. • Remove transdermal patch before defibrillation to prevent arcing. • Observe for tolerance to therapeutic effects; may necessitate increased dosage. • Transdermal effects may take 2 to 3 days to become apparent. Oral therapy may have to continue in interim.

clopidogrel bisulfate

Plavix

Adenosine diphosphate-induced platelet aggregation inhibitor

Antiplatelet agent

Pregnancy Risk Category: B

To reduce atherosclerotic events in patients with atherosclerosis documented by recent CVA, MI, or peripheral arterial disease —
Adults: 75 mg P.O. q.d.

- Use with caution in patients at risk for increased bleeding from trauma, surgery, or other pathologic conditions, and in patients with hepatic impairment.
- Platelet aggregation will not return to normal for at least 5 days after discontinuing clopidogrel.
- Usually used in patients who are hypersensitive or intolerant to aspirin or after stent placement.
- Know that use of NSAIDs may increase risk of GI bleeding.
- Safety has not been established for concomitant use of heparin or warfarin.

clorazepate dipotassium

Apo-Clorazepate†, Gen-XENE, Novoclopate†, Tranxene, Tranxene-SD, Tranxene-T-Tab

Benzodiazepine

Antianxiety agent/anticonvulsant/sedative-hypnotic

Pregnancy Risk Category: D

Controlled Substance Schedule: IV

Acute alcohol withdrawal — **Adults:** day 1: 30 mg P.O. initially, then 30 to 60 mg P.O. in divided doses; day 2: 45 to 90 mg P.O. in divided doses; day 3: 22.5 to 45 mg P.O. in divided doses; day 4: 15 to 30 mg P.O. in divided doses; then gradually reduce dose to 7.5 to 15 mg q.d. Maximum recommended daily dose 90 mg.

Adjunct in partial seizure disorder — **Adults and children > 12 yr:** Maximum recommended initial dose 7.5 mg P.O. t.i.d. Increase no more than 7.5 mg/wk to maximum 90 mg q.d. **Children 9 to 12 yr:** maximum recommended initial dose 7.5 mg P.O. b.i.d. Increase no more than 7.5 mg/wk to maximum 60 mg q.d.

- Reduce dosage in elderly or debilitated patients.
- Monitor liver, renal, and hematopoietic function studies periodically, as ordered, with repeated or prolonged therapy.
- Possibility of abuse and addiction exists. Don't withdraw abruptly after prolonged use; withdrawal symptoms may occur.
- Not recommended for children < 9 yr.
- Instruct patient to avoid alcohol.
- Tell patient to avoid activities requiring alertness until CNS effects are known.

85

†Canadian ‡Australian

DRUG/CLASS/ CATEGORY	INDICATIONS/ DOSAGES	KEY NURSING CONSIDERATIONS
clotrimazole Canestest, Gyne-Lotrimin, Lotrimin, Mycelex, Mycelex-7, Mycelex-G, Mycelex OTC *Synthetic imidazole derivative* *Antifungal* Pregnancy Risk Category: B	*Superficial fungal infections* — **Adults and children:** Apply thinly and massage into affected and surrounding area, morning and evening, for 2 to 4 wk. If no improvement occurs after 4 wk, reevaluate patient. *Vulvovaginal candidiasis* — **Adults:** 2 100-mg vaginal tablets inserted q.d. h.s. for 7 days, or 1 500-mg vaginal tablet q.d. h.s. for 1 day; or 1 applicatorful vaginal cream q.d. h.s. for 7 days. *Oropharyngeal candidiasis treatment* — **Adults and children ≥ 3 yr:** Dissolve lozenge over 15 to 30 min in mouth five times q.d. for 14 days. *Prevention of oropharyngeal candidiasis in immunocompromised patients* — **Adults and children:** Dissolve lozenge over 15 to 30 min in mouth t.i.d. for duration of chemotherapy or until steroid reduced to maintenance levels.	• Report irritation or sensitivity; discontinue if irritation occurs, and notify doctor. • Warn patient not to use occlusive wrappings or dressings. • Ensure that patient understands that frequent or persistent yeast infections may be symptom of more serious medical problem.
clozapine Clozaril *Tricyclic dibenzodiazepine derivative* *Antipsychotic* Pregnancy Risk Category: B	*Schizophrenia in severely ill patients unresponsive to other therapies* — **Adults:** initially, 12.5 mg P.O. q.d. or b.i.d. titrated upward at 25 to 50 mg q.d. (if tolerated) to 300 to 450 mg q.d. by end of 2 wk. Individual dosage based on clinical response, pa-	• Poses significant risk of agranulocytosis. • Ensure that weekly WBC counts and blood tests are performed. • Monitor closely for signs of infection. Protective isolation may be needed.

	tient tolerance, and adverse reactions. Don't increase subsequent dose more than once or twice weekly, and don't exceed 100 mg. Many patients respond to dose of 300 to 600 mg q.d., but some may need up to 900 mg. Don't exceed 900 mg q.d.	■ Must be withdrawn gradually over 1 to 2 wk. Monitor closely for recurrence of psychotic symptoms. ■ Don't dispense more than 1-wk supply of drug. ■ May cause seizures or transient fevers.

codeine phosphate
Paveral†
codeine sulfate
Opioid
Analgesic/antitussive
Pregnancy Risk Category: C
Controlled Substance
Schedule: II

Mild to moderate pain — **Adults:** 15 to 60 mg P.O., or 15 to 60 mg (phosphate) S.C., I.M., or I.V. q 4 to 6 hr, p.r.n. **Children > 1 yr:** 0.5 mg/kg P.O., S.C., or I.M. q 4 hr, p.r.n.
Nonproductive cough — **Adults:** 10 to 20 mg P.O. q 4 to 6 hr. Maximum 120 mg/day. **Children 6 to 12 yr:** 5 to 10 mg P.O. q 4 to 6 hr. Maximum 60 mg/day. **Children 2 to 6 yr:** 2.5 to 5 mg P.O. q 4 to 6 hr. Maximum 30 mg/day.

- ***I.V. use:*** Give by very slow direct injection into large vein.
- Don't mix with other solutions.
- For full analgesic effect, administer before patient has intense pain.
- Don't use as antitussive when cough is crucial diagnostic sign or is beneficial (as after thoracic surgery).
- Monitor respiratory and circulatory status.

colchicine
Colgout†, Colsalide,
Novocolchicine†
Colchicum autumnale
alkaloid
Antigout agent
Pregnancy Risk Category: C
(P.O.), D (I.V.)

Prevention of acute gout attacks as prophylactic or maintenance therapy — **Adults:** 0.5 or 0.6 mg P.O. q.d. Dose and its frequency may vary with severity and frequency of attacks.
Prevention of gout attacks in patients undergoing surgery — **Adults:** 0.5 or 0.6 mg P.O. t.i.d. 3 days before and 3 days after surgery.
Acute gout; acute gouty arthritis — **Adults:** 0.5 to 1.3 mg P.O.; then 0.5 or 0.6 mg q 1 to 2 hr until relief, nausea, vomiting, or diarrhea ensues or maximum dose of 8 mg reached. Or, 2 mg I.V.; then 0.5 mg I.V. q 6 hr, p.r.n. 24-hr maximum (one course of treatment) 4 mg.

- Obtain baseline lab studies before and during therapy.
- ***I.V. use:*** Give by slow I.V. push over 2 to 5 min.
- Do not administer I.M. or S.C.
- Give with meals to reduce GI effects.
- Monitor I&O and keep output at 2,000 ml q.d.
- First sign of acute overdose may be GI symptoms.

87

†Canadian ‡Australian

DRUG / CLASS / CATEGORY	INDICATIONS / DOSAGES	KEY NURSING CONSIDERATIONS
colestipol hydrochloride Colestid *Anion exchange resin* *Antilipemic* Pregnancy Risk Category: B	*Primary hypercholesterolemia* — **Adults:** granules: 5 to 30 g P.O. q.d. or in divided doses; tablets: 2 to 16 g/day given once or in divided doses.	• Monitor serum cholesterol and triglyceride levels regularly. • Monitor bowel habits. • Don't administer in dry form. Encourage diet high in fiber and fluids. • In patient also receiving cardiac glycoside, monitor serum levels of that drug.
corticotropin (adrenocorticotropic hormone, ACTH) ACTH, Acthar **repository corticotropin** Acthar Gel (H.P.)†, ACTH Gel, H.P. Acthar Gel *Anterior pituitary hormone* *Diagnostic aid/replacement hormone/multiple sclerosis and nonsuppurative thyroiditis treatment* Pregnancy Risk Category: C	*Diagnostic test of adrenocortical function* — **Adults:** 40 U I.V. infusion q 12 hr for 48 hr; or I.M. or I.V. 25 U aqueous form in 500 ml D_5W I.V. over 8 hr, between blood samplings. Individual dosages generally vary with adrenal glands' sensitivity to stimulation and with specific disease. Infants and younger children require larger doses per kg. *For therapeutic use* — **Adults:** 40 U aqueous form S.C. or I.M. in 4 divided doses; or 40 to 80 U q 24 to 72 hr (repository form).	• *I.V. use:* Use only aqueous form I.V. Dilute in 500 ml D_5W and infuse over 8 hr. • If using gel, warm to room temperature, draw into large needle, and give slowly as deep I.M. injection with 21G or 22G needle. • Unusual stress may call for additional use of rapidly acting corticosteroids. • May mask signs of chronic disease and decrease host resistance and ability to localize infection. • Record weight changes, fluid exchange, and resting BP until minimal effective dosage reached.

cortisone acetate

Cortate‡, Cortone Acetate

Glucocorticoid/mineralo-corticoid

Anti-inflammatory/replacement therapy

Pregnancy Risk Category: D

Adrenal insufficiency; allergy; inflammation — **Adults:** 25 to 300 mg P.O. or 20 to 300 mg I.M. q.d. Dosages highly individualized, depending on disease severity.

- To reduce GI irritation, give with milk or food.
- For better results and less toxicity, give once-daily dose in morning.
- I.M. route produces slow onset of action.
- Monitor serum electrolyte, blood glucose, and fluid imbalances.

co-trimoxazole (trimethoprim-sulfamethoxazole)

Apo-Sulfatrim†, Bactrim DS, Septra, SMZ-TMP, Sulfatrim

Sulfonamide and folate antagonist

Antibiotic

Pregnancy Risk Category: C (contraindicated at term)

Shigellosis or UTI caused by susceptible strains of E. coli, Proteus (indole positive or negative), Klebsiella, or Enterobacter — **Adults:** 160 mg trimethoprim/800 mg sulfamethoxazole (double-strength tablets) P.O. q 12 hr for 10 to 14 days in UTI and for 5 days in shigellosis. For uncomplicated cystitis or acute urethral syndrome, 1 double-strength tablet q 12 hr for 3 days. If indicated, I.V. infusion given: 8 to 10 mg/kg/day in 2 to 4 divided doses q 6, 8, or 12 hr for up to 14 days for severe UTI. Maximum 960 mg trimethoprim. **Children ≥ 2 mo:** 8 mg/kg/day P.O., in 2 divided doses q 12 hr (10 days for UTI; 5 days for shigellosis). If indicated, I.V. infusion given: 8 to 10 mg/kg/day in 2 to 4 divided doses q 6, 8, or 12 hr. Don't exceed adult dose.

Chronic bronchitis; upper respiratory tract infections — **Adults:** 160 mg trimethoprim/800 mg sulfamethoxazole P.O. q 12 hr for 10 to 14 days.

- Dosage for mg/kg/day based on trimethoprim component.
- Obtain specimen for culture and sensitivity tests before first dose.
- Adverse reactions, especially hypersensitivity reactions, rash, and fever, are more common in AIDS patients.
- Promptly report rash, sore throat, fever, or mouth sores (early signs of blood dyscrasia).
- *I.V. use:* Dilute infusion in D_5W. Don't mix with other drugs or solutions. Infuse slowly over 60 to 90 min. Don't give by rapid infusion or bolus injection. Don't refrigerate. Use within 6 hr.
- Never administer I.M.

(continued)

DRUG / CLASS / CATEGORY

co-trimoxazole
(continued)

INDICATIONS / DOSAGES

UTI in men with prostatitis — **Adults:** 160 mg trimethoprim/800 mg sulfamethoxazole P.O. b.i.d. for 3 to 6 mo.
Adjust-a-dose: In patients with renal failure, if creatinine clearance 15 to 30 ml/min, reduce daily dose by 50%. Drug isn't recommended for patients with creatinine clearance < 15 ml/min.

DRUG / CLASS / CATEGORY

cromolyn sodium (sodium cromoglycate)
Crolom, Intal, Intal Aerosol Spray, Intal Nebulizer Solution, Nasalcrom
Coumarin derivative
Mast cell stabilizer/antiasthmatic
Pregnancy Risk Category: B

INDICATIONS / DOSAGES

Mild to moderate persistent asthma —
Adults and children ≥ 5 yr: 2 metered sprays using inhaler q.i.d. at regular intervals. Or, 20 mg via nebulization q.i.d. at regular intervals.
Prevention and treatment of seasonal and perennial allergic rhinitis — **Adults and children > 5 yr:** 1 spray in each nostril t.i.d. or q.i.d., up to six times q.d.
Prevention of exercise-induced bronchospasm — **Adults and children ≥ 5 yr:** 2 metered sprays inhaled no more than 1 hr before anticipated exercise.
Conjunctivitis — **Adults and children ≥ 4 yr:** 1 to 2 drops in each eye 4 to 6 times q.d. at regular intervals.

KEY NURSING CONSIDERATIONS

- Except for ophthalmic solution, use only when acute asthma episode has been controlled, airway is clear, and patient can breathe independently.
- Dissolve powder in capsules for oral dose in hot water and further dilute with cold water before ingestion. Don't mix with fruit juice, milk, or food.
- Watch for recurrence of asthmatic symptoms when dosage decreased.

cyanocobalamin (vitamin B₁₂)

Anacobin†, Bedoz†, Crystamine, Crysti-12, Cyanoject
hydroxocobalamin (vitamin B₁₂)

Codroxomin, Hydrobexan, Hydro-Cobex, Hydro-Crysti-12, LA-12
Water-soluble vitamin
Vitamin/nutritional supplement
Pregnancy Risk Category: NR

Vitamin B₁₂ deficiency — **Adults:** 30 mcg hydroxocobalamin I.M. q.d. for 5 to 10 days, depending on severity. Maintenance: 100 to 200 mcg I.M. q mo. **Children:** 1 to 5 mg hydroxocobalamin spread over ≥ 2 wk in doses of 100 mcg I.M. depending on severity. Maintenance: 30 to 50 mcg/mo I.M.

Pernicious anemia; vitamin B₁₂ malabsorption — **Adults:** 100 mcg cyanocobalamin I.M. or S.C. q.d. for 6 to 7 days; then 100 mcg I.M. or S.C. q.o.d. over ≥ 2 wk; then 100 mcg I.M. or S.C. q mo for life.

Methylmalonic aciduria — **Neonates:** 1,000 mcg cyanocobalamin I.M. q.d.

- Use cautiously in anemic patients with co-existing cardiac, pulmonary, or hypertensive disease, and in those with severe vitamin B₁₂-dependent deficiencies.
- Use cautiously in premature infants.
- Determine reticulocyte count, hematocrit, B₁₂, iron, and folate levels before therapy.
- Don't mix in same syringe with other drugs.
- Incompatible with many drugs and solutions.
- Closely monitor potassium levels for first 48 hr.
- Protect vitamin B₁₂ from light. Do not refrigerate or freeze.
- In pernicious anemia, stress need to return for monthly injections; anemia will recur if not treated monthly.

cyclobenzaprine hydrochloride

Flexeril
TCA derivative
Skeletal muscle relaxant
Pregnancy Risk Category: B

Short-term treatment of muscle spasm — **Adults:** 10 mg P.O. t.i.d. Maximum 60 mg q.d.; maximum duration of treatment 2 to 3 wk.

- Be alert for nausea, headache, and malaise, which may occur with abrupt withdrawal after long-term use.
- Watch for symptoms of overdose, including cardiac toxicity. Notify doctor immediately and have physostigmine available.

DRUG/CLASS/ CATEGORY	INDICATIONS/ DOSAGES	KEY NURSING CONSIDERATIONS
cyclopentolate hydrochloride AK-Pentolate, Cyclogyl *Anticholinergic* *Cycloplegic/mydriatic* Pregnancy Risk Category: NR	*Diagnostic procedures requiring mydriasis and cycloplegia* — **Adults:** 1 or 2 drops of 0.5%, 1%, or 2% solution instilled into eye(s), followed by 1 or 2 drops in 5 to 10 min, if needed. **Children:** 1 drop of 0.5%, 1%, or 2% solution instilled into each eye, followed in 5 to 10 min with 1 drop 0.5% or 1% solution, if needed.	■ Physostigmine is antidote of choice. ■ Teach patient how to instill drug. ■ Warn patient to avoid hazardous activities until temporary blurring subsides.
cyclophosphamide Cycloblastin‡, Cytoxan, Cytoxan Lyophilized, Endoxan-Asta‡, Neosar, Procytox† *Alkylating agent* *Antineoplastic* Pregnancy Risk Category: D	*Breast and ovarian cancers; Hodgkin's disease; chronic lymphocytic leukemia; chronic myelocytic leukemia; acute lymphoblastic leukemia; acute myelocytic and monocytic leukemia; neuroblastoma; retinoblastoma; malignant lymphoma; multiple myeloma; mycosis fungoides; sarcoma* — **Adults and children:** initially, 40 to 50 mg/kg I.V. in divided doses over 2 to 5 days. Or, 10 to 15 mg/kg I.V. q 7 to 10 days, 3 to 5 mg/kg I.V. twice weekly, or 1 to 5 mg/kg P.O. q.d., depending on patient tolerance. Subsequent dosages adjusted according to response. *Minimal change nephrotic syndrome in children* — **Children:** 2.5 to 3 mg/kg P.O. q.d. for 60 to 90 days.	■ Parenteral form associated with carcinogenic, mutagenic, and teratogenic risks for personnel. ■ After reconstitution, administer by direct I.V. injection or infusion. For I.V. infusion, dilute with compatible solution such as D₅W. ■ Don't give drug h.s.; may increase the possibility of cystitis. If cystitis occurs, discontinue drug and notify doctor. Mesna may be given to lower the incidence and severity of bladder toxicity. ■ Monitor serum uric acid level. ■ Encourage voiding q 1 to 2 hr while awake and drinking ≥ 3 L fluid q.d.

cycloserine
Seromycin
Isoxazolidone/d-alanine analogue
Antitubercular
Pregnancy Risk Category: C

Adjunctive treatment in pulmonary or extrapulmonary TB — **Adults:** initially, 250 mg P.O. q 12 hr for 2 wk; then, if blood levels < 25 to 30 mcg/ml and no toxicity has developed, increase to 250 mg q 8 hr for 2 wk. If optimum blood levels still not achieved and no toxicity has developed, increase to 250 mg q 6 hr. Maximum 1 g/day. If CNS toxicity occurs, discontinue drug for 1 wk, then resume at 250 mg q.d. for 2 wk. If no serious toxic effects occur, increase dose in 250-mg increments q 10 days until blood level of 25 to 30 mcg/ml reached.

- Obtain specimen for culture and sensitivity tests before therapy begins and periodically thereafter to detect possible resistance.
- Observe for psychotic symptoms, hallucinations, and possible suicidal tendencies.
- Administer pyridoxine, anticonvulsants, tranquilizers, or sedatives, as ordered, to relieve adverse reactions.
- Monitor serum cycloserine levels, hematologic tests, and renal and liver function studies periodically, as ordered.
- Monitor for skin rash.

cyclosporine (cyclosporin)
Neoral, Sandimmune†, Sandimmune
Polypeptide antibiotic
Immunosuppressant
Pregnancy Risk Category: C

Prophylaxis of organ rejection in kidney, liver, or heart transplantation — **Adults and children:** 15 mg/kg P.O. 4 to 12 hr before transplantation and continued q.d. postoperatively for 1 to 2 wk. Then dose reduced 5% each wk to maintenance level of 5 to 10 mg/kg/day. Or, 5 to 6 mg/kg I.V. concentrate 4 to 12 hr before transplantation. Postoperatively, dose repeated q.d. until patient can tolerate oral form.

Adjust-a-dose: In patients with adverse reactions such as hypertension, elevated serum creatinine (30% above pretreatment level), or abnormal CBC and liver function tests, decrease dose by 25% to 50%.

- To increase palatability of oral solutions, mix with whole milk or fruit juice. Use glass container.
- Neoral and Sandimmune aren't bioequivalent. Less Neoral may be needed to yield the same blood concentration derived from Sandimmune.
- **I.V. use:** Administer cyclosporine I.V. concentrate at ⅓ oral dose and dilute before use. Dilute each ml of concentrate in 20 to 100 ml of D₅W or 0.9% NaCl for injection immediately before administration; infuse over 2 to 6 hr.
- Monitor cyclosporine blood levels, BUN, liver function tests, and serum creatinine levels.

DRUG / CLASS / CATEGORY	INDICATIONS / DOSAGES	KEY NURSING CONSIDERATIONS
cytarabine (ara-C, cytosine arabinoside) Alexant, Cytosar, Cytosar-U *Antimetabolite* *Antineoplastic* Pregnancy Risk Category: D	*Acute nonlymphocytic leukemia; acute lymphocytic leukemia; blast phase of chronic myelocytic leukemia —* **Adults and children:** 100 mg/m² q.d. by continuous I.V. infusion or 100 mg/m² I.V. q 12 hr. Given for 7 days and repeated q 2 wk. Maintenance: 1 mg/kg S.C. once or twice a wk. *Meningeal leukemia —* **Adults and children:** highly variable from 5 mg/m² to 75 mg/m² intrathecally. Frequency also varies from once a day for 4 days to once q 4 days.	▪ Give antiemetic before administering. ▪ Parenteral form has carcinogenic, mutagenic, and teratogenic risks for personnel. ▪ For I.V. infusion, dilute using 0.9% NaCl for injection or D₅W. ▪ For intrathecal administration, use preservative-free 0.9% NaCl solution. ▪ Maintain high fluid intake and give allopurinol to avoid urate nephropathy. ▪ Monitor uric acid level. Frequency and renal function studies, and CBC. ▪ Assess patient for neurotoxicity.
cytomegalovirus immune globulin (human), intravenous (CMV-IGIV) CytoGam *Immune globulin* *Immune serum* Pregnancy Risk Category: C	*To attenuate primary CMV disease in seronegative patients who received a kidney from CMV seropositive donor —* **Adults:** administered I.V. based on time after transplantation: within 72 hr, 150 mg/kg; 2 wk after, 100 mg/kg; 4 wk after, 100 mg/kg; 6 wk after, 100 mg/kg; 8 wk after, 100 mg/kg; 12 wk after, 50 mg/kg; 16 wk after, 50 mg/kg. Initial dose given at 15 mg/kg/hr. Increased to 30 mg/kg/hr after 30 min if no untoward reactions occur, then to 60 mg/kg/hr after another 30 min if no reactions. Volume maximum 75 ml/hr. Subsequent doses may be given at 15 mg/kg/hr for 15 min, increasing q 15 min in steps to 60 mg/kg/hr.	▪ **I.V. use:** Administer through separate I.V. line with constant infusion pump. If unable to administer through separate line, piggyback into preexisting line. Do not dilute more than 1:2 with diluent. ▪ Begin infusion within 6 hr of entering vial; finish within 12 hr. ▪ Monitor vital signs closely. ▪ For anaphylaxis or drop in BP, stop infusion, notify doctor, and be prepared to perform cardiac resuscitation and administer such drugs as diphenhydramine and epinephrine. ▪ Refrigerate at 36° to 46° F (2° to 8° C).

dacarbazine (DTIC)
DTIC†, DTIC-Dome
Alkylating agent (cell cycle-phase nonspecific)
Antineoplastic
Pregnancy Risk Category: C

Metastatic malignant melanoma — **Adults:** 2 to 4.5 mg/kg I.V. q.d. for 10 days; repeated q 4 wk as tolerated. Or 250 mg/m² I.V. q.d. for 5 days, repeated at 3-wk intervals.
Hodgkin's disease — **Adults:** 150 mg/m² I.V. q.d. (in combination with other agents) for 5 days, repeated q 4 wk; or 375 mg/m² on 1st day of combination, repeated q 15 days.

- Avoid extravasation during infusion. If I.V. solution infiltrates, discontinue immediately, apply ice to area for 24 to 48 hr, and notify doctor.
- To prevent bleeding, avoid all I.M. injections when platelet count < 100,000/mm³.
- Toxicity often accompanies therapeutic effects. Monitor CBC and platelet count.

daclizumab
Zenapax
Monoclonal antibody
Immunosuppressant
Pregnancy Risk Category: C

Prophylaxis of acute organ rejection in patients receiving renal transplants in combination with an immunosuppressive regimen that includes cyclosporine and corticosteroids — **Adults:** 1 mg/kg I.V. The standard course of therapy is five doses. Administer first dose no more than 24 hr before transplantation; remaining four doses are given at 14-day intervals.

- Use only under supervision of doctor experienced in immunosuppressive therapy and management of organ transplantation.
- Protect undiluted solution from direct light.
- Drug is used as part of an immunosuppressive regimen that includes corticosteroids and cyclosporine. Monitor for lipoproliferative disorders and opportunistic infections.
- Anaphylactoid reactions have been reported following administration of proteins. Drugs used in treatment of anaphylactic reactions should be immediately available.
- *I.V. use:* Do not use as direct I.V. injection. Dilute in 50 ml sterile 0.9% NaCl solution before administration. To avoid foaming, don't shake. Inspect for particulate matter or discoloration before use. If evidence of particulate matter or discoloration, don't use. Administer over 15 min *(continued)*

†Canadian ‡Australian

DRUG/CLASS/ CATEGORY	INDICATIONS/ DOSAGES	KEY NURSING CONSIDERATIONS
daclizumab (continued)		via central or peripheral line. Don't add or infuse other drugs simultaneously through same I.V. line.
		▪ Drug may be refrigerated at 36° to 46° F (2° to 8° C) for 24 hr and is stable at room temperature for 4 hr. Discard solution if not used within 24 hr.
		▪ Patient and family members should not receive vaccinations during daclizumab therapy unless approved by doctor.
dactinomycin (actinomycin D) Cosmegen Antibiotic antineoplastic (cell cycle-phase non-specific) Antineoplastic Pregnancy Risk Category: C	Dosage and indications vary. Check treatment protocol with doctor. Sarcoma; trophoblastic tumors in women; testicular cancer — Adults: 500 mcg (0.5 mg) I.V. q.d. for 5 days. Maximum 15 mcg/kg/day, or 400 to 600 mcg/m²/day for 5 days. After bone marrow recovery, may repeat course. Wilms' tumor; rhabdomyosarcoma; Ewing's sarcoma — Children: 10 to 15 mcg/kg or 450 mcg/m²/day I.V. for 5 days. Maximum 500 mcg/day. Or 2.5 mg/m² I.V. in equally divided daily doses over 7 days. After bone marrow recovery, may repeat course.	▪ I.V. use: Give by direct injection into vein or through tubing of free-flowing I.V. solution of 0.9% NaCl for injection or D_5W. For I.V. infusion, dilute with up to 50 ml D_5W or 0.9% NaCl for injection; infuse over 15 min.
		▪ Vesicant; if extravasation occurs, severe tissue necrosis may result. If infiltration occurs, apply cold compresses and notify doctor.
		▪ If skin contact occurs, irrigate with water for ≥ 15 min.
		▪ Monitor CBC, platelet counts, and renal and hepatic functions, as ordered. Observe for stomatitis, diarrhea, and leukopenia.

dalteparin sodium
Fragmin
*Low-molecular-weight
heparin*
Anticoagulant
Pregnancy Risk Category: B

*Prophylaxis against deep vein thrombosis in
patients undergoing abdominal surgery who
are at risk for thromboembolic complications* — **Adults:** 2,500 IU S.C. q.d., starting
1 to 2 hr before surgery and repeated q.d.
for 5 to 10 days postoperatively.

- Have patient assume sitting or supine position when administering. Give S.C. injection deeply. Rotate sites daily.
- Not interchangeable (unit for unit) with un-
fractionated heparin or other low-molecular-
weight heparin.
- Periodic, routine CBC and fecal occult
blood tests recommended. Regular monitoring of PT or activated PTT not required.
- Monitor closely for thrombocytopenia.
- Discontinue if thromboembolic event occurs despite dalteparin prophylaxis.

danaparoid sodium
Orgaran
Glycosaminoglycan
*Anticoagulant/antithrom-
botic*
Pregnancy Risk Category: B

*Prophylaxis against postoperative deep vein
thrombosis (DVT) in patients undergoing
elective hip replacement surgery* — **Adults:**
750 anti-Xa units S.C. b.i.d. starting 1 to 4
hr preoperatively, and then not sooner than
2 hr after surgery. Treatment continued for 7
to 14 days postoperatively or until risk of
DVT diminished.

- Never give I.M. To administer, have patient
lie down. Give S.C. injection deeply. Don't
rub afterward.
- Not interchangeable (unit for unit) with
heparin or low-molecular-weight heparin.
- Routine CBC and fecal occult blood tests
recommended during therapy.
- Has little effect on PT, PTT, fibrinolytic activity, and bleeding time.
- Monitor Hct and BP closely; decrease in
either may signal hemorrhage.
- If serious bleeding occurs, stop drug and
transfuse blood products, as ordered.

DRUG/CLASS/CATEGORY	INDICATIONS/DOSAGES	KEY NURSING CONSIDERATIONS
danazol Cyclomen, Danocrine *Androgen* *Antiestrogen/androgen* Pregnancy Risk Category: X	*Mild endometriosis* — **Women:** initially, 100 to 200 mg P.O. b.i.d. uninterrupted for 3 to 6 mo; may continue for 9 mo. Subsequent dosage based on patient response. *Moderate to severe endometriosis* — **Women:** 400 mg P.O. b.i.d. uninterrupted for 3 to 6 mo; may continue for 9 mo. *Fibrocystic breast disease* — **Women:** 100 to 400 mg P.O. q.d. in 2 divided doses uninterrupted for 2 to 6 mo.	▪ Unless contraindicated, instruct patient to use with diet high in calories and protein. ▪ Monitor closely for virilization signs. Some androgenic effects, such as voice deepening, may not be reversible on drug discontinuation. ▪ Periodic dosage decreases or gradual drug withdrawal preferred.
dantrolene sodium Dantrium *Hydantoin derivative* *Skeletal muscle relaxant* Pregnancy Risk Category: C	*Spasticity and sequelae secondary to severe chronic disorders (such as multiple sclerosis, cerebral palsy, spinal cord injury, CVA)* — **Adults:** 25 mg P.O. q.d. Increase gradually in 25-mg increments, up to 100 mg b.i.d. to q.i.d., to maximum 400 mg q.d. **Children:** initially, 0.5 mg/kg P.O. b.i.d.; increase to t.i.d., then q.i.d. Increase, as needed, by 0.5 mg/kg q.d. to 3 mg/kg b.i.d. to q.i.d., to maximum 100 mg q.i.d.	▪ Watch for hepatitis (fever and jaundice), severe diarrhea, severe weakness, or sensitivity reactions (fever and skin eruptions). Withhold dose and notify doctor if these occur. ▪ Prepare oral suspension for single dose by dissolving capsule contents in juice or other liquid. ▪ Obtain liver function tests at beginning of therapy. ▪ Caution patient about exposure to sunlight; photosensitivity may occur.
dapsone Avlosulfont, Dapsone 100‡ *Synthetic sulfone*	*All forms of leprosy (Hansen's disease)* — **Adults:** 100 mg P.O. q.d., indefinitely; give with rifampin 600 mg P.O. q.d. for 6 mo.	▪ Monitor for signs and symptoms of erythema nodosum reaction (malaise, fever, painful inflammatory induration in skin and mucosa, iritis, neuritis).

Antileprotic/antimalarial
Pregnancy Risk Category: C

Children: 1.4 mg/kg P.O. q.d. for minimum of 3 yr.
Dermatitis herpetiformis — **Adults:** 50 mg P.O. q.d.; increase to 300 mg q.d, p.r.n.

- Be prepared to reduce dose or stop drug with decreased Hgb or RBC or WBC count.
- If generalized, diffuse dermatitis occurs, notify doctor.
- Administer antihistamines, as ordered, to combat allergic dermatitis.

---

daunorubicin hydrochloride
Cerubidine†, Cerubidine‡
Antibiotic antineoplastic (cell cycle–phase nonspecific)
Antineoplastic
Pregnancy Risk Category: D

Dosage and indications vary.
Remission induction in acute nonlymphocytic (myelogenous, monocytic, erythroid) leukemia — **Adults:** in combination, 30 to 45 mg/m²/day I.V. on days 1, 2, and 3 of first course and on days 1 and 2 of subsequent courses with cytarabine infusions.
Remission induction in acute lymphocytic leukemia — **Adults:** in combination, 45 mg/m²/day I.V. on days 1, 2, and 3 of first course. **Children ≥ 2 yr:** 25 mg/m² I.V. on day 1 q wk. for up to 6 wk. if needed. **Children < 2 yr or body surface area < 0.5 m²:** dose calculated based on body weight (1 mg/kg).

- Take preventive measures (including adequate hydration) before treatment starts.
- *I.V. use:* Withdraw into syringe containing 10 to 15 ml 0.9% NaCl for injection. Inject into tubing of free-flowing I.V. solution of D₅W or 0.9% NaCl for injection over 2 to 3 min. Or, dilute in 50 ml 0.9% NaCl for injection, and infuse over 10 to 15 min, or dilute in 100 ml and infuse over 30 to 45 min. If extravasation occurs, stop infusion immediately, apply ice for 24 to 48 hr, and notify doctor.
- Monitor CBC, liver function tests, and pulse, as ordered; monitor ECG q mo during therapy. Monitor for nausea and vomiting, which may last 24 to 48 hr.
- Stop drug and notify doctor if signs of heart failure or cardiomyopathy develop.

DRUG/CLASS/ CATEGORY	INDICATIONS/ DOSAGES	KEY NURSING CONSIDERATIONS
delavirdine mesylate Rescriptor *Nonnucleoside reverse-transcriptase inhibitor* *Antiretroviral* Pregnancy Risk Category: C	*Treatment of HIV-1 infection when therapy is warranted* — **Adults:** 400 mg P.O. t.i.d. in combination with other appropriate antiretroviral agents.	• Drug-induced rash is more common in patients with lower CD4+ cell counts and usually occurs within first 3 wk of treatment. Rash is typically diffuse, maculopapular, erythematous, and often pruritic. Incidence of rash isn't significantly reduced by adjusted drug doses. Rash occurs mainly on upper body and proximal arms. Diphenhydramine, hydroxyzine, or topical corticosteroids may relieve symptoms. • Monitor renal and liver function tests carefully; effects in patients with hepatic or renal impairment have not been studied. • Always use drug in combination with appropriate antiretroviral therapy; resistance develops rapidly when used as monotherapy. • Monitor patient's fluid balance and weight.
demeclocycline hydrochloride Declomycin, Ledermycin‡ *Tetracycline antibiotic* *Antibiotic* Pregnancy Risk Category: D	*Infections caused by susceptible gram-positive and gram-negative organisms,* Rickettsia, M. pneumoniae, C. trachomatis; psittacosis; *granuloma inguinale* — **Adults:** 150 mg P.O. q 6 hr or 300 mg P.O. q 12 hr. **Children > 8 yr:** 6 to 12 mg/kg P.O. q.d. in divided doses q 6 to 12 hr. *Gonorrhea* — **Adults:** initially, 600 mg P.O.; then 300 mg P.O. q 12 hr for 4 days (total 3 g).	• Obtain specimen for culture and sensitivity tests before first dose. • Don't expose to light or heat; store in tightly capped container. • Monitor for superinfection. • Check tongue for signs of candidal infection. Stress good oral hygiene.

desipramine hydrochloride
Norpramin, Pertofran‡, Pertofrane
Dibenzazepine TCA
Antidepressant
Pregnancy Risk Category: C

Depression — **Adults:** 100 to 200 mg P.O. q.d. in divided doses, increased to maximum 300 mg q.d. Or give entire dose h.s. **Elderly and adolescents:** 25 to 100 mg P.O. q.d. in divided doses, increased gradually to maximum 150 mg q.d., if needed.

- Record mood changes. Monitor for suicidal tendencies, and allow only minimum drug supply.
- Produces fewer anticholinergic effects than other TCAs. Such effects can occur rapidly.
- Discontinue gradually several days before surgery.

desmopressin acetate
DDAVP, Minirin‡, Stimate
Posterior pituitary hormone
Antidiuretic/hemostatic
Pregnancy Risk Category: B

Nonnephrogenic diabetes insipidus; temporary polyuria and polydipsia with pituitary trauma — **Adults:** 0.1 to 0.4 ml intranasally q.d. in 1 to 3 doses. Adjust morning and evening doses separately for adequate diurnal rhythm of water turnover. Or, give injectable form 0.5 to 1 ml I.V. or S.C. q.d., usually in 2 divided doses. **Children 3 mo to 12 yr:** 0.05 to 0.3 ml intranasally q.d. in 1 or 2 doses.

- Overdose may cause oxytocic or vasopressor activity. Withhold drug and notify doctor.
- Intranasal use can cause changes in nasal mucosa resulting in erratic, unreliable absorption. Report worsening condition to doctor; may prescribe injectable DDAVP.
- Adjust fluid intake to reduce risk of water intoxication and sodium depletion, especially in children and elderly patients.

dexamethasone (injectable)
Dexdron, Hexadrol
dexamethasone acetate
Dalalone D.P., Decadron-LA, Dexasone-L.A.
dexamethasone sodium phosphate
Dalalone, Decadron Phosphate, Dexasone

Cerebral edema — **Adults:** initially, 10 mg (phosphate) I.V.; then 4 to 6 mg I.M. q 6 hr until symptoms subside (usually 2 to 4 days); then taper over 5 to 7 days.
Inflammatory conditions; allergic reactions; neoplasias — **Adults:** 0.75 to 9 mg/day P.O. or 0.5 to 9 mg/day (phosphate) I.M. or 4 to 16 mg (acetate) I.M. into joint or soft tissue q 1 to 3 wk; or 0.8 to 1.6 mg (acetate) into lesions q 1 to 3 wk.

- For better results and less toxicity, give once-daily dose in morning with food.
- Inspect skin for petechiae.
- Monitor weight, BP, serum electrolytes, and blood glucose.
- Watch for depression or psychotic episodes, especially with high-dose therapy.
- *I.V. use:* When giving as direct injection, inject undiluted over at least 1 min.

(continued)

DRUG/CLASS/ CATEGORY	INDICATIONS/ DOSAGES	KEY NURSING CONSIDERATIONS
dexamethasone *(continued)* *Glucocorticoid* *Anti-inflammatory/immuno-suppressant* Pregnancy Risk Category: C	*Shock* — **Adults:** 1 to 6 mg/kg (phosphate) I.V. as single dose; or 40 mg I.V. q 2 to 6 hr, p.r.n.; continue only until patient stabilized.	
dexamethasone (topical) Aeroseb-Dex, Decaderm, Decaspray **dexamethasone sodium phosphate** *Corticosteroid* *Anti-inflammatory* Pregnancy Risk Category: C	*Inflammation associated with corticosteroid-responsive dermatoses* — **Adults and children:** Clean area; apply sparingly t.i.d. to q.i.d. For aerosol use on scalp, shake can gently and apply to dry scalp after shampooing. Slide applicator tube under hair to touch scalp. Spray (about 2 sec) while moving tube to all affected areas, keeping it under hair and in contact with scalp. Spot-spray inadequately covered areas. Don't massage drug into scalp or spray forehead or near eyes.	• Gently wash skin before applying. Rub in gently, leaving thin coat. Don't apply near eyes, mucous membranes, or in ear canal. • Notify doctor if skin infection, striae, atrophy, or fever develops. • When using aerosol around face, cover patient's eyes and warn against inhaling spray. To avoid freezing tissues, don't spray > 1 to 2 sec or closer than 6" (15 cm). • Continue treatment for several days after lesions clear, as ordered.
dexamethasone (ophthalmic) Maxidex Ophthalmic Suspension **dexamethasone sodium phosphate**	*Uveitis; iridocyclitis; inflammatory conditions of eyelids, conjunctiva, cornea, anterior or segment of globe; corneal injury from chemical or thermal burns or penetration of foreign bodies; allergic conjunctivitis; suppression of graft rejection after kerato-plasty* — **Adults and children:** 1 to 2 drops suspension or solution or 1.25 to 2.5 cm	• Use cautiously in patients with corneal abrasions that may be infected (especially with herpes). • May need to increase glaucoma medications. • Monitor for corneal ulceration. • Tell patient to shake suspension well before use.

Decadron Phosphate Ophthalmic, Maxidex Ophthalmic
Corticosteroid
Ophthalmic anti-inflammatory
Pregnancy Risk Category: C

ointment into conjunctival sac. In severe disease, drops may be used hourly, tapering to discontinuation as condition improves. In mild conditions, drops may be used up to 6 times daily or ointment applied t.i.d. or q.i.d. As condition improves, dosage tapered to b.i.d., then q.d.

- Teach patient how to administer drug.
- Warn patient to stop drug and call doctor if visual acuity changes or visual field diminishes.
- Treatment may extend from days to weeks.

dextroampheta-mine sulfate
Dexedrine, Dexedrine Spansule, Oxydess II, Spancap #1
Amphetamine
CNS stimulant/short-term adjunctive anorexigenic/ sympathomimetic amine
Pregnancy Risk Category: C
Controlled Substance
Schedule: II

Narcolepsy — **Adults:** 5 to 60 mg P.O. q.d. in divided doses. **Children 6 to 12 yr:** 5 mg P.O. q.d., with 5-mg increments weekly, p.r.n. **Children ≥ 12 yr:** 10 mg P.O. q.d., with 10-mg increments weekly, p.r.n. Give first dose on awakening; additional doses (one or two) at intervals of 4 to 6 hr.
Short-term adjunct in exogenous obesity — **Adults and children ≥ 12 yr:** 5 to 30 mg P.O. q.d. 30 to 60 min before meals in divided doses of 5 to 10 mg. Or, 1 10- or 15-mg sustained-release capsule q.d. in morning.
Attention deficit disorder with hyper-activity — **Children 3 to 5 yr:** 2.5 mg P.O. q.d., with 2.5-mg increments weekly, p.r.n. **Children ≥ 6 yr:** 5 mg P.O. q.d. or b.i.d., with 5-mg increments weekly, p.r.n.

- Don't use to prevent fatigue.
- Make sure obese patient is on weight-reduction program.
- If tolerance to anorexigenic effect develops, discontinue drug and notify doctor.
- Advise patient to avoid activities requiring alertness until CNS effects are known.
- Instruct patient to report excessive stimulation.
- Fatigue may occur as drug wears off.

†Canadian ‡Australian

DRUG / CLASS / CATEGORY	INDICATIONS / DOSAGES	KEY NURSING CONSIDERATIONS
dextrose (d-glucose) *Carbohydrate* *TPN component/caloric/ fluid volume replacement* Pregnancy Risk Category: C	*Fluid replacement and caloric supplementation* — **Adults and children:** Dosage varies. Peripheral I.V. infusion of 2.5% to 10% solution or central I.V. infusion of 20% solution for minimal fluid needs. 25% solution for acute hypoglycemia in neonates or infants. 50% solution for insulin-induced hypoglycemia. Solution of 10% to 70% diluted in admixtures, for TPN given through central vein.	• *I.V. use:* Control infusion rate carefully; maximum rate 0.5 g/kg/hr. Use infusion pump when infusing with amino acids for TPN. • Use central veins to infuse dextrose solutions with concentration > 10%. • Monitor serum glucose carefully. • Never stop hypertonic solutions abruptly. • Monitor I&O and weight carefully. • Check vital signs frequently.
diazepam Apo-Diazepam†, Diazepam Intensol, Valium, Zetran *Benzodiazepine* *Antianxiety agent/skeletal muscle relaxant/amnesic agent/anticonvulsant/ sedative-hypnotic* Pregnancy Risk Category: D Controlled Substance Schedule: IV	*Anxiety* — **Adults:** 2 to 10 mg P.O. 2 to 4 times q.d., or 15 to 30 mg extended-release capsules P.O. q.d. Or, 2 to 10 mg I.M. or I.V. q 3 to 4 hr, p.r.n. **Elderly:** 2 to 2.5 mg once or twice q.d.; increased gradually. **Children ≥ 6 mo:** 1 to 2.5 mg P.O. three to four times q.d., increased gradually, p.r.n. *Muscle spasm* — **Adults:** 2 to 10 mg P.O. two to four times q.d. or 15 to 30 mg extended-release capsules q.d. Or, 5 to 10 mg I.M. or I.V. Initially; then 5 to 10 mg I.M. or I.V. q 3 to 4 hr, p.r.n. **Children > 30 days to 5 yr:** 1 to 2 mg I.M. or I.V. slowly, repeated q 3 to 4 hr, p.r.n. **Children ≥ 5 yr:** 5 to 10 mg I.M. or I.V. q 3 to 4 hr, p.r.n.	• Monitor respirations q 5 to 15 min and before each repeated I.V. dose. Have emergency resuscitation equipment and oxygen at bedside. • Don't mix injectable form with other drugs. • Don't store parenteral solution in plastic syringes. • *I.V. use:* Give no faster than 5 mg/min. • Check daily for phlebitis at injection site. • I.V. route most reliable parenteral route; I.M. use not recommended because absorption is variable and injection painful. • Avoid extravasation. Don't inject into small veins.

Status epilepticus and severe recurrent seizures — **Adults:** 5 to 10 mg I.V. (preferred) or I.M. Repeat q 10 to 15 min, p.r.n., to maximum 30 mg. Repeat q 2 to 4 hr, p.r.n. **Children > 30 days to 5 yr:** 0.2 to 0.5 mg I.V. slowly q 2 to 5 min to maximum 5 mg. Repeat q 2 to 4 hr, p.r.n. **Children ≥ 5 yr:** 1 mg I.V. q 2 to 5 min to maximum 10 mg. Repeat q 2 to 4 hr, p.r.n.

diazoxide Hyperstat IV *Peripheral vasodilator Antihypertensive* Pregnancy Risk Category: C	*Hypertensive crisis* — **Adults and children:** 1 to 3 mg/kg by I.V. bolus undiluted (to maximum 150 mg) q 5 to 15 min until adequate response occurs. Repeat at 4- to 24-hr intervals, p.r.n.	• **I.V. use:** Monitor BP and ECG continuously. Keep patient supine during and 1 hr after infusion. Protect I.V. solutions from light. • Avoid extravasation. • Monitor fluid balance and blood glucose.

diclofenac potassium Cataflam **diclofenac sodium** Fenac‡, Voltaren, Voltaren SR† *NSAID Antarthritic/anti-inflammatory* Pregnancy Risk Category: B	*Ankylosing spondylitis* — **Adults:** 25 mg P.O. q.i.d. (and h.s., p.r.n.). *Osteoarthritis* — **Adults:** 50 mg P.O. b.i.d. or t.i.d., or 75 mg P.O. b.i.d. (sodium form only). *Rheumatoid arthritis* — **Adults:** 50 mg P.O. t.i.d. or q.i.d. Or, 75 mg P.O. b.i.d. (sodium form only) or 50 to 100 mg P.R. h.s. as substitute for last P.O. dose of day. Maximum 225 mg q.d. *Analgesia and primary dysmenorrhea* — **Adults:** 50 mg P.O. t.i.d. (potassium form only).	• Can decrease renal blood flow and lead to reversible renal impairment. Monitor patient closely. • Monitor serum transaminase periodically during therapy. • May mask symptoms of infection. • To minimize GI distress, instruct patient to take with milk or meals. • Tell patient not to crush, chew, or break enteric-coated tablets.

DRUG/CLASS/CATEGORY	INDICATIONS/DOSAGES	KEY NURSING CONSIDERATIONS
dicyclomine hydrochloride Antispas, Bentyl, Neoquess, Spasmoban† *Anticholinergic* *Antimuscarinic/GI antispasmodic* Pregnancy Risk Category: B	*Irritable bowel syndrome; other functional GI disorders* — **Adults:** initially, 20 mg P.O. q.i.d., increased to 40 mg q.i.d., or 20 mg I.M. q 4 to 6 hr.	• Don't give S.C. or I.V. • Give 30 min to 1 hr before meals and h.s. Bedtime dose can be larger; administer at least 2 hr after last meal. • Monitor vital signs and urine output. • Prepare to adjust dosage according to patient's needs and response, as ordered.
didanosine (ddI) Videx *Purine analogue* *Antiviral* Pregnancy Risk Category: B	*Treatment of HIV infection when antiretroviral therapy warranted* — **Adults ≥ 60 kg (132 lb):** 200 mg (tablets) P.O. q 12 hr; or 250 mg buffered powder P.O. q 12 hr. **Adults < 60 kg:** 125 mg (tablets) P.O. q 12 hr; or 167 mg buffered powder P.O. q 12 hr. **Children:** 120 mg/m² P.O. q 12 hr. *Adjust-a-dose:* Patients with reduced renal function and those on dialysis require dosage adjustment.	• Administer on empty stomach. • Pediatric powder for oral solution must be prepared by pharmacist before dispensing. • Associated with high incidence of diarrhea. • Don't use fruit juice or other acidic beverages to dissolve powder.
diflunisal Dolobid *NSAID, salicylic acid derivative* *Nonnarcotic analgesic/antipyretic/anti-inflammatory* Pregnancy Risk Category: C	*Mild to moderate pain; osteoarthritis; rheumatoid arthritis* — **Adults:** 500 to 1,000 mg P.O. q.d. in 2 divided doses, usually q 12 hr. Maximum 1,500 mg q.d. **Adults > 65 yr:** half of usual adult dose.	• Don't give to children or teenagers with chickenpox or flulike illness because of risk of Reye's syndrome. • Tell patient to take with water, milk, or meals.

digoxin
Digoxin, Lanoxicaps,
Lanoxin, Novodigoxin†
Cardiac glycoside
Antiarrhythmic/inotropic
Pregnancy Risk Category: C

Heart failure; PSVT; atrial fibrillation and flutter — **Adults:** loading dose 0.5 to 1 mg I.V. or P.O. in divided doses over 24 hr; maintenance: 0.125 to 0.5 mg I.V. or P.O. q.d. (average: 0.25 mg). **Adults > 65 yr:** 0.125 mg P.O. q.d. as maintenance dose. **Premature neonates:** loading dose 0.015 to 0.025 mg/kg I.V. in 3 divided doses over 24 hr; maintenance: 0.01 mg/kg q.d., divided q 12 hr. **Neonates:** loading dose 0.025 to 0.035 mg/kg P.O., divided q 8 hr over 24 hr; I.V. loading dose 0.02 to 0.03 mg/kg: maintenance: 0.01 mg/kg P.O. q.d., divided q 12 hr. **Children 1 mo to 2 yr:** loading dose 0.035 to 0.06 mg/kg P.O. in 3 divided doses over 24 hr; I.V. loading dose 0.03 to 0.05 mg/kg; maintenance: 0.01 to 0.02 mg/kg P.O. q.d., divided q 12 hr. **Children > 2 yr:** loading dose 0.02 to 0.04 mg/kg P.O. q.d., divided q 8 hr over 24 hr. I.V. loading dose, 0.015 to 0.035 mg/kg; maintenance dose, 0.012 mg/kg P.O. q.d., divided q 12 hr.
Adjust-a-dose: Reduce loading and maintenance doses in patients with impaired renal function.

- Before therapy, obtain baseline data (apical pulse, HR, BP, and electrolytes) and ask about use of cardiac glycosides within previous 2 to 3 wk.
- Before administering, take apical-radial pulse for full min. Record and report significant changes. If changes occur, check BP and obtain ECG.
- Excessive slowing of pulse ($\leq$ 60 beats/min) may signal digitalis toxicity. Withhold drug and notify doctor.
- *I.V. use:* Infuse slowly over at least 5 min.
- Encourage consumption of potassium-rich foods.
- Smaller doses given in impaired renal function or to frail patients.

DRUG/CLASS/ CATEGORY	INDICATIONS/ DOSAGES	KEY NURSING CONSIDERATIONS
digoxin immune Fab (ovine) Digibind *Antibody fragment* *Cardiac glycoside antidote* Pregnancy Risk Category: C	*Potentially life-threatening digoxin or digitoxin intoxication* — **Adults and children:** I.V. dosage varies according to amount of digoxin or digitoxin to be neutralized. Each vial binds about 0.5 mg of digoxin or digitoxin. Average dosage, 6 vials (228 mg). However, if toxicity resulted from acute digoxin ingestion and neither serum digoxin level nor estimated ingestion amount known, 20 vials (760 mg) may be needed. See package insert for complete, specific dosage instructions.	▪ Use only for life-threatening overdose in shock or cardiac arrest or with ventricular arrhythmias, progressive bradycardia, or secnd- or third-degree AV block not responsive to atropine. ▪ *I.V. use:* Reconstitute 38-mg vial with 4 ml sterile water for injection. Gently roll vial to dissolve powder. Reconstituted solution contains 9.5 mg/ml. May give by direct injection if cardiac arrest seems imminent. Or, dilute with 0.9% NaCl for injection to appropriate volume and give by intermittent infusion over 30 min through 0.22-micron membrane filter. ▪ Monitor serum potassium closely. ▪ Interferes with digitalis immunoassay measurements; standard serum digoxin levels misleading until drug cleared from body (about 2 days).
dihydroergotamine mesylate D.H.E. 45, Dihydergot† *Ergot alkaloid* *Vasoconstrictor* Pregnancy Risk Category: X	*To prevent or abort vascular or migraine headache* — **Adults:** 1 mg I.M. or I.V. Repeat q 1 to 2 hr, p.r.n., to total of 2 mg I.V. or 3 mg I.M. per attack. Maximum weekly dose 6 mg.	▪ Most effective when used at first sign of migraine or soon after onset. ▪ *I.V. use:* Directly inject solution into vein over 3 min. ▪ Be alert for ergotamine rebound. ▪ Protect ampules from heat and light.

diltiazem hydrochloride

Apo-Diltiaz†, Cardizem, Cardizem CD, Cardizem SR, Dilacor-XR, Tiazac

Calcium channel blocker
Antianginal
Pregnancy Risk Category: C

Vasospastic angina (Prinzmetal's [variant] angina); classic chronic stable angina pectoris — **Adults:** 30 mg P.O. t.i.d. or q.i.d. before meals and h.s. Increase gradually to maximum 360 mg/day in divided doses. Or, 120 or 180 mg (extended-release capsules). Adjust dose, p.r.n. to maximum 480 mg q.d.

Hypertension — **Adults:** 60 to 120 mg P.O. b.i.d. (sustained-release). Adjust dose to effect. Maximum 360 mg/day. Or, 180 to 240 mg q.d. (extended-release) initially. Adjust dose, p.r.n.

Atrial fibrillation or flutter; PSVT — **Adults:** 0.25 mg/kg as I.V. bolus injection over 2 min. If response inadequate, 0.35 mg/kg I.V. after 15 min followed by continuous infusion of 10 mg/hr. Some patients respond well to rates of 5 mg/hr; maximum 15 mg/hr.

- **I.V. use:** Infusions longer than 24 hr not recommended.
- Monitor BP and HR during initiation of therapy and dosage adjustments.
- If systolic BP < 90 or HR < 60, withhold dose and notify doctor.
- Tell patient to avoid hazardous activities during initiation of therapy.
- Advise patient that S.L. nitroglycerin may be taken concomitantly, p.r.n, if anginal symptoms acute.

dimenhydrinate

Dimetabs, Dinate, Dramamine

Ethanolamine-derivative antihistamine
Antihistamine (H₁-receptor antagonist)/antiemetic/ antivertigo agent
Pregnancy Risk Category: B

Prevention and treatment of motion sickness — **Adults and children ≥ 12 yr:** 50 to 100 mg P.O. q 4 to 6 hr; 50 mg I.M., p.r.n.; or 50 mg I.V. diluted in 10 ml NaCl for injection, injected over 2 min. Maximum 400 mg q.d. **Children 6 to 12 yr:** 25 to 50 mg P.O. q 6 to 8 hr, not to exceed 150 mg in 24 hr. **Children 2 to 6 yr:** 12.5 to 25 mg P.O. q 6 to 8 hr, not to exceed 75 mg in 24 hr. **Children > 2 yr:** 1.25 mg/kg or 37.5 mg/m² I.M. q.i.d. Maximum 300 mg q.d.

- Most I.V. products contain benzyl alcohol, associated with fatal "gasping syndrome" in premature and low-birth-weight infants. May mask symptoms of ototoxicity, brain tumor, or intestinal obstruction.
- **I.V. use:** Before giving, dilute each ml of drug with 10 ml sterile water for injection, D₅W, or 0.9% NaCl for injection. Give by direct injection over not less than 2 min. Avoid mixing parenteral preparation with other drugs.

109

DRUG/CLASS/ CATEGORY	INDICATIONS/ DOSAGES	KEY NURSING CONSIDERATIONS
dinoprostone Prepidil, Prostin E₂ *Prostaglandin* *Oxytocic* Pregnancy Risk Category: C	*To abort second-trimester pregnancy; to evacuate uterus in missed abortion, intra-uterine fetal deaths up to 28 wk of gestation, or benign hydatidiform mole* — **Adults:** 20-mg suppository inserted high into posterior vaginal fornix. Repeat q 3 to 5 hr until abortion complete. *Ripening of unfavorable cervix in pregnant patients at or near term* — **Adults:** gel contents of 1 syringe given intravaginally; if cervix unfavorable after 6 hr, repeat. Don't give > 1.5 mg within 24-hr period.	▪ After administration, have patient remain supine for 10 min. ▪ When drug used as abortifacient, may pre-treat patient with antiemetic and antidiar-rheal. ▪ Treat dinoprostone-induced fever with wa-ter or alcohol sponging and increased flu-id intake, not with aspirin. ▪ Abortion should be complete within 30 hr when suppository used.
diphenhydramine hydrochloride Allerdryl,† Benadryl, Hy-dramine, Nytol Maximum Strength, Sominex *Ethanolamine-derivative antihistamine* *Antihistamine/antiemetic/ antivertigo agent/antitussive/sedative-hypnotic/anti-dyskinetic (anticholinergic)* Pregnancy Risk Category: B	*Rhinitis; allergy symptoms; motion sickness; Parkinson's disease* — **Adults and children ≥ 12 yr:** 25 to 50 mg P.O. t.i.d. or q.i.d.; or, 10 to 50 mg deep I.M. or I.V. Maximum I.M. or I.V. dose 400 mg q.d. **Children < 12 yr:** 5 mg/kg q.d. P.O., deep I.M., or I.V. in divided doses q.i.d. Maximum 300 mg q.d. *Sedation* — **Adults:** 25 to 50 mg P.O. or deep I.M., p.r.n. *Nonproductive cough* — **Adults:** 25 mg P.O. q 4 to 6 hr (maximum 150 mg q.d.). **Children 6 to 12 yr:** 12.5 mg P.O. q 4 to 6 hr (maximum 75 mg q.d.). **Children 2 to 6 yr:** 6.25 mg P.O. q 4 to 6 hr (maximum 25 mg/day).	▪ Children < 12 yr should use only as direct-ed by doctor. ▪ Alternate injection sites to prevent irrita-tion. Administer I.M. injection deeply into large muscle. ▪ Tell patient to take 30 min before travel to prevent motion sickness. ▪ Instruct patient to take with food or milk to reduce GI distress. ▪ Tell patient to use sunscreen and to avoid overexposure to sunlight.

diphenoxylate hydrochloride and atropine sulfate

Logen, Lomanate, Lomotil, Lonox

Opiate
Antidiarrheal
Pregnancy Risk Category: C
Controlled Substance
Schedule: V

Acute, nonspecific diarrhea — **Adults:** initially, 5 mg P.O. q.i.d.; then adjusted, p.r.n. **Children 2 to 12 yr:** 0.3 to 0.4 mg/kg liquid form P.O. q.d. in 4 divided doses. For maintenance, initial dose reduced, p.r.n., up to 75%.

- Use cautiously in children ≥ 2 yr; in patients with hepatic disease, narcotic dependence, or acute ulcerative colitis; and in pregnant patients. Stop therapy immediately and notify doctor if abdominal distention or other signs of toxic megacolon develop.
- Monitor fluid and electrolyte balance. Correct fluid and electrolyte disturbances before starting drug. Dehydration, especially in young children, may increase risk of delayed toxicity.
- Drug is not indicated for treating antibiotic-induced diarrhea.
- Drug is unlikely to be effective if no response occurs within 48 hr.
- Risk of physical dependence increases with high dosage and long-term use. Atropine sulfate helps discourage abuse.

diphtheria and tetanus toxoids, adsorbed

Toxoid
Diphtheria and tetanus prophylaxis agent
Pregnancy Risk Category: C

Primary immunization — **Adults and children ≥ 7 yr:** adult strength, 0.5 ml I.M. 4 to 8 wk apart for 2 doses and 3rd dose 6 to 12 mo after 2nd dose. Booster, 0.5 ml I.M. q 10 yr. **Infants 6 wk to 1 yr:** pediatric strength, 0.5 ml I.M. ≥ 4 wk apart for 3 doses. Give booster dose 6 to 12 mo after 3rd injection. **Children 1 to 6 yr:** pediatric strength, 0.5 ml I.M. ≥ 4 wk apart for 2 doses. Give booster dose 6 to 12 mo after 2nd injection. If final immunizing dose given after seventh birthday, use adult strength.

- Obtain history of allergies and reaction to immunization.
- Before injection, verify strength (pediatric or adult) of toxoid to use.
- Keep epinephrine 1:1,000 available to treat anaphylaxis.
- Give in site not recently used for vaccines or toxoids.

111

†Canadian ‡Australian

DRUG/CLASS/ CATEGORY	INDICATIONS/ DOSAGES	KEY NURSING CONSIDERATIONS
diphtheria and tetanus toxoids and acellular pertussis vaccine Acel-Imune, DTaP, Tripedia **diphtheria and tetanus toxoids and whole-cell pertussis vaccine (DTP, DPT)** DTwP, Tri-Immunol *Combination toxoid and vaccine* *Diphtheria, tetanus, and pertussis prophylaxis agent* Pregnancy Risk Category: C	*Primary immunization* — **Children 6 wk to 6 yr:** 0.5 ml I.M. 4 to 8 wk apart for 3 doses and 4th dose 1 yr later. Booster, 0.5 ml I.M. when starting school, unless 4th dose in series administered after fourth birthday; then, booster not necessary at time of school entrance. Not advised for adults or children > 6 yr. Products containing acellular pertussis vaccine may now be used for any dose in DTP immunization.	▪ Obtain history of allergies and reaction to immunization. ▪ Keep epinephrine 1:1,000 available to treat anaphylaxis. ▪ Shake before using. Store refrigerated. ▪ Administer only by deep I.M. injection, preferably in thigh or deltoid muscle. Don't give S.C. ▪ Acellular vaccine may be associated with lower incidence of local pain and fever.
dipivefrin Propine *Sympathomimetic* *Antiglaucoma agent* Pregnancy Risk Category: B	*IOP reduction in chronic open-angle glaucoma* — **Adults:** for initial glaucoma therapy, 1 drop of 0.1% solution q 12 hr. Adjust dosage based on patient response as determined by tonometric readings.	▪ Often used concomitantly with other antiglaucoma drugs. ▪ May cause fewer adverse reactions than conventional epinephrine therapy.

dipyridamole I.V. Persantine, Persantin‡, Persantine *Pyrimidine analogue* *Coronary vasodilator/* *platelet aggregation* *inhibitor* Pregnancy Risk Category: B	*Inhibition of platelet adhesion in prosthetic heart valves* — **Adults:** 75 to 100 mg P.O. q.i.d. *Alternative to exercise in CAD evaluation during thallium (²⁰¹Tl) myocardial perfusion scintigraphy* — **Adults:** 0.57 mg/kg as I.V. infusion at constant rate over 4 min (0.142 mg/kg/min). *Acute coronary insufficiency* — **Adults:** 10 ml I.V. or I.M.	• If patient develops GI distress, give 1 hr before meals or with meals. • *I.V. use:* If using as diagnostic agent, dilute in 0.45% or 0.9% NaCl solution or D₅W in at least 1:2 ratio for total volume of 20 to 50 ml. Inject ²⁰¹Tl within 5 min after completing dipyridamole infusion. • Observe for signs of bleeding or other adverse reactions.
dirithromycin Dynabac *Macrolide* *Antibiotic* Pregnancy Risk Category: C	*Acute bacterial exacerbations of chronic bronchitis or secondary bacterial infection of acute bronchitis due to M. catarrhalis or S. pneumoniae; uncomplicated skin and skin-structure infections due to S. aureus (methicillin-susceptible strains)* — **Adults and children ≥ 12 yr:** 500 mg P.O. q.d. for 7 days. *Community-acquired pneumonia due to L. pneumophila, M. pneumoniae, or S. pneumoniae* — **Adults and children ≥ 12 yr:** 500 mg P.O. q.d. for 14 days.	• Obtain culture and sensitivity results to ensure organism is sensitive to drug. Not recommended for empiric use. • Don't use in patients with known, suspected, or potential bacteremias. • Administer with food or within 1 hr of food intake. • Monitor for superinfection. • Safety in children < 12 yr not established.
disopyramide Rythmodan† **disopyramide phosphate** Norpace, Norpace CR, Rythmodan-LA†	*Ventricular tachycardia and ventricular arrhythmias (those severe enough to be life-threatening)* — **Adults > 50 kg (110 lb):** 150 mg q 6 hr with conventional capsules or 300 mg q 12 hr with extended-release preparation. **Adults ≤ 50 kg:** 100 mg P.O. q 6 hr or 200 mg q 12 hr	• Check apical pulse before administering. Notify doctor if < 60 or > 120. • Discontinue drug and notify doctor if heart block develops, QRS complex widens by more than 25%, or QT interval lengthens by more than 25% above baseline. *(continued)*

DRUG/CLASS/ CATEGORY	INDICATIONS/ DOSAGES	KEY NURSING CONSIDERATIONS
disopyramide *(continued)* *Pyridine-derivative anti-arrhythmic* *Antiarrhythmic* Pregnancy Risk Category: C	as extended-release capsules. **Children <1 yr:** 10 to 30 mg/kg P.O. q.d. **Children 1 to 4 yr:** 10 to 20 mg/kg P.O. q.d. **Children 4 to 12 yr:** 10 to 15 mg/kg P.O. q.d. **Children 12 to 18 yr:** 6 to 15 mg/kg P.O. q.d. *Note:* For pediatric dosages, divide into equal amounts and give q 6 hr. **Adjust-a-dose:** In patients with advanced renal insufficiency, if creatinine clearance is 30 to 40 ml/min, give 100 mg q 8 hr; 15 to 30 ml/min, 100 mg q 12 hr; < 15 ml/min, 100 mg q 24 hr.	• Watch for recurrence of arrhythmias and check for adverse reactions; notify doctor if any occur. • Correct electrolyte abnormalities before therapy begins, as ordered.
disulfiram Antabuse *Aldehyde dehydrogenase inhibitor* *Alcoholic deterrent* Pregnancy Risk Category: NR	*Adjunct in management of chronic alco-holism —* **Adults:** 250 to 500 mg P.O. as single dose in morning for 1 to 2 wk or in evening if drowsiness occurs. Maintenance, 125 to 500 mg P.O. q.d. (average dose 250 mg) until permanent self-control estab-lished. Treatment may continue for mo or yr.	• Use only under close medical and nursing supervision. Never administer until patient has abstained from alcohol for ≥ 12 hr. Patient should clearly understand conse-quences of drug and give permission for its use. Use only in patients who are coop-erative, well motivated, and receiving sup-portive psychiatric therapy. • Complete physical exam and lab studies, including CBC, SMA-12, and transaminase level, should precede therapy and be re-peated regularly, as ordered.

dobutamine hydrochloride
Dobutrex
Adrenergic, beta₁ agonist
Inotropic agent
Pregnancy Risk Category: B

To increase cardiac output in short-term treatment of cardiac decompensation caused by depressed contractility, such as during refractory heart failure; as adjunct in cardiac surgery — **Adults:** 2.5 to 15 mcg/kg/min I.V. infusion. Rates up to 40 mcg/kg/min may be needed (rare).

- Administer after cardiac glycoside.
- Continuously monitor ECG, BP, PAWP, cardiac condition, and urine output.
- Before starting therapy, correct hypovolemia with plasma volume expanders, as ordered.
- *I.V. use:* Give through large vein. Use infusion pump. Avoid extravasation.
- Dilute concentrate for injection before administration. Don't exceed maximum concentration of 5 mg/ml.

docetaxel
Taxotere
Taxoid
Antineoplastic
Pregnancy Risk Category: D

Treatment of patients with locally advanced or metastatic breast cancer who have progressed during anthracycline-based therapy or have relapsed during anthracycline-based adjuvant therapy — **Adults:** 60 to 100 mg/m² I.V. over 1 hr q 3 wk.

- Monitor liver function studies.
- Premedicate with oral corticosteroids, such as dexamethasone 16 mg P.O. (8 mg b.i.d.) q.d. for 5 days starting 1 day before docetaxel administration.
- Wear gloves during preparation and administration. If solution contacts skin, wash immediately and thoroughly with soap and water. Mark all waste materials with CHEMOTHERAPY HAZARD labels.
- Bone marrow toxicity most frequent and dose-limiting toxic effect. Frequent blood count monitoring necessary during therapy.
- Monitor for hypersensitivity reactions.

DRUG/CLASS/ CATEGORY	INDICATIONS/ DOSAGES	KEY NURSING CONSIDERATIONS
docusate calcium Surfak **docusate sodium** Colace, Genasoft *Surfactant* *Emollient laxative* Pregnancy Risk Category: C	*Stool softener* — **Adults and children > 12 yr:** 50 to 500 mg P.O. q.d. until bowel movements normal. **Children < 3 yr:** 10 to 40 mg docusate sodium P.O. q.d. **Children 3 to 6 yr:** 20 to 60 mg docusate sodium P.O. q.d. **Children 6 to 12 yr:** 40 to 120 mg docusate sodium P.O. q.d.	▪ Give liquid in milk, fruit juice, or infant formula to mask bitter taste. ▪ Before administering, determine if patient has adequate fluid intake, exercise routine, and diet. ▪ Teach patient about dietary sources of bulk. ▪ Instruct patient to use only occasionally and not for > 1 wk without doctor's knowledge.
dolasetron mesylate Anzemet *Selective serotonin 5-HT$_3$– receptor agonist* *Antinauseant/antiemetic* Pregnancy Risk Category: B	*Prevention of nausea and vomiting associated with cancer chemotherapy* — **Adults:** 100 mg P.O. given as single dose 1 hr before chemotherapy; or 1.8 mg/kg (or a fixed dose of 100 mg) as single I.V. dose 30 min before chemotherapy. **Children 2 to 16 yr:** 1.8 mg/kg P.O. 1 hr before chemotherapy; or 1.8 mg/kg as single I.V. dose 30 min before chemotherapy. Injectable formulation can be mixed with apple juice and administered P.O. Maximum 100 mg. *Prevention of postoperative nausea and vomiting* — **Adults:** 100 mg P.O. ≤ 2 hr before surgery; 12.5 mg as single I.V. dose about 15 min before cessation of anesthesia. **Children 2 to 16 years:** 1.2 mg/kg P.O. ≤ 2 hours before surgery, up to maximum	▪ Administer with caution in patients who have or may develop prolonged cardiac conduction intervals, such as those with electrolyte abnormalities, history of arrhythmias, or cumulative high-dose anthracycline therapy. ▪ Drug isn't recommended for use in children < 2 yr. ▪ Injection for oral administration is stable in apple or apple-grape juice for 2 hr at room temperature. ▪ *I.V. use:* Injection can be infused as rapidly as 100 mg/30 sec or diluted in 50 ml compatible solution and infused over 15 min. ▪ Report nausea and vomiting to doctor.

of 100 mg; or 0.35 mg/kg (up to 12.5 mg) as single I.V. dose about 15 min before cessation of anesthesia. Injectable formulation can be mixed with apple juice and administered P.O.
Treatment of postoperative nausea and vomiting — **Adults:** 12.5 mg as single I.V. dose as soon as nausea or vomiting presents. **Children 2 to 16 years:** 0.35 mg/kg, up to maximum of 12.5 mg, as single I.V. dose as soon as nausea or vomiting presents.

- Monitor for symptoms of active or occult GI bleeding.

donepezil hydrochloride
Aricept
Acetylcholinesterase inhibitor
CNS agent for Alzheimer's disease
Pregnancy Risk Category: C

Mild to moderate dementia of Alzheimer's type — **Adults:** initially, 5 mg P.O. q.d. h.s. After 4 to 6 wk, may increase to 10 mg q.d.

dopamine hydrochloride
Intropin, Revimine†
Adrenergic
Inotropic, vasopressor
Pregnancy Risk Category: C

To treat shock and correct hemodynamic imbalances; to improve perfusion to vital organs; to increase cardiac output; to correct hypotension — **Adults:** initially, 1 to 5 mcg/kg/min by I.V. infusion. Titrate dose to desired hemodynamic or renal response; may increase infusion by 1 to 4 mcg/kg/min at 10- to 30-min intervals.

- If volume deficit exists, replace fluid before giving drug.
- Frequently monitor ECG, BP, cardiac output, CVP, PAWP, pulse rate, urine output, and color and temperature of extremities.
- *I.V. use:* Don't mix with alkaline solutions. Use central line or large vein to minimize risk of extravasation.

DRUG / CLASS / CATEGORY	INDICATIONS / DOSAGES	KEY NURSING CONSIDERATIONS
dorzolamide hydrochloride Trusopt *Sulfonamide* *Antiglaucoma agent* Pregnancy Risk Category: C	Treatment of increased IOP in patients with ocular hypertension or open-angle glaucoma — **Adults:** 1 drop in conjunctival sac of affected eye t.i.d.	▪ If patient receiving > 1 topical ophthalmic drug, administer drugs ≥ 10 min apart.
doxazosin mesylate Cardura *Alpha-adrenergic blocker* *Antihypertensive* Pregnancy Risk Category: C	*Essential hypertension* — **Adults:** 1 mg P.O. q.d.; determine effect on standing and supine BP at 2 to 6 hr and 24 hr after dosing. If necessary, increase to 2 mg q.d. Adjust dosage slowly. May increase to 4 mg q.d., then 8 mg. Maximum, 16 mg. *Benign prostatic hyperplasia* — **Adults:** initially, 1 mg P.O. q.d. in morning or evening; may increase to 2 mg and, thereafter, 4 mg and 8 mg q.d., p.r.n. Recommended adjustment interval 1 to 2 wk.	▪ Monitor BP closely. ▪ If syncope occurs, place patient in recumbent position and treat supportively. Transient hypotensive response doesn't contraindicate continued therapy. ▪ Orthostatic hypotension most common after first dose but also can occur during dosage adjustment or interruption of therapy.
doxepin hydrochloride Adapin, Deptran‡, Novo-Doxepin‡, Sinequan, Triadapin‡ *TCA* *Antidepressant* Pregnancy Risk Category: NR	*Depression or anxiety* — **Adults:** initially, 25 to 75 mg P.O. q.d. in divided doses to maximum 300 mg q.d. Or, give entire maintenance dose q.d. with maximum 150 mg P.O.	▪ Record mood changes. Monitor patient for suicidal tendencies, and allow only minimal drug supply. ▪ Discontinue gradually several days before surgery. ▪ Dilute oral concentrate with 120 ml (4 oz) of water, milk, or juice (not grape juice).

doxorubicin hydrochloride

Adriamycin†, Adriamycin PFS, Adriamycin RDF, Rubex

Antineoplastic antibiotic (cell cycle–phase nonspecific)

Antineoplastic

Pregnancy Risk Category: D

Dosage and indications vary. Check treatment protocol with doctor.

Bladder, breast, lung, ovarian, stomach, and thyroid cancers; Hodgkin's disease; acute lymphoblastic and myeloblastic leukemia; Wilms' tumor; neuroblastoma; lymphoma; sarcoma — **Adults:** 60 to 75 mg/m² I.V. as single dose q 3 wk; or 30 mg/m² I.V. in single daily dose, days 1 to 3 of 4-wk cycle. Or, 20 mg/m² I.V. once weekly. Maximum cumulative dose 550 mg/m².

Adjust-a-dose: In patients with myelosuppression or impaired cardiac or hepatic function, dosage may be reduced. Be prepared to decrease dosage if serum bilirubin level rises. Give 50% of dosage when bilirubin 1.2 to 3 mg/100 ml; give 25% of dosage when bilirubin > 3 mg/100 ml.

- Never give I.M. or S.C.
- Perform cardiac function studies (including ECG) before treatment and periodically throughout.
- May be given concomitantly with doxorubicin if accumulated doxorubicin dose has reached 300 mg/m².
- Don't place I.V. line over joints or in extremities with poor venous or lymphatic drainage. If extravasation occurs, discontinue and notify doctor. Monitor area closely. Early consultation with plastic surgeon may be advisable.
- If vein streaking occurs, slow administration rate. If welts occur, stop administration and report to doctor.
- Monitor CBC and hepatic function tests, as ordered; monitor ECG monthly. If tachycardia develops, be prepared to stop drug or slow infusion rate and notify doctor.
- If signs of heart failure develop, stop drug and notify doctor. In many cases, heart failure can be prevented by limiting cumulative dose to 550 mg/m² (400 mg/m² when patient also receiving or has received cyclophosphamide or radiation therapy to cardiac area).

119

DRUG / CLASS / CATEGORY	INDICATIONS / DOSAGES	KEY NURSING CONSIDERATIONS
doxycycline calcium Vibramycin **doxycycline hyclate** Doryx, Doxy-Caps, Doxycin†, Monodox, Vibramycin **doxycycline hydrochloride** Cyclidox‡, Doryx‡, Doxylin†, Vibramycin‡, Vibra-Tabs 50‡ **doxycycline monohydrate** Monodox, Vibramycin *Tetracycline* Antibiotic Pregnancy Risk Category: D	*Infections caused by susceptible gram-positive and gram-negative organisms* Rickettsia, M. pneumoniae, C. trachomatis, *and* B. burgdorferi (Lyme disease), psittacosis; granuloma inguinale — **Adults and children > 8 yr weighing ≥ 45 kg (99 lb):** 100 mg P.O. q 12 hr on 1st day; then 100 mg P.O. q.d.; or 200 mg I.V. on 1st day in one or two infusions; then 100 to 200 mg I.V. q.d. **Children > 8 yr weighing < 45 kg:** 4.4 mg/kg P.O. or I.V. q.d., in divided doses q 12 hr on 1st day; then 2.2 to 4.4 mg/kg q.d. in 1 or 2 divided doses. Give I.V. infusion slowly (minimum 1 hr). Infusion must be completed within 12 hr (within 6 hr in lactated Ringer's solution or dextrose 5% in lactated Ringer's solution). *Uncomplicated urethral, endocervical, or rectal infections caused by* C. trachomatis *or* U. urealyticum — **Adults:** 100 mg P.O. b.i.d. for at least 7 days (10 days for epididymitis). *Pelvic inflammatory disease* — **Adults:** 100 mg I.V. q 12 hr and continued for at least 2 days after symptomatic improvement; thereafter, 100 mg P.O. q 12 hr for total course of 14 days.	▪ Obtain specimen for culture and sensitivity tests before first dose. ▪ Check expiration date. Outdated or deteriorated tetracyclines have been associated with reversible nephrotoxicity (Fanconi's syndrome). ▪ Administer with milk or food if adverse GI reactions develop. ▪ Don't expose to light or heat. Protect from sunlight during infusion. ▪ Check tongue for signs of fungal infection. Stress good oral hygiene.

dronabinol

Marinol

Cannabinoid

Antiemetic/appetite stimulant

Pregnancy Risk Category: C

Controlled Substance

Schedule: II

Nausea and vomiting associated with cancer chemotherapy — **Adults:** 5 mg/m² P.O. 1 to 3 hr before chemotherapy. Then same dose q 2 to 4 hr after chemotherapy for total of 4 to 6 doses per day. If needed, increase in 2.5-mg/m² increments to maximum 15 mg/m² per dose.

Anorexia and weight loss in patients with AIDS — **Adults:** 2.5 mg P.O. b.i.d. before lunch and dinner. If unable to tolerate, decrease dose to 2.5 mg daily in evening or h.s. May gradually increase to maximum 20 mg/day.

- Principal active substance in *Cannabis sativa* (marijuana); can produce physical and psychological dependence and has high abuse potential.
- CNS effects intensify at higher dosages.
- Effects may persist for days after treatment ends.

droperidol

Inapsine

Dopamine blocker/butyrophenone derivative

Antipsychotic/neuroleptic

Pregnancy Risk Category: C

Premedication — **Adults and children > 12 yr:** 2.5 to 10 mg I.M. 30 to 60 min preoperatively. **Children 2 to 12 yr:** 1 to 1.5 mg per 9 to 11 kg (20 to 25 lb) of body weight I.M. **Adjust-a-dose:** In debilitated patients, the elderly, and those who have received other depressant drugs, use reduced dose.

For induction as adjunct to general anesthesia — **Adults and children > 12 yr:** 2.5 mg per 9 to 11 kg of body weight I.V. For maintenance, 1.25 to 2.5 mg, usually I.V. **Children 2 to 12 yr:** 1 to 1.5 mg per 9 to 11 kg of body weight I.V.

Use without general anesthetic in diagnostic procedures — **Adults and children > 12 yr:** 2.5 to 10 mg I.M. 30 to 60 min before pro-

- Use cautiously in patients with hepatic or renal dysfunction and in breast-feeding patients.
- Use with caution in patients with suspected or diagnosed pheochromocytoma because severe hypertension and tachycardia can occur.
- Have fluids and other measures to manage hypotension readily available.
- Monitor for signs and symptoms of neuroleptic malignant syndrome (fever, altered consciousness, extrapyramidal symptoms, tachycardia).
- Administer I.V. doses slowly.

(continued)

121

†Canadian ‡Australian

DRUG/CLASS/ CATEGORY	INDICATIONS/ DOSAGES	KEY NURSING CONSIDERATIONS
droperidol *(continued)*	cedure. May give additional doses of 1.25 to 2.5 mg, usually I.V. *Adjunct to regional anesthesia when additional sedation required* — **Adults:** 2.5 to 5 mg I.M. or slow I.V.	
econazole nitrate Ecostatin, Spectazole *Synthetic imidazole derivative* *Antifungal* Pregnancy Risk Category: C	*Tinea pedis, tinea cruris, tinea corporis, tinea versicolor; cutaneous candidiasis* — **Adults and children:** Rub into affected areas q.d. for ≥ 2 wk. *Cutaneous candidiasis* — **Adults and children:** Rub into affected areas b.i.d.	▪ Clean affected area before applying. ▪ Don't use occlusive dressings.
efavirenz Sustiva *Nonnucleoside, reverse transcriptase inhibitor* *Antiretroviral* Pregnancy Risk Category: C	*Treatment of HIV-1 infection* — **Adults:** 600 mg P.O. q.d. **Children ≥ 3 yr weighing ≥ 40 kg (88 lb):** 600 mg P.O. q.d. **Children ≥ 3 yr weighing 10 to < 40 kg (22 to < 88 lb):** those weighing 10 to < 15 kg (22 to < 33 lb), 200 mg P.O. q.d.; those weighing 15 to < 20 kg (33 to < 44 lb), 250 mg P.O. q.d.; those weighing 20 to < 25 kg (44 to < 55 lb), 300 mg P.O. q.d.; those weighing 25 to < 32.5 kg (55 to < 72 lb), 350 mg P.O. q.d.; those weighing 32.5 to < 40 kg (72 to < 88 lb), 400 mg P.O. q.d	▪ Use cautiously in patients with hepatic impairment or in those also receiving hepatotoxic drugs. Monitor liver function tests in patients with history of hepatitis B or C and in those also taking ritonavir. ▪ Rule out pregnancy before starting therapy. ▪ Use only with other antiretroviral agents because resistant viruses emerge rapidly when used alone. ▪ Administer at bedtime to decrease CNS adverse effects. ▪ Give with water, juice, milk, or soda. Drug may be given without regard to meals.

- Rash is the most common side effect. Report immediately if rash occurs.

Note: Give above doses with a protease inhibitor or nucleoside analogue reverse transcriptase inhibitors.

enalaprilat
Vasotec I.V.
enalapril maleate
Amprace‡, Renitec‡, Vasotec
ACE inhibitor
Antihypertensive
Pregnancy Risk Category: C
(D in second and third trimesters)

Hypertension — **Adult:** patient not on diuretics: initially 2.5 to 5 mg P.O. q.d., then adjust according to response. Dosage range 10 to 40 mg q.d. as single dose or 2 divided doses. Or, 1.25 mg I.V. infusion q 6 hr over 5 min. Patient on diuretics: initially 2.5 mg P.O. q.d. Or, 0.625 mg I.V. over 5 min; repeat in 1 hr, p.r.n., then 1.25 mg I.V. q 6 hr.
To switch from I.V. to oral therapy —
Adults: initially, 5 mg P.O. q.d.; if patient was receiving 0.625 mg I.V. q 6 hr, then 2.5 mg P.O. q.d. Adjust dosage to response.
To convert from oral to I.V. therapy —
Adults: 1.25 mg I.V. over 5 min q 6 hr.
Adjust-a-dose: In hypertensive patients with renal failure who have creatinine clearance > 30 ml/min, initiate therapy at 2.5 mg P.O. q.d. and gradually adjust.

- Monitor potassium intake and serum potassium level.
- Monitor CBC with differential.
- *I.V. use:* Inject slowly over at least 5 min, or dilute in 50 ml compatible solution and infuse over 15 min.
- Monitor BP response.
- Advise patient to report adverse reactions.
- Advise caution in hot weather and during repositioning or exercise to avoid light-headedness and syncope.

---

enoxaparin sodium
Lovenox
Low-molecular-weight heparin
Anticoagulant
Pregnancy Risk Category: B

To prevent pulmonary embolism and deep vein thrombosis after hip or knee replacement surgery — **Adults:** 30 mg S.C. q 12 hr for 7 to 10 days. Give initial dose between 12 and 24 hr postoperatively if hemostasis established.

- Never administer I.M. Don't massage after S.C. injection. Watch for signs of bleeding. Rotate sites and keep record.
- Don't expel gas bubble from syringe before injection.
- If possible, don't give I.M. injections.

123

DRUG/CLASS/ CATEGORY	INDICATIONS/ DOSAGES	KEY NURSING CONSIDERATIONS
epinephrine (adrenaline) Adrenalin, Bronkaid Mist, Bronkaid Mistometer†, Primatene Mist **epinephrine bitartrate** AsthmaHaler Mist, Bronitin Mist, Bronkaid Suspension Mist, Medihaler-Epi **epinephrine hydrochloride** Adrenalin Chloride, Asthma-Nefrin†, EpiPen, EpiPen Jr., Racepinephrine, Sus-Phrine, Vaponefrin *Adrenergic* *Bronchodilator/vasopressor/cardiac stimulant* Pregnancy Risk Category: C	*Bronchospasm; hypersensitivity reactions; anaphylaxis* — **Adults:** 0.1 to 0.5 ml of 1:1,000 S.C. or I.M. Repeat q 10 to 15 min, p.r.n. Or, 0.1 to 0.25 ml of 1:1,000 I.V. slowly over 5 to 10 min. **Children:** 0.01 ml (10 mcg) of 1:1,000/kg S.C.; repeat q 20 min to 4 hr, p.r.n. Or, 0.004 to 0.005 ml/kg of 1:200 (Sus-Phrine) S.C.; repeat q 8 to 12 hr, p.r.n. *Acute asthmatic attacks* — **Adults and children ≥ 4 yr:** 160 to 250 mcg (metered aerosol), equivalent to 1 inhalation, repeated once if necessary after 1 min; don't give subsequent doses for at least 3 hr. Or, 1% (1:100) solution epinephrine or 2.25% solution racepinephrine by hand-bulb nebulizer as 1 to 3 deep inhalations, repeated q 3 hr, p.r.n. *To restore cardiac rhythm in cardiac arrest* — **Adults:** usual dose 0.5 to 1 mg I.V. May repeat q 3 to 5 min, p.r.n. Higher-dose epinephrine may be used: 3 to 5 mg (about 0.1 mg/kg) repeated q 3 to 5 min. **Children:** usual dose 0.01 mg/kg (0.1 ml/kg 1:10,000 injection) I.V. Usual initial dose through ET tube 0.1 mg/kg (0.1 ml/kg 1:1,000 injection) diluted in 1 to 2 ml 0.45% or 0.9% NaCl solution. Subsequent I.V. or intratra-	• Drug of choice in emergency treatment of acute anaphylactic reactions. • *I.V. use:* Don't mix with alkaline solutions. • When giving I.V., monitor BP, HR, and ECG when therapy starts and frequently thereafter. • Avoid I.M. injection of parenteral suspension into buttocks. Gas gangrene may occur. • Massage site after I.M. injection. • Observe closely for adverse reactions. Notify doctor if these develop. • If > 1 inhalation ordered, tell patient to wait at least 2 min before repeating procedure. • If patient also uses steroid inhaler, instruct to use bronchodilator first, then wait about 5 min before using steroid. • If necessary, teach patient with history of acute hypersensitivity reactions how to self-inject drug at home.

cheal doses 0.1 to 0.2 mg/kg (0.1 to 0.2 ml/kg of 1:1,000 injection). May repeat q 3 to 5 min.

---

epinephrine hydrochloride (ophthalmic)
Epifrin, Glaucon
epinephryl borate
Epinal, Eppy/N
Adrenergic
Topical anesthetic (adjunct)/topical antihemorrhagic/antiglaucoma agent
Pregnancy Risk Category: C

Open-angle glaucoma — **Adults:** 1 or 2 drops 1% or 2% solution q.d. or b.i.d. Adjust dosage according to tonometric readings.

- Can be injected into anterior chamber to produce rapid mydriasis during cataract removal, or can be used to control local bleeding during surgery.
- Don't substitute one salt if another ordered; these salts not interchangeable.
- Monitor BP and other vital signs.
- Apply light finger pressure on lacrimal sac for 1 min after instilling drops. Don't touch dropper tip to eye or surrounding tissues.

---

epinephrine hydro-chloride (topical)
Adrenalin Chloride
Adrenergic
Anesthetic (adjunct)/antihemorrhagic
Pregnancy Risk Category: NR

Nasal congestion; local superficial bleeding — **Adults and children ≥ 6 yr:** instill 1 or 2 drops of solution.

- Instruct patient to use only when needed and not to exceed recommended dosage.

---

epoetin alfa (erythropoietin)
Epogen, Procrit
Glycoprotein
Antianemic
Pregnancy Risk Category: C

Anemia due to reduced production of endogenous erythropoietin caused by end-stage renal disease — **Adults:** dosage individualized. Initially, 50 to 100 U/kg I.V. 3 times/wk. (Can administer S.C. or I.V. in nondialysis patients with chronic renal failure or patients re-

- Monitor BP before therapy. BP may rise, especially when Hct increases in early therapy. Monitor blood count, as ordered. Hct may rise and cause excessive clotting.
- *I.V. use:* Give by direct injection without

(continued)

†Canadian ‡Australian.

DRUG/CLASS/ CATEGORY	INDICATIONS/ DOSAGES	KEY NURSING CONSIDERATIONS
epoetin alfa *(continued)*	ceiving continuous peritoneal dialysis.) Reduce dosage when target Hct reached or if Hct rises > 4 points in any 2-wk period. Increase dosage if Hct doesn't increase by 5 to 6 points after 8 wk of therapy. Maintenance dosage highly individualized. *Adjunctive treatment of HIV-infected patients with anemia secondary to zidovudine therapy* — **Adults:** 100 U/kg I.V. or S.C. 3 times/wk for 8 wk or until target Hgb level reached. If response unsatisfactory after 8 wk, may increase dose by 50 to 100 U/kg I.V. or S.C. 3 times/wk. After 4 to 8 wk, may increase dosage further in increments of 50 to 100 U/kg 3 times/wk, to maximum 300 U/kg I.V. or S.C. 3 times/wk. *Anemia secondary to cancer chemotherapy* — **Adults:** 150 U/kg S.C. 3 times/wk for 8 wk or until target Hgb level reached.	dilution. Solution contains no preservatives. Discard unused portion. Don't mix with other drugs. • When used in HIV-infected patients, be prepared to individualize dosage based on response. Dosage recommendations are for patients with endogenous erythropoietin levels ≤ 500 U/L and cumulative zidovudine doses of ≤ 4.2 g/wk. • Give iron supplementation starting no later than when treatment starts and continuing throughout therapy. • Response depends on amount of endogenous erythropoietin in plasma. Patients with ≥ 500 U/L usually have transfusion-dependent anemia and probably won't respond. Those with levels < 500 U/L usually respond well.
eptifibatide Integrilin *Cyclic heptapeptide Platelet aggregation inhibitor* Pregnancy Risk Category: B	*Treatment of patients with acute coronary syndrome (unstable angina or non-Q-wave MI), including patients to be managed medically and those undergoing percutaneous coronary intervention* — **Adults:** I.V. bolus of 180 mcg/kg (up to maximum dose of 22.6 mg) as soon as possible following di-	• Drug intended for use with heparin and aspirin. • If patient is to undergo CABG surgery, stop infusion before surgery. • Minimize use of arterial and venous punctures, I.M. injections, urinary catheters, nasotracheal tubes, and nasogastric tubes,

and avoid use of noncompressible I.V. sites (such as subclavian or jugular veins).
- If patient's platelet count < 100,000/mm³, discontinue eptifibatide and heparin.
- *I.V. use:* May give drug in same I.V. line as alteplase, atropine, dobutamine, heparin, lidocaine, meperidine, metoprolol, midazolam, morphine, nitroglycerin, verapamil, 0.9% NaCl, and D_5W and 0.9% NaCl; line may also contain up to 60 mEq/L of potassium chloride.
- Withdraw bolus dose from 10-ml vial into syringe and administer by I.V. push over 1 to 2 min. Administer I.V. infusion undiluted directly from 100-ml vial using infusion pump.

agnosis, followed by continuous I.V. infusion of 2 mcg/kg/min (up to maximum infusion rate of 15 mg/hr) for up to 72 hr. Infusion rate may be decreased to 0.5 mcg/kg/min during percutaneous coronary intervention. Infusion should then be continued for additional 20 to 24 hr after procedure for up to 96 hr of therapy.

Treatment of patients not presenting with acute coronary syndrome who are undergoing percutaneous coronary intervention — **Adults:** I.V. bolus of 135 mcg/kg administered immediately before procedure, followed by continuous infusion of 0.5 mcg/kg/min for 20 to 24 hr.

---

ergotamine tartrate

Ergotrate Mono‡, Ergomar, Ergostat, Gynergen†, Medihaler Ergotamine

Ergot alkaloid
Vasoconstrictor
Pregnancy Risk Category: X

Vascular or migraine headache — **Adults:** initially, 2 mg P.O. or S.L., then 1 to 2 mg P.O. q hr or S.L. q ½ hr, to maximum 6 mg q.d. and 10 mg weekly. Or, aerosol inhaler: 1 spray (360 mcg) initially, repeated q 5 min, p.r.n., to maximum of 6 sprays (2.16 mg)/24 hr or 15 sprays (5.4 mg)/wk.

- Most effective when used during prodromal stage of headache or as soon as possible after onset.
- Obtain dietary history to determine if condition associated with certain foods.
- Be alert for ergotamine rebound.
- With long-term use, instruct patient to check for and report coldness in extremities or tingling in fingers and toes.

---

erythromycin

Akne-Mycin, Erycette, EryDerm, Ergel, Ery-Sol Erythromycin

Inflammatory acne vulgaris — **Adults and children:** apply in thin film to affected areas b.i.d.

- Wash, rinse, and dry affected areas before application.

(continued)

†Canadian ‡Australian.

127

DRUG / CLASS / CATEGORY	INDICATIONS / DOSAGES	KEY NURSING CONSIDERATIONS
erythromycin *(continued)* *Topical antibiotic* Pregnancy Risk Category: C		▪ Prolonged use may be necessary when treating acne vulgaris; may result in overgrowth of nonsusceptible organisms.
erythromycin (ophthalmic) Ilotycin Ophthalmic Ointment *Erythromycin* *Ophthalmic antibiotic* Pregnancy Risk Category: NR	*Acute and chronic conjunctivitis, trachoma, other eye infections* — **Adults and children:** 1-cm length applied directly to infected eye up to six times q.d. *Prophylaxis of ophthalmia neonatorum due to N. gonorrhoeae or C. trachomatis* — **Neonates:** ribbon of ointment about 1 cm long applied in lower conjunctival sac of each eye shortly after birth.	▪ For prophylaxis of ophthalmia neonatorum, apply ≤1 hr after birth. Used in neonates born either by vaginal delivery or cesarean section. Gently massage eyelids for 1 min to spread ointment. ▪ For use only when sensitivity studies show drug effective against infecting organisms. ▪ Store at room temperature in tightly closed, light-resistant container.
erythromycin base E-Mycin, Eramycin, Eryc, Robimycin **erythromycin estolate** Ilosone **erythromycin ethylsuccinate** EryPed, EryPed 200 **erythromycin lactobionate**	*Acute pelvic inflammatory disease caused by N. gonorrhoeae* — **Adults:** 500 mg I.V. (or lactobionate) q 6 hr for 3 days, then 250 mg (base, estolate, stearate) or 400 mg ethylsuccinate) P.O. q 6 hr for 7 days. *Mild to moderate severe respiratory tract, skin, soft-tissue infections* — **Adults:** 250 to 500 mg (base, estolate, stearate) P.O. q 6 hr; or 400 to 800 mg (ethylsuccinate) P.O. q 6 hr; or 15 to 20 mg/kg I.V. q.d. (lactobionate) continuous infusion or divided doses q 6 hr for 10 days. **Children:** 30 to 50 mg/kg (oral	▪ Obtain urine specimen for culture and sensitivity tests before first dose. ▪ Monitor hepatic function. ▪ When giving suspension, note concentration. ▪ **I.V. use:** Reconstitute according to directions; dilute each 250 mg in at least 100 ml 0.9% NaCl solution. Infuse over 1 hr. Don't give erythromycin lactobionate with other drugs. ▪ Monitor for superinfection. ▪ For best absorption, instruct patient to

Erythrocin
erythromycin stearate
Erythrocin Stearate
Erythromycin
Antibiotic
Pregnancy Risk Category: B

erythromycin salts) P.O. q.d., divided doses q 6 hr; or 15 to 20 mg/kg I.V. q.d., divided doses q 4 to 6 hr for 10 days.

take oral form with full glass of water 1 hr before or 2 hr after meals. May take with food if GI upset occurs. Coated tablets may be taken with meals. Caution not to drink fruit juice with drug and not to swallow chewable tablets whole.

- Instruct patient to report adverse reactions.

---

esmolol hydrochloride
Brevibloc
Beta$_1$-adrenergic blocker
Antiarrhythmic
Pregnancy Risk Category: C

Supraventricular tachycardia; to control ventricular rate in atrial fibrillation or flutter in perioperative, postoperative, or other emergent circumstances; noncompensatory sinus tachycardia when HR requires specific interventions — **Adults:** loading dose: 500 mcg/kg/min by I.V. infusion over 1 min, then 4-min maintenance infusion of 50 mcg/kg/min. If no adequate response in 5 min, repeat loading dose and follow with maintenance infusion of 100 mcg/kg/min for 4 min. Repeat loading dose and increase maintenance infusion by 50-mcg/kg/min increments. Maximum maintenance infusion for tachycardia 200 mcg/kg/min.
Perioperative, postoperative tachycardia or hypertension — **Adults:** perioperative treatment of tachycardia or hypertension: 80 mg (about 1 mg/kg) I.V. bolus over 30 sec; then 150 mcg/kg/min I.V. infusion, p.r.n. Adjust rate, p.r.n., to maximum 300 mcg/kg/min.

- *I.V. use:* Don't give by I.V. push; use infusion control device. May use 10-mg/ml single-dose vials without diluting, but always dilute injection concentrate (250 mg/ml) to maximum concentration of 10 mg/ml before infusion. Remove 20 ml from 500 ml of D$_5$W, lactated Ringer's solution, or 0.45% or 0.9% NaCl solution, and add two ampules esmolol (final concentration 10 mg/ml).
- Solutions incompatible with diazepam, furosemide, sodium bicarbonate, and thiopental sodium.
- Monitor ECG and BP continuously during infusion; hypotension possible.
- Hypotension usually can be reversed within 30 min by decreasing dose or, if necessary, stopping infusion. Notify doctor.
- Instruct patient to report adverse reactions promptly.

129

†Canadian ‡Australian.

DRUG / CLASS / CATEGORY	INDICATIONS / DOSAGES	KEY NURSING CONSIDERATIONS
estazolam ProSom *Benzodiazepine Hypnotic* Pregnancy Risk Category: X Controlled Substance Schedule: IV	*Insomnia* — **Adults:** 1 mg P.O. h.s. Some patients may require 2 mg. **Elderly:** 1 mg P.O. h.s. Use higher doses with extreme care.	• Avoid prolonged administration. • Monitor liver and renal functions and CBC. • Patient should avoid activities that require mental alertness or physical coordination. • Warn patient that alcohol can cause additive depressant effects.
esterified estrogens Estratab, Menest, Neo-Estrone† Estrone† *Estrogen Estrogen replacement/anti-neoplastic* Pregnancy Risk Category: X	*Inoperable prostate cancer* — **Men:** 1.25 to 2.5 mg P.O. t.i.d. *Breast cancer* — **Men and postmenopausal women:** 10 mg P.O. t.i.d. for 3 or more mo. *Female hypogonadism* — **Women:** 2.5 to 7.5 mg q.d. in divided doses in cycles of 20 days on, 10 days off. *Female castration; primary ovarian failure* — **Women:** 1.25 mg q.d. in cycles of 3 wk on, 1 wk off. Adjust for symptoms.	• Discontinue at least 1 mo before procedures associated with prolonged immobilization or thromboembolism. • Warn patient to immediately report adverse reactions. • Tell diabetic patient to report elevated blood glucose. • Teach patient how to perform routine breast self-exam.
estradiol (oestradiol) Climara, Estrace, Estraderm **estradiol cypionate** depGynogen, Depo-Estradiol, E-Cypionate, Estrofem **estradiol valerate (oestradiol valerate)**	*Vasomotor menopause symptoms; female hypogonadism; female castration; primary ovarian failure* — **Adults:** 1 to 2 mg P.O. q.d. in cycles of 21 days on and 7 days off, or cycles of 5 days on and 2 days off, or 1 transdermal system (Estraderm) delivering 0.05 mg/24 hr, or as system (Climara) delivering either 0.05 mg/	• Ensure that patient undergoes physical exam before and during therapy. • Ask patient about allergies, especially to foods or plants. • Never give I.V. • Apply transdermal patch to clean, dry, hairless, intact skin on abdomen or but-

Climara Patch, Delestrogen, Dioval, Estradiol L.A., Estra-L 20, Estra-L 40, Femogex, Gynogen L.A., Menaval-20, Primogyn Depot‡

Estrogen

Estrogen replacement/antineoplastic

Pregnancy Risk Category: X

24 hr or 0.1 mg/24 hr and applied q wk in cycles of 3 wk on and 1 wk off. Or, 1 to 5 mg (cypionate) I.M. q 3 to 4 wk, or 10 to 20 mg (valerate) I.M. q 4 wk, p.r.n.

Palliative treatment of advanced, inoperable breast cancer — **Men and postmenopausal women:** 10 mg P.O. (estradiol) t.i.d. for 3 mo.

Palliative treatment of advanced inoperable prostate cancer — **Men:** 30 mg I.M. (val.) q 1 to 2 wk, or 1 to 2 mg P.O. (estradiol) t.i.d.

tocks. Don't apply to areas where clothing can loosen patch.
- Rotate application sites.
- Warn patient to immediately report adverse reactions.
- Tell diabetic patient to report elevated blood glucose.

---

estradiol/morethin-drone acetate transdermal system

CombiPatch

Estrogen

Estrogen replacement/antineoplastic

Pregnancy Risk Category: X

Moderate-to-severe vasomotor menopausal symptoms, vulvar and vaginal atrophy, hypoestrogenemia caused by hypogonadism, castration, or primary ovarian failure in women with intact uterus — **Adults:** *Continuous combined regimen:* 9-cm² patch worn continuously on lower abdomen. Remove old system and apply new system twice weekly during 28-day cycle. May increase to 16-cm² patch. *Continuous sequential regimen:* apply as sequential regimen in combination with estradiol transdermal system (such as Alora, Esclim, Estra-derm, Vivelle). 0.05-mg estradiol transdermal patch worn for first 14 days of 28-day cycle; replace system twice weekly. For rest of 28-day cycle, replace 9-cm² patch system to lower abdomen. May increase to 16-cm² patch, p.r.n.

- Use cautiously in patients with impaired liver function, asthma, epilepsy, migraine, and cardiac or renal dysfunction. Also use cautiously in breast-feeding patients.
- Women not currently receiving continuous estrogen or estrogen/progestin therapy may start therapy at any time.
- Women receiving continuous hormone replacement therapy should complete current cycle of therapy before beginning estradiol therapy. First day of withdrawal bleeding is appropriate time to initiate therapy.
- Apply patch system to smooth (fold-free), clean, dry, nonirritated area of skin on lower abdomen, avoiding the waistline. Rotate application sites with an interval of at least 1 wk between applications to same site.
- Monitor patient's BP regularly.

131

DRUG/CLASS/ CATEGORY	INDICATIONS/ DOSAGES	KEY NURSING CONSIDERATIONS
estrogens, conjugated (estrogenic substances, conjugated; oestrogens, conjugated) C.E.S.†, Premarin, Premarin Intravenous *Estrogen Estrogen replacement/antineoplastic/antiosteoporotic* Pregnancy Risk Category: X	*Abnormal uterine bleeding (hormonal imbalance)* — **Women:** 25 mg I.V. or I.M., repeated in 6 to 12 hr, p.r.n. *Female castration; primary ovarian failure* — **Women:** 1.25 mg P.O. q.d. in cycles of 3 wk on and 1 wk off. *Osteoporosis* — **Postmenopausal women:** 0.625 mg P.O. q.d. in cyclic regimen (3 wk on, 1 wk off).	• *I.V. use:* When giving by direct injection, administer slowly to avoid flushing reaction. • When giving I.M., inject deeply into large muscle. Rotate injection sites to prevent muscle atrophy. • Warn patient to immediately report adverse reactions. • Tell diabetic patient to report elevated blood glucose so that antidiabetic medication dosage can be adjusted.
estropipate (piperazine estrone sulfate) Ogen, OrthoEST *Estrogen Estrogen replacement* Pregnancy Risk Category: X	*Primary ovarian failure; female castration; female hypogonadism* — **Women:** 1.25 to 7.5 mg P.O. q.d. for first 3 wk, followed by rest period of 8 to 10 days. If bleeding doesn't occur by end of rest period, repeat cycle. *Vasomotor menopausal symptoms* — **Women:** 0.625 mg to 5 mg P.O. q.d. in cyclic method of 3 wk on, 1 wk off. *Prevention of osteoporosis* — **Women:** 0.625 mg P.O. q.d. for 25 days of 31-day cycle.	• Ensure that patient undergoes thorough physical exam before therapy starts. Patients on long-term therapy should have exams yearly. Periodically monitor serum lipid levels, BP, weight, and hepatic function. • Warn patient to immediately report adverse reactions. • Teach patient how to perform routine breast self-exams.
etanercept Enbrel *Fusion protein Antineoplastic*	*Reduction of signs and symptoms of moderately to severely active rheumatoid arthritis in patients with inadequate response to one or more disease-modifying antirheu-*	• Don't give live vaccines during therapy. • Reconstitute aseptically with 1 ml of supplied sterile bacteriostatic water for injection, USP (0.9% benzyl alcohol). Inject

Pregnancy Risk Category: B	matic drugs in combination with methotrexate or in patients who do not respond adequately to methotrexate alone — **Adults:** 25 mg S.C. twice weekly.

ethacrynate sodium Edecrin Sodium **ethacrynic acid** Edecrin *Loop diuretic* *Diuretic* Pregnancy Risk Category: B	*Acute pulmonary edema* — **Adults:** 50 mg or 0.5 to 1 mg/kg I.V. Usually only 1 dose necessary, though second dose may be required. *Edema* — **Adults:** 50 to 200 mg P.O. daily. Refractory cases may require up to 200 mg b.i.d. **Children:** initial dose 25 mg P.O., increased cautiously in 25-mg increments q.d. until desired effect achieved.	diluent slowly into vial. Do not filter reconstituted solution. ▪ Injection sites should be at least 1 inch apart. Rotate sites regularly. ▪ *I.V. use:* Reconstitute vacuum vial with 50 ml D_5W or 0.9% NaCl. Give slowly through tubing of running infusion over several min. ▪ Don't give S.C. or I.M. ▪ If dose > 1 I.V. necessary, use new injection site to avoid thrombophlebitis. ▪ Monitor I&O, weight, BP, serum electrolytes, and blood uric acid levels. ▪ Watch for signs of hypokalemia.

ethambutol hydrochloride Etibit, Myambutol *Semisynthetic antituberculotic* *Antituberculotic* Pregnancy Risk Category: C	*Adjunctive treatment in pulmonary TB* — **Adults and children > 13 yr:** initial treatment for patients who haven't received previous antitubercular therapy, 15 mg/kg P.O. as single dose q.d. **Retreatment:** 25 mg/kg P.O. q.d. as single dose for 60 days (or until bacteriologic smears and cultures become negative) with at least one other antitubercular; then decrease to 15 mg/kg/day as single dose.	▪ Obtain AST and ALT levels before therapy and monitor levels q 3 to 4 wk. ▪ Always administer with other antituberculotics to prevent development of resistant organisms. ▪ Tell patient to report adverse effects, especially blurred vision, red-green color blindness, or changes in urinary elimination. ▪ Reassure that visual disturbances should disappear few wk to mo after drug stopped.

ethinyl estradiol (ethinyloestradiol)	*Palliative treatment of metastatic breast cancer (at least 5 yr after menopause)* — **Women:** 1 mg P.O. t.i.d. for at least 3 mo.	▪ Warn patient to immediately report adverse reactions. *(continued)*

†Canadian ‡Australian.

DRUG/CLASS/ CATEGORY	INDICATIONS/ DOSAGES	KEY NURSING CONSIDERATIONS
ethinyl estradiol *(continued)* Estinyl Estrogen Estrogen replacement/anti-neoplastic Pregnancy Risk Category: X	*Female hypogonadism —* **Women:** 0.05 mg P.O. q.d. to t.i.d. 2 wk each mo, followed by 2 wk of progesterone therapy; continued for 3 to 6 mo dosing cycles, followed by 2 mo off. *Vasomotor menopausal symptoms —* **Women:** 0.02 to 0.05 mg P.O. q.d. for cycles of 3 wk on and 1 wk off. *Palliative treatment of metastatic inoperable prostate cancer —* **Men:** 0.15 to 2 mg P.O. q.d.	▪ Tell diabetic patient to report elevated blood glucose. ▪ Explain to patient on cyclic therapy for postmenopausal symptoms that, although withdrawal bleeding may occur during wk off drug, fertility isn't restored. ▪ Teach women how to perform breast self-exams.
ethinyl estradiol *monophasic:* w/desogestrel — Desogen; w/ethynodiol diacetate — Demulen 1/35, w/levonorgestrel — Nordette; w/norethindrone — Genora 1/35; w/norethindrone acetate — Loestrin 21 1/20; w/norgestimate — Ortho-Cyclen; w/norgestrel — Ovral; w/norethindrone acetate and ferrous fumarate — Loestrin Fe 1/20; *biphasic:* w/norethindrone — Jenest-28; *triphasic:* w/levonorgestrel — Triphasil; w/norethin-	*Contraception —* **Adults:** *Monophasic oral contraceptives —* 1 tablet P.O. q.d., starting on day 5 of menstrual cycle. With 20- and 21-tablet pkg, new dosing cycle begins 7 days after last tablet taken. With 28-tablet pkg, dose is 1 tablet q.d. without interruption. *Biphasic oral contraceptives —* 1 color tablet P.O. q.d. for 10 days; then next color tablet for 11 days. With 21-tablet package, new dosing cycle begins 7 days after last tablet taken. With 28-tablet package, dose is 1 tab q.d. without interruption. *Triphasic oral contraceptives —* 1 tablet P.O. q.d. in sequence specified by brand. With 21-tablet package, new dosing cycle begins 7 days after last tablet taken. With 28-tablet	▪ Triphasic contraceptives may cause fewer adverse reactions, such as breakthrough bleeding and spotting. ▪ Monitor serum lipid levels, BP, weight, and hepatic function. ▪ Oral contraceptives affect many lab tests. ▪ Monitor blood glucose. ▪ Warn patient to immediately report adverse reactions. ▪ Advise patient of increased risks associated with simultaneous use of cigarettes and oral contraceptives. ▪ Instruct patient to take tablets at same time each day; nighttime dosing may reduce nausea and headaches. ▪ Advise patient to use additional method of birth control, such as condoms or di-

drone — Ortho-Novum
7/7/7; w/norgestimate —
Ortho Tri-Cyclen
mestranol
monophasic: w/norethin-
drone — Genora 1/50
Estrogen and progestin
Oral contraceptive
Pregnancy Risk Category: X

package, dose is 1 tablet q.d. without inter-
ruption.
Acne vulgaris — **Adults:** 1 tablet P.O. q.d.,
using the 28-tablet package of Ortho Tri-
Cyclen. Dosage schedule for acne should
follow same guidelines for Ortho Tri-Cyclen
as when used as an oral contraceptive.

- Stress importance of Papanicolaou tests
  and annual gynecologic exams.

---

etidronate disodium
Didronel
Pyrophosphate analogue
Antihypercalcemic
Pregnancy Risk Category: C

*Symptomatic Paget's disease of bone (os-
teitis deformans) —* **Adults:** 5 to 10 mg/kg
P.O. q.d. (no > 6 mo) or 11 to 20 mg/kg P.O.
q.d. (no > 3 mo) in single dose 2 hr before
meal with water or juice.
*Heterotopic ossification after total hip re-
placement —* **Adults:** 20 mg/kg P.O. q.d. for
1 mo before total hip replacement and for
3 mo afterward.
Malignancy-associated hypercalcemia —
Adults: 7.5 mg/kg I.V. q.d. for 3 consecutive
days; period of ≥ 7 days should elapse between courses of I.V. therapy. Maintenance
dosage 20 mg/kg P.O. q.d. for 30 days, initiated day after last I.V. dosage. May use for
maximum of 90 days.

- **I.V. use:** Dilute daily dose in ≥ 250 ml
  0.9% NaCl solution or D_5W and infuse
  over ≥ 2 hr.
- Don't give with food, milk, or antacids;
  may reduce absorption.
- Some patients may receive I.V. drug for up
  to 7 days. Risk of hypokalemia increases
  after 3 days.
- Monitor renal function before and during
  therapy, as ordered.
- To orthotic effect, review serum alkaline
  phosphatase and urinary hydroxyproline
  excretion. Serum phosphate may rise, especially in patients receiving higher doses.
  Phosphate level usually returns to normal
  2 to 4 wk after drug discontinued.

---

etodolac
Lodine

Acute and chronic management of pain —
Adults: 200 to 400 mg P.O. q 6 to 8 hr,
p.r.n., not to exceed 1,200 mg q.d. For pa-

- Can lead to reversible renal impairment.
- To minimize GI discomfort, instruct patient
  to take with milk or meals.

(continued)

135

†Canadian   ‡Australian.

DRUG/CLASS/ CATEGORY	INDICATIONS/ DOSAGES	KEY NURSING CONSIDERATIONS
etodolac (continued) Nonsteroidal antiinflammatory Antarthritic Pregnancy Risk Category: C	tients ≤ 60 kg (132 lb), total daily dose shouldn't exceed 20 mg/kg.	▪ Teach patient about signs and symptoms of GI bleeding; tell him to contact doctor immediately if any occurs. ▪ Advise patient to avoid alcohol and aspirin.
etoposide (VP-16) VePesid **etoposide phosphate** Etopophos Podophyllotoxin (cell cycle-phase specific, G_2 and late S phase) Antineoplastic Pregnancy Risk Category: D	*Testicular cancer* — **Adults:** 50 to 100 mg/m² I.V. on 5 consecutive days q 3 to 4 wk; or 100 mg/m² on days 1, 3, and 5 q 3 to 4 wk. *Small-cell carcinoma of lung* — **Adults:** 35 mg/m²/day I.V. for 4 days; or 50 mg/m²/day I.V. for 5 days. Oral dose: twice I.V. dose, rounded to nearest 50 mg. **Adjust-a-dose:** In patients with creatinine clearance 15 to 50 ml/min, give 75% initial recommended dose; in those with creatinine clearance < 15 ml/min, consider further dose reduction.	▪ Monitor BP q 15 min. If systolic pressure < 90, stop infusion and notify doctor. ▪ Have emergency drugs and equipment available in case of anaphylaxis. ▪ **I.V. use:** Give etoposide by slow I.V. infusion (over ≥ 30 min) to prevent severe hypotension. May give etoposide phosphate over 5 to 210 min. Don't administer etoposide through membrane-type in-line filter. ▪ Dilute etoposide for infusion in either D_5W or 0.9% NaCl solution to concentration of 0.2 or 0.4 mg/ml. May give etoposide phosphate without further dilution, or may dilute to concentration as low as 0.1 mg/ml in either D_5W or 0.9% NaCl.
famciclovir Famvir Synthetic acyclic guanine derivative	*Acute herpes zoster infection (shingles)* — **Adults:** 500 mg P.O. q 8 hr for 7 days. *Recurrent episodes of genital herpes* — **Adults:** 125 mg P.O. b.i.d. for 5 days. Start	▪ May take without regard to meals. ▪ Inform patient that drug won't cure genital herpes but can decrease symptom length

Antiviral
Pregnancy Risk Category: B

and severity.
- Teach patient how to prevent spread of herpes infection.
- Urge patient to report early symptoms.

as soon as symptoms occur.
Adjust-a-dose: Dose reduction required in patients with renal failure.

---

famotidine
Pepcid, Pepcid AC, Pepcidine‡
H₂-receptor antagonist
Antiulcer agent
Pregnancy Risk Category: B

Duodenal ulcer (short-term treatment) —
Adults: acute therapy: 40 mg P.O. h.s. or 20 mg P.O. b.i.d. Maintenance: 20 mg P.O. q.d. h.s.
Benign gastric ulcer (short-term) —
Adults: 40 mg P.O. q.d. h.s. for 8 wk.
Gastroesophageal reflux disease (GERD) —
Adults: 20 mg P.O. b.i.d. up to 6 wk. For esophagitis caused by GERD, 20 to 40 mg b.i.d. up to 12 wk.
Prevention or treatment of heartburn —
Adults: 10 mg (Pepcid AC only) P.O. 1 hr before meals (prevention) or 10 mg (Pepcid AC only) P.O. with water for symptoms. Maximum 20 mg daily. Don't take daily for > 2 wk.
Hospitalized patients with intractable ulcerations or hypersecretory conditions or those who cannot take oral medication — **Adults:** 20 mg I.V. q 12 hr.

- ***I.V. use:*** To prepare injection, dilute 2 ml (20 mg) with compatible I.V. solution to total volume of 5 or 10 ml; inject over at least 2 min. Or, give by intermittent I.V. infusion. Dilute 20 mg (2 ml) in 100 ml compatible solution and infuse over 15 to 30 min. Stable for 48 hr at room temperature after dilution.
- Prescription drug most effective taken h.s.
- With doctor's knowledge, allow patient to take antacids concomitantly, especially at start of therapy when pain severe.
- Urge patient to avoid cigarette smoking.

---

felodipine
Agon SR‡, Plendil, Plendil ER‡, Renedil†
Calcium channel blocker

Hypertension — **Adults:** initially, 5 mg P.O. q.d. Adjust according to patient response, generally at intervals not less than 2 wk. Usual dose 5 to 10 mg q.d.; maximum: 20 mg q.d. **Elderly > 65 yr:** initially, 2.5 mg P.O.

- Monitor BP for response.
- Monitor for peripheral edema.
- Tell patient to swallow tablets whole and not to crush or chew them.

(continued)

137

†Canadian †Australian.

DRUG / CLASS / CATEGORY	INDICATIONS / DOSAGES	KEY NURSING CONSIDERATIONS
felodipine (continued) Antihypertensive Pregnancy Risk Category: C	q.d. Maximum: 10 mg q.d. *Adjust-a-dose:* In patient with impaired hepatic function, give 2.5 mg P.O. q.d.	• Tell patient to continue taking even when he feels better and to check with doctor or pharmacist before taking other drugs, including OTC drugs.
fenofibrate (micronized) Tricor Fibric acid derivative Antihyperlipidemic Pregnancy Risk Category: C	Adjunct to diet for treatment of patients with very high serum triglyceride levels (types IV and V hyperlipidemia) who are at risk of pancreatitis and who don't respond adequately to determined dietary effort— **Adults:** initially, 67 mg P.O. q.d. Dose may be increased following repeat serum triglyceride estimations at 4- to 8-week intervals to maximum dose of three capsules q.d. (201 mg). *Adjust-a-dose:* Minimize dose in patients with severe renal impairment. Initiate therapy at a dose of 67 mg/day and increase only after effects on renal function and triglyceride levels have been evaluated at this dose. No modification is needed for patients with moderate renal impairment.	• Obtain baseline lipid levels and liver function tests before starting therapy. Perform periodic monitoring of liver function during therapy. Discontinue therapy if enzyme levels persist > three times normal limit. • Monitor for symptoms of pancreatitis, myositis, rhabdomyolysis, cholelithiasis, and renal failure. Be alert for occurrence of myalgia, muscle tenderness, or weakness, especially in the presence of malaise or fever. • Beta blockers, estrogens, and thiazide diuretics may increase plasma triglyceride levels; continued use of these agents should be evaluated.
fenoldopam mesylate Corlopam	Short-term (up to 48 hr) hospital management of severe hypertension when rapid but quickly reversible reduction of blood pressure is indicated, including malignant hyper-	• Drug causes dose-related tachycardia. • Drug contains sodium metabisulfite, which may cause allergic-type reactions.

Dopamine receptor agonist
Antihypertensive
Pregnancy Risk Category: B

tension with deteriorating end-organ function — **Adults:** initiate infusion rates at 0.025 to 0.3 mcg/kg/min and titrate upward or downward to achieve desired BP no more frequently than q 15 min. Recommended increments for titration are 0.05 to 0.1 mcg/kg/min.

- Monitor serum electrolytes and watch for hypokalemia.
- **I.V. use:** Administer by continuous I.V. infusion using infusion pump. Don't use bolus dose. Check BP and HR q 15 min until patient is stable.

fenoprofen calcium

Nalfon, Nalfon 200

Nonsteroidal anti-inflammatory
Nonnarcotic
Pregnancy Risk Category: NR

Rheumatoid arthritis; osteoarthritis — **Adults:** 300 to 600 mg P.O. t.i.d. to q.i.d. Maximum 3.2 g q.d.

Mild to moderate pain — **Adults:** 200 mg P.O. q 4 to 6 hr, p.r.n.

Fever — **Adults:** single P.O. doses up to 400 mg.

- May lead to reversible renal impairment.
- Inform patient that full therapeutic effect for arthritis may take 2 to 4 wk.
- Instruct patient to take 30 min before or 2 hr after meals. If adverse GI reactions occur, may be taken with milk or meals.
- Tell patient to contact doctor immediately if GI bleeding occurs.
- Warn patient to avoid alcohol and aspirin.

fentanyl citrate

Sublimaze

fentanyl transdermal system

Duragesic

fentanyl transmucosal

Fentanyl Oralet

Opioid agonist
Analgesic/adjunct to anesthesia/anesthetic
Pregnancy Risk Category: C

Preoperative — **Adults:** 50 to 100 mcg I.M. 30 to 60 min before surgery. Or, 5 mcg/kg as oralet unit, 20 to 40 min before need.

Adjunct to general anesthetic — **Adults:** low-dose general anesthetic, 2 mcg/kg I.V. Moderate-dose therapy, 2 to 20 mcg/kg I.V.; then 25 to 100 mcg I.V., p.r.n. High-dose therapy, 20 to 50 mcg/kg I.V.; then 25 mcg to half of initial loading dose I.V., p.r.n.

Adjunct to regional anesthesia — **Adults:** 50 to 100 mcg I.M. or I.V. over 1 to 2 min, p.r.n.

Induction and maintenance of anesthesia —

- Monitor circulatory and respiratory status and urinary function carefully.
- Keep narcotic antagonist and resuscitation equipment available when giving I.V.
- Give before onset of intense pain.
- Periodically monitor postoperative vital signs and bladder function.
- Remove foil overwrap of oralet just before administration. Have patient place oralet in mouth and suck (not chew or swallow) it.
- Remove oralet unit using handle after it's
(continued)

†Canadian ‡Australian

139

DRUG / CLASS / CATEGORY	INDICATIONS / DOSAGES	KEY NURSING CONSIDERATIONS
fentanyl *(continued)* Controlled Substance Schedule: II	**Children 2 to 12 yr:** 2 to 3 mcg/kg I.V. *Postoperative —* **Adults:** 50 to 100 mcg I.M. q 1 to 2 hr, p.r.n. *Management of chronic pain —* **Adults:** 1 transdermal system applied to upper torso skin area not irritated or irradiated. Start with 25-mcg/hr system; adjust dosage as needed and tolerated. May wear system for 72 hr; some may need applied q 48 hr.	consumed, patient shows adequate effect, or patient shows signs of respiratory depression. Place any remaining portion in plastic overwrap and dispose as appropriate for Schedule II drugs or flush in toilet. • Transdermal form not recommended for postoperative pain.
ferrous fumarate Femiron, Feostat, Fumasorb, Fumerin, Novofumar† *Oral iron supplement* *Hematinic* Pregnancy Risk Category: A	*Iron deficiency —* **Adults:** 50 to 100 mg elemental iron P.O. t.i.d. **Children:** 4 to 6 mg/kg/day of elemental iron P.O. in 3 divided doses.	• GI upset may be related to dose. Between-meal doses preferable, but can be given with some foods. • Check for constipation. • Oral iron may turn stools black. • Monitor Hgb, Hct, and reticulocyte count.
ferrous gluconate Fergon, Simron *Oral iron supplement* *Hematinic* Pregnancy Risk Category: A	*Iron deficiency —* **Adults:** 50 to 100 mg elemental iron P.O. t.i.d. **Children:** 4 to 6 mg/ kg/ day elemental iron P.O. in 3 divided doses.	• GI upset may be dose-related. Between-meal doses preferable, but can be given with some foods. • Check for constipation. • May turn stools black. • Monitor Hgb, Hct, and reticulocyte count.
ferrous sulfate Apo-Ferrous Sulfate†, Feosol, Mol-Iron	*Iron deficiency —* **Adults:** 50 to 100 mg elemental iron P.O. t.i.d. **Children:** 4 to 6	• GI upset may be related to dose. Between-meal doses preferable, but can be given with some foods. Enteric-coated products

ferrous sulfate, dried
Feosol
Oral iron supplement
Hematinic
Pregnancy Risk Category: A

mg/kg/day elemental iron P.O. in 3 divided doses.

- reduce GI upset but decrease amount of iron absorbed.
- Oral iron may turn stools black. Although harmless, could mask melena.
- Monitor Hgb, Hct, and reticulocyte count, as ordered.

fexofenadine
Allegra
H_1-receptor antagonist
Antihistaminic
Pregnancy Risk Category: C

Seasonal allergic rhinitis — **Adults and children ≥ 12 yr:** 60 mg P.O. b.i.d.
Adjust-a-dose: In patients with impaired renal function or those on dialysis, give 60 mg P.O. q.d.

- Use with caution in breast-feeding women.
- Caution patient not to perform hazardous activities if drowsiness occurs.
- Instruct patient not to exceed prescribed dosage and to take only when needed.

filgrastim (granulocyte colony-stimulating factor; G-CSF)
Neupogen
Biologic response modifier
Colony-stimulating factor
Pregnancy Risk Category: C

To decrease incidence of infection in patients with nonmyeloid malignant disease receiving myelosuppressive antineoplastic agents —
Adults and children: 5 mcg/kg/day I.V. or S.C. as 1 dose given ≥ 24 hr after cytotoxic chemotherapy. May increase by 5 mcg/kg for each chemotherapy cycle depending on duration and severity of nadir of absolute neutrophil count.

To decrease incidence of infection in patients with nonmyeloid malignant disease receiving myelosuppressive antineoplastic agents followed by bone marrow transplantation —
Adults and children: 10 mcg/kg/day I.V. or S.C. ≥ 24 hr after cytotoxic chemotherapy and bone marrow infusion. Adjust dosage according to neutrophil response.

- Obtain baseline CBC and platelet count before therapy, then twice weekly during therapy, as ordered.
- **I.V. use:** Dilute in 50 to 100 ml D_5W and give by intermittent infusion over 15 to 60 min or continuous infusion over 24 hr. If final concentration will be 2 to 15 mcg/ml, add albumin at concentration of 2 mg/ml (0.2%).
- Once dose withdrawn, don't reenter vial. Discard unused portion. Vials are for single-dose use and contain no preservatives.
- Refrigerate at 36° to 46° F (2° to 8° C). Don't freeze; avoid shaking. Store at room temperature up to 6 hr; discard after 6 hr.

(continued)

141

DRUG / CLASS / CATEGORY	INDICATIONS / DOSAGES	KEY NURSING CONSIDERATIONS
filgrastim *(continued)*	*Congenital neutropenia* — **Adults:** 6 mcg/kg S.C. b.i.d. Dosage adjusted to response.	• Transiently increased neutrophil count common 1 or 2 days after therapy starts. Give daily for up to 2 wk or until ANC returns to 10,000/mm³ after expected chemotherapy-induced neutrophil nadir.
finasteride Propecia, Proscar *Steroid (synthetic 4-azasteroid) derivative Androgen synthesis inhibitor* Pregnancy Risk Category: X	*Symptomatic BPH* — **Adults:** 5 mg (Proscar) P.O. q.d. *Treatment of male pattern hair loss in men only* — **Adults:** 1 mg (Propecia) P.O. q.d.	• Monitor patients with large residual urine volume or severely diminished urine flow. May not be candidates for drug. • Evaluate sustained increases in serum prostate-specific antigen; could signal non-compliance.
flecainide acetate Tambocor *Benzamide derivative local anesthetic Ventricular antiarrhythmic* Pregnancy Risk Category: C	*PSVT, paroxysmal atrial fibrillation, flutter in patients without structural heart disease; life-threatening ventricular arrhythmias* — **Adults:** For PSVT, 50 mg P.O. q 12 hr. May increase in increments of 50 mg b.i.d. q 4 days until efficacy achieved. Maximum 300 mg/day. For life-threatening ventricular arrhythmias, 100 mg P.O. b.i.d. Increase in increments of 50 mg b.i.d. q 4 days until efficacy achieved. Maximum 400 mg q.d. ***Adjust-a-dose:*** In renally impaired patients, give 100 mg P.O. q 12 hr, with dose adjustments made at intervals > 4 days.	• Monitor renally impaired patients for adverse cardiac effects and toxicity. • Stress importance of taking drug exactly as prescribed. • Instruct patient to report adverse reactions promptly and to limit fluid and sodium intake.

fluconazole
Diflucan
Bis-triazole derivative
Antifungal
Pregnancy Risk Category: C

Oropharyngeal and esophageal candidiasis — **Adults:** 200 mg P.O. or I.V. on 1st day, then 100 mg q.d. Continue for at least 2 wk after symptoms resolve. **Children:** 6 mg/kg on 1st day, then 3 mg/kg for at least 2 wk.
Vaginal candidiasis — **Adults:** 150 mg P.O. as single dose.
Systemic candidiasis — **Adults:** up to 400 mg P.O. or I.V. q.d. Continue for at least 2 wk after symptoms resolve.
Cryptococcal meningitis — **Adults:** 400 mg P.O. or I.V. on 1st day, then 200 mg q.d. Continue 10 to 12 wk after CSF cultures negative.
Adjust-a-dose: In patients with creatinine clearance < 50 ml/min, reduce dosage.

- *I.V. use:* Give by continuous infusion no faster than 200 mg/hr. Use infusion pump. To prevent air embolism. Don't connect in series with other infusions. Don't add other drugs to solution.
- Periodically monitor liver function during prolonged therapy, as ordered.
- If mild rash occurs, monitor closely. If lesions progress, stop drug and notify doctor.
- Incidence of adverse reactions greater in patients with HIV.

flucytosine (5-FC, 5-fluorocytosine)
Ancobon, Ancotil†
Fluorinated pyrimidine
Antifungal
Pregnancy Risk Category: C

Severe fungal infections caused by susceptible strains of Candida *and* Cryptococcus — **Adults > 50 kg (110 lb):** 50 to 150 mg/kg q.d. P.O. q 6 hr. **Adults < 50 kg:** 1.5 to 4.5 g/m²/day P.O. in 4 divided doses.
Adjust-a-dose: In patients with renal impairment, increase dosing intervals to q 12 to 48 hr, depending on creatinine clearance.

- Obtain hematologic tests and renal and liver function studies, as ordered.
- Give capsules over 15 min to reduce adverse GI reactions.
- Monitor fluid I&O; report marked change.
- Instruct patient to report adverse reactions promptly.
- Inform patient that therapeutic response may take weeks or months.

fludrocortisone acetate
Florinef

Adrenal insufficiency (partial replacement); salt-losing adrenogenital syndrome — **Adults:** 0.1 to 0.2 mg P.O. q.d. Decrease to 0.05 mg q.d. if transient hypertension oc-

- Used with cortisone or hydrocortisone in adrenal insufficiency.
- Monitor BP and serum electrolytes.

(continued)

143

†Canadian ‡Australian

flumazenil 144

DRUG / CLASS / CATEGORY	INDICATIONS / DOSAGES	KEY NURSING CONSIDERATIONS
fludrocortisone acetate *(continued)* *Mineralocorticoid/glucocorticoid* *Mineralocorticoid replacement therapy* Pregnancy Risk Category: C	curs. **Children:** 0.05 to 0.1 mg P.O. q.d. *Orthostatic hypotension in diabetic patients; orthostatic hypotension —* **Adults:** 0.1 to 0.4 mg P.O. q.d.	• Weigh patient daily; report sudden gain. • Unless contraindicated, give low-sodium diet that's high in potassium and protein. • Tell patient to report worsening symptoms, such as hypotension, weakness, cramping, and palpitations.
flumazenil Romazicon *Benzodiazepine antagonist* *Antidote* Pregnancy Risk Category: C	*Complete or partial reversal of sedative effects of benzodiazepines after anesthesia or short diagnostic procedures (conscious sedation) —* **Adults:** 0.2 mg I.V. over 15 sec. If patient doesn't reach desired level of consciousness after 45 sec, repeat at 1-min intervals until total dose of 1 mg given (initial dose plus 4 additional doses), p.r.n. Most patients respond after 0.6 to 1 mg. In case of resedation, may repeat after 20 min; however, don't give > 1 mg at one time and not > 3 mg/hr. *Suspected benzodiazepine overdose —* **Adults:** 0.2 mg I.V. over 30 sec. If desired level of consciousness not reached after 30 sec, 0.3 mg given over 30 sec. If poor response, 0.5 mg given over 30 sec; repeat 0.5-mg doses, p.r.n., at 1-min intervals until	• *I.V. use:* Administer by direct injection or dilute with compatible solution. Discard unused drug that has been drawn into syringe or diluted within 24 hr. • Administer into I.V. line in large vein with free-flowing I.V. solution to minimize pain at injection site. Compatible solutions include D₅W, lactated Ringer's for injection, and 0.9% NaCl. • Monitor patient closely for possible resedation after reversal of benzodiazepine effects (flumazenil's duration of action shorter than that of all benzodiazepines). Duration of monitoring depends on which drug being reversed. Monitor closely after long-acting benzodiazepines or after high doses of short-acting benzodiazepines. Severe resedation unlikely in patients

total dose of 3 mg given. Most patients respond to total doses between 1 and 3 mg; rarely, patients who respond partially after 3 mg may require additional doses, up to 5 mg total. If no response in 5 min after receiving 5 mg, sedation unlikely to be caused by benzodiazepines. In case of resedation, may repeat dose after 20 min; however, don't give > 1 mg at one time and not > 3 mg/hr.

showing no signs of resedation 2 hr after 1-mg flumazenil.
- Tell patient to avoid alcohol, CNS depressants, and OTC drugs for 24 hr.
- Know that patient won't recall information given in postprocedure period; drug doesn't reverse amnesic effects of benzodiazepines.

---

flunisolide
AeroBid, AeroBid-M,
Nasalide (nasal inhalant)
Glucocorticoid
Anti-inflammatory/
antiasthmatic
Pregnancy Risk Category: C

Persistent asthma — **Adults:** 2 inhalations (500 mcg) b.i.d. Maximum total 2,000 mcg q.d. (8 inhalations/day). **Children 6 to 15 yr:** 2 inhalations (500 mcg) b.i.d. Don't exceed 4 inhalations/day.
Seasonal or perennial rhinitis: **Adults:** 2 sprays (50 mcg) in each nostril b.i.d. If needed, increase to 2 sprays in each nostril t.i.d. **Children 6 to 14 yr:** 1 spray in each nostril t.i.d. or 2 sprays in each nostril b.i.d.

- Warn patient that drug won't relieve emergency asthma attacks.
- If patient is using a bronchodilator, teach to use several min before flunisolide.
- Instruct patient to wait 1 min before repeating inhalation and to hold breath several seconds to enhance drug action.
- Withdraw slowly, as ordered, in patients who've received long-term oral corticosteroids.

---

fluocinonide
Lidemol†, Lidex, Lidex-E,
Topsyn
Topical adrenocorticoid
Anti-inflammatory
Pregnancy Risk Category: C

Inflammation associated with corticosteroid-responsive dermatoses — **Adults and children:** clean area; apply cream, gel, ointment, or topical solution sparingly b.i.d. or q.i.d.

- Gently wash skin before applying. Rub in gently, leaving thin coat. When treating hairy sites, part hair and apply directly to lesion. Don't apply near eyes, mucous membranes, or in ear canal.
- Notify doctor if skin infection, striae, atrophy, or fever develops.

(continued)

145

DRUG / CLASS / CATEGORY	INDICATIONS / DOSAGES	KEY NURSING CONSIDERATIONS
fluocinonide *(continued)*		- Systemic absorption likely with use of occlusive dressings, prolonged treatment, or extensive body-surface treatment. Watch for symptoms. - Continue treatment for several days after lesions clear, as ordered.
fluorouracil (5-fluorouracil, 5-FU) Adrucil, Efudex, Fluoroplex *Antimetabolite (cell cycle-phase specific, S phase)* *Antineoplastic* Pregnancy Risk Category: D (injection), X (topical)	*Colon, rectal, breast, stomach, pancreatic cancers* — **Adults:** 12 mg/kg I.V. q.d. for 4 days; if no toxicity, 6 mg/kg on days 6, 8, 10, and 12; then single weekly maintenance dose of 10 to 15 mg/kg I.V. begun after toxicity from first course subsides. Maximum single dose 800 mg/day. *Palliative treatment of advanced colorectal cancer* — **Adults:** 425 mg/m² I.V. q.d. for 5 days. Give with 20 mg/m² leucovorin I.V. Repeat at 4-wk intervals for 2 additional courses; repeat at intervals of 4 to 5 wk if tolerated. *Multiple actinic (solar) keratoses; superficial basal cell carcinoma* — **Adults:** Apply cream or topical solution b.i.d. Usual duration of treatment 2 to 6 wk.	- Toxicity may be delayed for 1 to 3 wk. - Use plastic I.V. containers to give continuous infusions. Don't refrigerate. Protect from sunlight. - Monitor CBC and platelet counts. Watch for ecchymoses, petechiae, easy bruising, and anemia. Monitor I&O, and renal and hepatic function tests. - Ingestion and systemic absorption of topical form may cause serious adverse reactions. Application to large ulcerated areas may cause systemic toxicity. - Watch for stomatitis or diarrhea. Discontinue and notify doctor if diarrhea occurs. - Encourage diligent oral hygiene to prevent superinfection of denuded mucosa.
fluoxetine hydrochloride Prozac, Prozac 20‡	*Depression; obsessive-compulsive disorder* — **Adults:** initially, 20 mg P.O. in morning; increase dosage according to re-	- Warn patient to avoid hazardous activities until CNS effects known.

Selective serotonin reuptake inhibitor
Antidepressant
Pregnancy Risk Category: B

sponse. May give b.i.d. in morning and at noon. Gradually increase, as needed and tolerated, to 60 to 80 mg q.d.

Treatment of binge-eating and vomiting behavior in moderate to severe bulimia nervosa — **Adults:** 60 mg/day P.O. in morning.

- Tell patient to consult doctor before taking other medications and to avoid alcohol.
- Tell patient not to take in afternoon because of possible nervousness and insomnia.
- Tell patient to promptly report rash or hives, anxiety or nervousness, anorexia, or suspicion of pregnancy.

---

fluoxymesterone
Android-F, Halotestin
Androgen
Androgen replacement/ antineoplastic
Pregnancy Risk Category: X
Controlled Substance
Schedule: III

Hypogonadism caused by testicular deficiency — **Adults:** 5 to 20 mg P.O. q.d. in single dose or in 3 or 4 divided doses.

Delayed puberty — **Males:** 2.5 to 20 mg q.d.

Palliation of breast cancer in women — **Adults:** 10 to 40 mg P.O. q.d. in 3 or 4 divided doses. All dosages individualized and reduced to minimum when effect noted.

- Instruct patient to take with food or meals if GI upset occurs.
- Tell women to report menstrual irregularities or irregular bleeding and to stop drug.
- Urge female patient to report androgenic effects immediately.
- Watch for hypoglycemia in diabetic patients; check blood glucose.
- If liver function results abnormal, notify doctor; therapy should be stopped.

---

fluphenazine decanoate
Modecate†‡, Prolixin Decanoate
fluphenazine enanthate
Prolixin Enanthate
fluphenazine hydrochloride
Moditen HCl†, Permitil Concentrate, Prolixin, Prolixin

Psychotic disorders — **Adults:** initially, 0.5 to 10 mg (hydrochloride) P.O. q.d. in divided doses q 6 to 8 hr; may increase cautiously to 20 mg. Maintenance: 1 to 5 mg P.O. q.d. For I.M. doses, give ⅓ to ½ of oral doses. Usual I.M. dose 1.25 mg. Use doses above 10 mg/day with caution. Use lower doses for elderly patients (1 to 2.5 mg q.d.). Or, 12.5 to 25 mg of long-acting esters (decanoate or enanthate) I.M. or S.C. q 1 to 6 wk; maintenance: 25 to 100 mg, p.r.n.

- Watch for neuroleptic malignant syndrome.
- Monitor therapy with bilirubin tests, CBC and liver function, and periodic renal function and ophthalmic tests, as ordered.
- Check dosage order carefully.
- Dilute liquid concentrate with water, fruit juice, milk, or semisolid food.
- Oral liquid and parenteral forms can cause contact dermatitis.
- Withhold dose and notify doctor if patient

(continued)

147

DRUG/CLASS/ CATEGORY	INDICATIONS/ DOSAGES	KEY NURSING CONSIDERATIONS
fluphenazine *(continued)* Concentrate *Phenothiazine* *Antipsychotic* Pregnancy Risk Category: NR		• develops blood dyscrasia or persistent extrapyramidal reactions. • Warn patient to avoid hazardous activities until CNS effects known. • Instruct patient to relieve dry mouth with sugarless gum or hard candy. • Tell patient of possible urine discoloration.
flurazepam hydrochloride Apo-Flurazepam†, Dalmane, Novoflupam *Benzodiazepine* *Sedative-hypnotic* Pregnancy Risk Category: X Controlled Substance Schedule: IV	*Insomnia* — **Adults:** 15 to 30 mg P.O. h.s. **Elderly > age 65:** 15 mg P.O. h.s.	• Check hepatic and renal function and CBC during long-term therapy. • Assess mental status before initiating. • Encourage patient to keep taking even if insomnia occurs on first night. • Instruct patient to avoid alcohol use. • Caution patient not to perform activities that require alertness or physical coordination. • Prevent hoarding or self-overdosing.
flurbiprofen Ansaid, Apo-Flurbiprofen†, Froben†, Froben SR† *Nonsteroidal anti-inflammatory/phenylalkanoic acid derivative* *Antiarthritic* Pregnancy Risk Category: B	*Rheumatoid arthritis; osteoarthritis* — **Adults:** 200 to 300 mg P.O. q.d., divided b.i.d., t.i.d., or q.i.d. Where available, patients maintained on 200 mg q.d. may switch to one 200-mg extended-release capsule P.O. q.d., taken in evening after food. **Elderly:** may require a lower dose.	• Tell patient to take with food, milk, or antacid if GI upset occurs. • Teach patient signs and symptoms of GI bleeding and tell him to contact doctor immediately if they occur. • Advise patient to avoid alcohol and aspirin. • Tell patient taking extended-release capsules to swallow them whole.

flurbiprofen sodium Ocufen Liquifilm *Nonsteroidal anti-inflammatory* *Ophthalmic anti-inflammatory/antimiotic* Pregnancy Risk Category: C	*Inhibition of intraoperative miosis* — **Adults:** 1 drop instilled into affected eye approximately q ½ hr, beginning 2 hr before surgery. Total of 4 drops given.	• Wound healing may be delayed. • Alert doctor immediately if visual acuity decreases or visual field diminishes.
flutamide Euflex†, Eulexin *Nonsteroidal antiandrogen* *Antineoplastic* Pregnancy Risk Category: D	*Metastatic prostate cancer (stage B₂, C, D₂) in combination with lutenizing hormone-releasing hormone analogues such as leuprolide acetate* — **Adults:** 250 mg P.O. q 8 hr.	• Monitor liver function tests and CBC periodically, as ordered. • Must be taken continuously with agent used for medical castration (such as leuprolide acetate) for full benefit of therapy.
fluticasone propionate (inhalation) Flixotide†, Flovent Inhalation Aerosol, Flovent Rotadisk *Corticosteroid* *Anti-inflammatory* Pregnancy Risk Category: C	*Maintenance treatment of asthma as prophylactic therapy and for patients requiring oral corticosteroid treatment for chronic asthma* — *Flovent Inhalation Aerosol:* **Adults and children ≥ 12 yr:** in those previously taking bronchodilators alone, initially, inhaled dose of 88 mcg b.i.d. to maximum of 440 mcg b.i.d. **Patients previously taking inhaled corticosteroids:** initially, inhaled dose of 88 to 220 mcg b.i.d. to maximum of 440 mcg b.i.d. **Patients previously taking oral corticosteroids:** inhaled dose of 880 mcg b.i.d. *Flovent Rotadisk:* **Adults and adolescents:** in patients previously taking bronchodilators alone, initially, inhaled dose	• Bronchospasm may occur with an immediate increase in wheezing after dosing. If bronchospasm occurs following dosing with fluticasone inhalation aerosol, treat immediately with a fast-acting inhaled bronchodilator. • Because of risk of systemic absorption of inhaled corticosteroids, observe for evidence of systemic corticosteroid effects. • Monitor patient, especially postoperatively or during periods of stress, for evidence of inadequate adrenal response. • During withdrawal from oral corticosteroids, patients may experience symptoms *(continued)*

149

†Canadian ‡Australian

DRUG / CLASS / CATEGORY	INDICATIONS / DOSAGES	KEY NURSING CONSIDERATIONS
fluticasone propionate (inhalation) *(continued)* Cutivate *Corticosteroid* *Topical anti-inflammatory* Pregnancy Risk Category: C	of 100 mcg b.i.d. to maximum of 500 mcg b.i.d. **Patients previously taking inhaled corticosteroids:** initially, inhaled dose of 100 to 250 mcg b.i.d. to maximum of 500 mcg b.i.d. **Patients previously taking oral corticosteroids:** inhaled dose of 1,000 mcg b.i.d. **Children 4 to 11 yr:** for patients previously on bronchodilators alone or on inhaled corticosteroids, initially, inhaled dose of 50 mcg b.i.d. to maximum of 100 mcg b.i.d.	of systemically active corticosteroid withdrawal (joint or muscular pain, lassitude, and depression) despite maintenance or even improvement of respiratory function. ■ For patients starting therapy who are also receiving oral corticosteroids, reduce dose of prednisone to no more than 2.5 mg/day on weekly basis, beginning after at least 1 wk of therapy with fluticasone. ■ Not intended for the relief of acute bronchospasm.
fluticasone propionate (topical) Cutivate *Corticosteroid* *Topical anti-inflammatory* Pregnancy Risk Category: C	*Inflammatory and pruritic manifestations associated with corticosteroid-responsive dermatoses* — **Adults:** apply sparingly to affected area b.i.d.; rub in gently and completely.	■ Don't mix with other bases or vehicles; may affect potency. ■ One-time coverage of adult body requires 12 to 26 g. Don't use > 50 g weekly. ■ Discontinue, as ordered, if local irritation or systemic infection, absorption, or hypersensitivity occurs.
fluticasone propionate (nasal) Flonase *Corticosteroid* *Topical anti-inflammatory* Pregnancy Risk Category: C	*Seasonal and perennial allergic rhinitis* — **Adults:** initially, 2 sprays (50 mcg each spray) in each nostril q.d. Or, 1 spray in each nostril b.i.d. After several days, may reduce dose to 1 spray in each nostril q.d. Maximum daily dose 2 sprays in each nostril. **Children ≥ 12 yr:** initially, 1 spray (50 mcg) in each nostril	■ Don't use after recent nasal septal ulcers, nasal surgery, or nasal trauma until healing occurs. ■ Monitor for signs of immediate hypersensitivity reactions or contact dermatitis after intranasal administration. ■ Drug effectiveness depends on regular use.

- Tell patient to notify doctor if exposed to chickenpox or measles.

---

q.d. If no response or symptoms severe, increase to 2 sprays in each nostril. Depending on response, may decrease dose to 1 spray in each nostril q.d. Maximum daily dose 2 sprays in each nostril.

fluvastatin sodium
Lescol
Hydroxymethylglutaryl-coenzyme A (HMG-CoA) reductase inhibitor
Cholesterol-lowering agent/antilipemic
Pregnancy Risk Category: X

Reduction of LDL and total cholesterol levels in patients with primary hypercholesterolemia (types IIa and IIb) — **Adults:** initially, 20 mg P.O. h.s. Increase to maximum 40 mg q.d., p.r.n.

- Initiate only after diet and other nonpharmacologic measures fail.
- Obtain liver function test results when therapy starts and periodically thereafter.
- Watch for signs of myositis.
- Teach patient about proper dietary management, weight control, and exercise.
- Tell patient to avoid alcohol and that drug contraindicated during pregnancy.

fluvoxamine maleate
Luvox
Selective serotonin reuptake inhibitor
Anticompulsive agent
Pregnancy Risk Category: C

Obsessive-compulsive disorder — **Adults:** initially, 50 mg P.O. q.d. h.s., increased in 50-mg increments q 4 to 7 days until maximum benefit achieved. Maximum 300 mg q.d. Give total daily doses of more than 100 mg in 2 divided doses.

- Record mood changes. Watch for suicidal tendencies; provide minimal drug supply.
- Warn patient not to engage in hazardous activities until CNS effects known.
- Tell patient to notify doctor if allergic reaction occurs.
- Advise patient not to discontinue until directed by doctor.

folic acid
Folvite, Novofolacid†
Folic acid derivative
Vitamin supplement
Pregnancy Risk Category: NR

Recommended daily allowance (RDA) — **Birth to 3 yr:** 25 to 50 mcg. **Children 4 to 6 yr:** 75 mcg. **Children 7 to 10 yr:** 100 mcg. **Adolescent and adult men:** 150 to 200 mcg. **Adolescent and adult women:** 150 to

- Don't mix with other medications in same syringe when giving I.M.
- Patients with small-bowel resections and

(continued)

†Canadian ‡Australian

DRUG / CLASS / CATEGORY	INDICATIONS / DOSAGES	KEY NURSING CONSIDERATIONS
folic acid *(continued)*	180 mcg. **Pregnant women:** 400 mcg. **Breast-feeding women:** 260 to 280 mcg. *Megaloblastic or macrocytic anemia secondary to folic acid or other nutritional deficiency, hepatic disease, alcoholism, intestinal obstruction, excessive hemolysis —* **Adults and children > 4 yr:** 0.4 mg to 1 mg P.O., S.C., or I.M. q.d. After correction of anemia secondary to folic acid deficiency, proper diet and RDA supplements necessary to prevent recurrence. **Children < 4 yr:** up to 0.3 mg P.O., S.C., or I.M. q.d. **Pregnant and breast-feeding women:** 0.8 mg P.O., S.C., or I.M. q.d. *Prevention of megaloblastic anemia during pregnancy to prevent fetal damage —* **Adults:** up to 1 mg P.O., S.C., or I.M. q.d. throughout pregnancy.	▪ intestinal malabsorption may require parenteral administration. ▪ Protect from light and heat; store at room temperature. ▪ Monitor CBC to measure drug effectiveness. ▪ Patients undergoing renal dialysis are at risk for folate deficiency. ▪ Many drugs, such as oral contraceptives and alcohol, can cause folate deficiencies. Teach patient about dietary sources of folic acid, such as yeast, whole grains, leafy vegetables, beans, nuts, and fruit. ▪ Inform patient that overcooking and canning destroy folate. ▪ Tell patient to take only under medical supervision.
fomivirsen sodium Vitravene *Human CMV inhibitor* *Antiviral (ophthalmic)* Pregnancy Risk Category: C	*Local treatment of CMV retinitis in patients with AIDS who are intolerant of or have a contraindication to other treatment or who were insufficiently responsive to previous treatment —* **Adults:** induction dose 330 mcg (0.05 ml) by intravitreal injection every other wk for two doses. Subsequent maintenance	▪ For use by intravitreal injection only. ▪ Provides localized therapy limited to treated eye. Monitor patient for extraocular CMV disease or disease in other eye. ▪ Know that ocular inflammation (uveitis) is more common during induction dosing.

	dose 330 mcg (0.05 ml) by intravitreal injection once q 4 wk after induction.	• Monitor light perception and optic nerve head perfusion postinjection. • Monitor for increased IOP.

foscarnet sodium (phosphonoformic acid)
Foscavir
Pyrophosphate analogue
Antiviral
Pregnancy Risk Category: C

CMV retinitis in patients with AIDS — **Adults:** initially, 60 mg/kg I.V. as induction treatment in patients with normal renal function. Give I.V. over 1 hr q 8 hr for 2 to 3 wk, depending on clinical response. Follow with maintenance infusion of 90 to 120 mg/kg q.d., given over 2 hr.
Mucocutaneous acyclovir-resistant herpes simplex virus infection — **Adults:** 40 mg/kg I.V. Give I.V. infusion over 1 hr q 8 to 12 hr for 2 to 3 wk.
Adjust-a-dose: Reduce dosage in renally impaired patients.

• *I.V. use:* Use infusion pump. To minimize renal toxicity, ensure adequate hydration before and during infusion.
• Can alter serum electrolytes; monitor levels. Assess for tetany and seizures associated with abnormal electrolyte levels.
• Monitor Hgb and Hct.
• Advise patient to report perioral tingling, numbness in extremities, and paresthesia.
• Instruct patient to alert nurse if discomfort occurs at I.V. insertion site.

fosinopril sodium
Monopril
ACE inhibitor
Antihypertensive
Pregnancy Risk Category: C (D in second and third trimesters)

Hypertension — **Adults:** initially, 10 mg P.O. q.d. Adjusted based on BP response at peak and trough levels. Usual dose 20 to 40 mg, up to 80 mg q.d. May be divided.
Heart failure — **Adults:** initially, 10 mg P.O. q.d. Increase over several wk to maximum 40 mg P.O. q.d.

• Monitor potassium intake and serum potassium level.
• Monitor CBC with differential.
• Monitor BP for effect.
• Advise patient to report signs or symptoms of infection.
• Instruct patient to use caution in hot weather and during exercise.

fosphenytoin sodium
Cerebyx
Hydantoin derivative

Status epilepticus — **Adults:** 15 to 20 mg phenytoin sodium equivalent (PE)/kg I.V. at 100 to 150 mg PE/min as loading dose; then 4 to 6 mg PE/kg/day I.V. as maintenance

• Always prescribe and dispense in PE units. Don't adjust recommended doses

(continued)

†Canadian ‡Australian

153

DRUG/CLASS/CATEGORY	INDICATIONS/DOSAGES	KEY NURSING CONSIDERATIONS
fosphenytoin sodium *(continued)* Anticonvulsant Pregnancy Risk Category: D	dose. (Phenytoin may be used instead of fosphenytoin as maintenance, using appropriate dose.) *Prevention and treatment of seizures during neurosurgery* — **Adults:** loading dose 10 to 20 mg PE/kg I.M. or I.V. at infusion rate not exceeding 150 mg PE/kg/day I.V. Maintenance dose: 4 to 6 mg PE/kg/day I.V. *Short-term substitution for oral phenytoin* — **Adult:** same total daily dose equivalent as oral phenytoin sodium therapy as single daily dose I.M. or I.V. at infusion rate not exceeding 150 mg PE/min. May require more frequent dosing.	• when substituting fosphenytoin for phenytoin, and vice versa. • Before I.V. infusion, dilute in 5% dextrose or 0.9% NaCl solution to concentration ranging from 1.5 to 25 mg PE/ml. • Monitor ECG, BP, and respirations. • Severe CV complications most common in elderly or gravely ill patients. • If rash appears, discontinue and notify doctor. • Abrupt withdrawal may trigger status epilepticus. • Warn patient that sensory disturbances may occur with I.V. use.
furosemide (frusemide‡) Apo-Furosemide†, Lasix, Myrosemide, Novosemide†, Urex‡ Loop diuretic Diuretic/antihypertensive Pregnancy Risk Category: C	*Acute pulmonary edema* — **Adults:** 40 mg I.V. injected slowly over 1 to 2 min; then 80 mg I.V. in 1 to 1½ hr, if needed. *Edema* — **Adults:** 20 to 80 mg P.O. q.d. in morning, second dose in 6 to 8 hr; carefully titrate up to 600 mg q.d., if needed. Or 20 to 40 mg I.M. or I.V., increased by 20 mg q 2 hr until desired response achieved. Give I.V. dose slowly over 1 to 2 min. **Infants and children:** 2 mg/kg P.O. q.d., increased by 1 to 2 mg/kg in 6 to 8 hr, if needed; carefully titrate to 6 mg/kg q.d., if needed.	• *I.V. use:* Give by direct injection over 1 to 2 min. Or, dilute with D₅W, 0.9% NaCl, or lactated Ringer's solution, and infuse no faster than 4 mg/min to avoid ototoxicity. Use prepared infusion solution within 24 hr. • Monitor weight, BP, and HR routinely. • If oliguria or azotemia develops or worsens, may need to discontinue. • Monitor I&O, and serum electrolyte, BUN, blood uric acid, and carbon dioxide levels frequently.

- May be poorly absorbed P.O. in severe heart failure. May need to be given I.V. even if patient receiving other oral medications.

Hypertension — **Adults:** 40 mg P.O. b.i.d. Adjust dosage according to response.	

gabapentin Neurontin *1-aminomethyl cyclohexon-acetic acid* *Anticonvulsant* Pregnancy Risk Category: C	*Adjunctive treatment of partial seizures with and without secondary generalization in adults with epilepsy* — **Adults:** initially, 300 mg P.O. h.s. on day 1; 300 mg P.O. b.i.d. on day 2; then 300 mg P.O. t.i.d. on day 3. Increase, as needed and tolerated, to 1,800 mg q.d. in 3 divided doses. Doses up to 3,600 mg q.d. have been well tolerated. **Adjust-a-dose:** In patients with renal failure, adjust dose based on creatinine clearance.	■ Give first dose at bedtime to minimize drowsiness, dizziness, fatigue, and ataxia. ■ Discontinue or substitute alternative drug gradually, over at least 1 wk, as ordered. ■ Don't suddenly withdraw other anticonvulsants. ■ Warn patient to avoid driving and operating heavy machinery until CNS effects known.

ganciclovir Cytovene *Synthetic nucleoside* *Antiviral* Pregnancy Risk Category: C	*CMV retinitis in immunocompromised patients, including those with AIDS and normal renal function* — **Adults:** induction: 5 mg/kg I.V. q 12 hr for 14 to 21 days; maintenance: 5 mg/kg I.V. q.d. for 7 days each wk, or 6 mg/kg q.d. for 5 days each wk. Or, 1,000 mg P.O. t.i.d. with food; or 500 mg P.O. q 3 hr while awake (6 times q.d.). Adjust dosage for impaired renal function based on creatinine clearance. *Prevention of CMV disease in advanced HIV infection and normal renal function* — **Adults:** 1,000 mg P.O. t.i.d. with food. *Prevention of CMV disease in transplant recipients with normal renal function —*	■ **I.V. use:** Give infusion at constant rate over at least 1 hr. Too-rapid infusions cause increased toxicity. Use infusion pump. Don't give as bolus. ■ Solution alkaline; use caution when preparing. ■ Don't administer S.C. or I.M. ■ Obtain neutrophil and platelet counts every 2 days during twice-daily dosing and at least weekly thereafter. ■ Explain importance of adequate hydration during therapy. ■ Instruct patient to report adverse reactions promptly.

(continued)

†Canadian ‡Australian

DRUG/CLASS/ CATEGORY	INDICATIONS/ DOSAGES	KEY NURSING CONSIDERATIONS
ganciclovir *(continued)*	**Adults:** 5 mg/kg I.V. q 12 hr for 7 to 14 days, then 5 mg/kg q.d. for 7 days each wk, or 6 mg/kg q.d. for 5 days each wk. ***Adjust-a-dose:*** Dosage adjustment necessary for patients with creatinine clearance < 70 ml/min. See package insert for very specific dosage adjustments.	
gemcitabine hydrochloride Gemzar *Nucleoside analogue (cell cycle–phase specific, S and G_1 phase)* *Antineoplastic* Pregnancy Risk Category: D	*Locally advanced or metastatic adenocarcinoma of pancreas and patients treated previously with fluorouracil —* **Adults:** 1,000 mg/m² I.V. over 30 min q wk ≤ 7 wk, unless toxicity. Monitor patients before each dose with CBC (including differential) and platelet count. If bone marrow suppression, adjust therapy. Give full dose if absolute granulocyte count (AGC) ≥ 1,000/mm³ and platelet count ≥ 100,000/mm³. If AGC 500/mm³ to 999/mm³ or platelet count 50,000/mm³ to 9,999/mm³, give 75% of dose. Withhold dose if AGC < 500/mm³ or platelet count < 50,000/mm³. Follow treatment course of 7 wk with 1 wk rest. Subsequent dosage cycles consist of 1 infusion q wk for 3 of 4 consecutive wk. Base dosage adjustments for subsequent cycles on AGC and platelet count nadirs and degree of nonhematologic toxicity.	• Obtain baseline and periodic renal and hepatic lab tests, as ordered. • **I.V. use:** Reconstitution at concentration > 40 mg/ml not recommended. May further dilute resulting concentration with 0.9% NaCl injection, to as low as 0.1 mg/ml, if needed. Solution should be clear to light straw-colored and free from particulates. Stable for 24 hr at room temperature. Don't refrigerate reconstituted drug. • Prolonging infusion time beyond 60 min or giving drug more frequently than once weekly may increase toxicity. • Careful hematologic monitoring, especially of neutrophil and platelet counts, required. Monitor closely. Expect dosage modification according to toxicity and degree of myelosuppression. Age, gender, and renal impairment may predispose to toxicity.

- Instruct patient to take ½ hr before breakfast and dinner.
- Teach patient proper dietary management of serum lipids.
- Advise patient to avoid hazardous activities until CNS effects known.
- Tell patient to report signs of bile duct obstruction.

gemfibrozil
Lopid
Fibric acid derivative
Antilipemic
Pregnancy Risk Category: C

Types IV and V hyperlipidemia unresponsive to diet and other drugs; reduction of CAD risk in patients with type IIb hyperlipidemia who can't tolerate or are refractory to bile acid sequestrants or niacin — **Adults:** 1,200 mg P.O. q.d. in 2 divided doses, 30 min before morning and evening meals.

gentamicin sulfate (systemic)
Cidomycin†, Garamycin, Gentamicin Sulfate ADD-Vantage, Jenamicin
Aminoglycoside
Antibiotic
Pregnancy Risk Category: NR

Serious infections caused by susceptible organisms — **Adults:** 3 mg/kg q.d. in divided doses I.M. or I.V. infusion q 8 hr. For life-threatening infections, up to 5 mg/kg q.d. in 3 to 4 divided doses; reduce to 3 mg/kg q.d. as soon as indicated. **Children:** 6 to 7.5 mg/kg q.d. in divided doses q 8 hr I.M. or by I.V. infusion. **Neonates > 1 wk or infants:** 7.5 mg/kg q.d. in divided doses q 8 hr.
Meningitis — **Adults:** systemic therapy as above; or 4 to 8 mg intrathecally q.d. **Children and infants > 3 mo:** systemic therapy as above; or 1 to 2 mg intrathecally q.d.
Endocarditis prophylaxis for GI or GU procedure or surgery — **Adults:** 1.5 mg/kg I.M. or I.V. 30 min before procedure or surgery. Maximum 80 mg. **Children:** 2 mg/kg I.M. or I.V. 30 min before procedure or surgery. Maximum 80 mg. After 8 hr, give half of initial dose.

- Evaluate hearing before and during therapy. Notify doctor of tinnitus, vertigo, or hearing loss.
- **I.V. use:** For intermittent I.V. infusion, dilute with 50 to 200 ml D_5W or 0.9% NaCl injection and infuse over 30 min to 2 hr. After infusion, flush line with 0.9% NaCl or D_5W.
- Obtain blood for peak drug level 1 hr after I.M. injection and 30 min to 1 hr after I.V. infusion; for trough levels, draw blood just before next dose. Don't collect blood in heparinized tube.
- Monitor renal function (output, specific gravity, urinalysis, BUN, creatinine, and creatinine clearance). Notify doctor of signs of decreasing renal function.
- Drug given with ampicillin (vancomycin in penicillin-allergic patients) for endocarditis prophylaxis.

DRUG/CLASS/ CATEGORY	INDICATIONS/ DOSAGES	KEY NURSING CONSIDERATIONS
gentamicin sulfate (topical) Garamycin, G-Myticin *Aminoglycoside* *Topical antibiotic* Pregnancy Risk Category: C	*Treatment and prophylaxis of superficial skin infections caused by susceptible bacteria* — **Adults and children > 1 yr:** rub in small amount gently t.i.d. or q.i.d, with or without gauze dressing.	• Clean affected area before applying. Remove crusts before application for impetigo contagiosa. • Prolonged use may result in overgrowth of nonsusceptible organisms.
gentamicin sulfate (ophthalmic) Garamycin Ophthalmic, Genoptic, Gentacidin, Gentak, Ocu-Mycin *Aminoglycoside* *Ophthalmic antibiotic* Pregnancy Risk Category: C	*External ocular infections caused by susceptible organisms, especially P. aeruginosa, Proteus, K. pneumoniae, E. coli, other gram-negative organisms* — **Adults and children:** 1 to 2 drops instilled in eye q 4 hr. In severe infections, up to 2 drops q hr. Or, apply ointment to lower conjunctival sac b.i.d. or t.i.d.	• Have culture taken before giving drug. Therapy may begin before results known. • Apply light finger pressure on lacrimal sac for 1 min after instilling drops. • If ophthalmic form given with systemic form, monitor serum gentamicin levels. • Solution not for injection into conjunctiva or anterior chamber of eye.
glatiramer acetate for injection (formerly copolymer 1) Copaxone *Acetate salts of synthetic peptides containing amino acids* *Immune response modifier* Pregnancy Risk Category: B	*To reduce frequency of relapses in patients with relapsing-remitting multiple sclerosis* — **Adults:** 20 mg S.C. q.d.	• Use diluent provided. Gently swirl lyophilized material and diluent and allow to stand at room temperature until completely dissolved (about 5 min). • Use immediately; drug does not contain preservatives. Discard unused drug. • Immediate postinjection, transient and self-limiting reactions (flushing, chest pain, palpitations, anxiety, dyspnea, throat constriction, urticaria) may occur.

glimepiride
Amaryl
Sulfonylurea
Antidiabetic
Pregnancy Risk Category: C

Adjunct to diet and exercise to lower blood glucose in type 2 diabetes mellitus when hyperglycemia can't be managed by diet and exercise alone — **Adults:** initially, 1 to 2 mg P.O. q.d. with first main meal of day; maintenance: 1 to 4 mg P.O. q.d. After reaching 2 mg, increase dosage in increments up to 2 mg q 1 to 2 wk, based on blood glucose response. Maximum: 8 mg/day.

Adjunct to insulin therapy in type 2 diabetes mellitus when hyperglycemia can't be managed by diet and exercise in conjunction with oral hypoglycemic agents — **Adults:** 8 mg P.O. q.d. with first main meal of day; used in combination with low-dose insulin.
Adjust-a-dose: In renally impaired patients, initial dose 1 mg P.O. q.d. Adjust upward, p.r.n.

- Monitor fasting blood glucose periodically to determine therapeutic response. Also monitor glycosylated Hgb, usually every 3 to 6 mo, to more precisely assess long-term glycemic control.
- Instruct patient to take with first meal of day.
- Advise patient that drug relieves symptoms but doesn't cure diabetes. Explain potential risks and advantages of drug and other treatment methods.
- Stress importance of adhering to diet and therapeutic regimen. Tell patient and family how and when to perform blood glucose self-monitoring, and teach how to recognize hyperglycemia and hypoglycemia.

glipizide
Glucotrol, Glucotrol XL,
Minidiab‡
Sulfonylurea
Antidiabetic
Pregnancy Risk Category: C

Adjunct to diet to lower blood glucose in type 2 diabetes mellitus — **Adults:** generally 5 mg P.O. q.d. Usual maintenance: 10 to 15 mg P.O. q.d. Maximum, 40 mg q.d. Divide doses above 15 mg, except extended-release tablets. For these tablets, 5 mg P.O. q.d. Adjust in 5-mg increments q 3 mo for glycemic control. Maximum daily dose 20 mg.
To replace insulin therapy — **Adults:** if insulin dosage > 20 units q.d., start at usual

- Give about 30 min before meals.
- During increased stress, patient may need insulin therapy.
- Patients switching from insulin therapy to oral antidiabetic require blood glucose monitoring at least t.i.d. before meals.
- Instruct patient about disease and importance of adhering to diet and therapeutic regimen. Tell how and when to perform blood glucose self-monitoring and teach

(continued)

159

DRUG/CLASS/ CATEGORY	INDICATIONS/ DOSAGES	KEY NURSING CONSIDERATIONS
glipizide *(continued)*	dose plus 50% of insulin. If insulin dose < 20 units, may stop insulin on initiating glipizide. ***Adjust-a-dose:*** For liver disease, initial dose 2.5 mg P.O. q.d. Extended-release tablets: initially, 5 mg P.O. q.d.; titrate cautiously.	signs and symptoms of hypoglycemia and hyperglycemia.
glucagon *Antihypoglycemic Antidiabetic/diagnostic agent* Pregnancy Risk Category: B	*Hypoglycemia* — **Adults and children > 20 kg (44 lb):** 0.5 to 1 mg S.C., I.M., or I.V.; may repeat q 5 to 20 min for 2 doses, p.r.n. In deep coma, also give glucose 10% to 50% I.V. When response, give more carbohydrate immediately. **Children ≤ 20 kg:** 0.025 mg S.C., I.M., or I.V. may repeat within 25 min. In deep coma, also give glucose 10% to 50% I.V. When response, give more carbohydrate immediately. *Note:* May repeat in 15 min, if necessary. Must give I.V. glucose if patient fails to respond. When patient responds, must give supplemental carbohydrate immediately. *Diagnostic aid for radiologic examination* — **Adults:** 0.25 to 2 mg I.V. or I.M. before radiologic procedure.	▪ *I.V. use:* Use only diluent supplied by manufacturer when preparing doses of 2 mg or less. For larger doses, dilute with sterile water for injection. ▪ For I.V. drip infusion, use dextrose solution. ▪ Arouse patient from coma as quickly as possible and give additional carbohydrates orally to prevent secondary hypoglycemic reactions. ▪ Unstable hypoglycemic diabetics may not respond to glucagon; give dextrose I.V. instead, as ordered. ▪ Instruct patient and family in proper glucagon administration and hypoglycemia recognition.
glyburide (glibenclamide) DiaBeta, Euglucon†, Gly-	*Adjunct to diet to lower blood glucose in type 2 diabetes* — **Adults:** initially, 2.5 to 5 mg regular tablets P.O. q.d. with breakfast.	▪ Micronized glyburide not bioequivalent to regular glyburide tablets.

nase PresTab, Micronase

Sulfonylurea

Antidiabetic

Pregnancy Risk Category: C

In debilitated, malnourished, or elderly patients, start at 1.25 mg q.d. Usual maintenance: 1.25 to 20 mg q.d. as single dose or in divided doses or may use micronized formulation. Initial dose 1.5 to 3 mg q.d. In sensitive patients, start at 0.75 mg q.d. Usual maintenance: 0.75 to 12 mg/day. Patients receiving > 6 mg/day may respond better with b.i.d. dosing.

To replace insulin therapy — **Adults:** If insulin dose > 40 U/day, may start at 5 mg q.d. plus 50% of insulin dose; if < 20 U/day, give 2.5 to 5 mg/day; if 20 to 40 U/day, give 5 mg/day. In all patients, substitute glyburide and discontinue insulin abruptly. For micronized tablets, if insulin dose > 40 U/day, give 3 mg P.O. with 50% reduction in insulin; if 20 to 40 U/day, give 3 mg P.O. as single daily dose; if < 20 U/day, give 1.5 to 3 mg/day as single dose.

Adjust-a-dose: In patients more sensitive to antidiabetic agents or those with adrenal or pituitary insufficiency, initially 1.25 mg q.d.

- Instruct patient about nature of disease, importance of adhering to diet, therapeutic regimen, weight reduction, exercise, and personal hygiene programs, and avoiding infection. Explain how and when to perform blood glucose self-monitoring and teach how to recognize and intervene for hypoglycemia and hyperglycemia.
- Instruct patient to report hypoglycemic episodes to doctor immediately.
- Teach patient to carry candy or other simple sugars to treat mild hypoglycemic episodes.
- Patients switching from insulin to oral antidiabetic require blood glucose monitoring at least t.i.d. before meals. May require hospitalization during transition.
- Caution patient not to change dosage without doctor's consent and to report abnormal blood or urine glucose results.

---

glycerin

Fleet Babylax, Sani-Supp

Trihydric alcohol

Laxative (osmotic)/lubricant

Pregnancy Risk Category: C

Constipation — **Adults and children ≥ 6 yr:** 2 to 3 g as rectal suppository or 5 to 15 ml as enema. **Children 2 to 6 yr:** 1 to 1.7 g as rectal suppository or 2 to 5 ml as enema.

- Used mainly to reestablish normal toilet habits in laxative-dependent patients.
- Advise patient to retain drug for at least 15 min. Usually acts within 1 hr. Entire suppository need not melt to be effective.
- Warn patient about adverse GI reactions.

DRUG/CLASS/CATEGORY	INDICATIONS/DOSAGES	KEY NURSING CONSIDERATIONS
goserelin acetate Zoladex *Synthetic decapeptide Luteinizing hormone–releasing hormone (LHRH; GnRH) analogue* Pregnancy Risk Category: X (endometriosis), D (breast cancer)	*Endometriosis: palliative treatment of advanced prostate cancer —* **Adults:** 3.6 mg S.C. q 28 days into upper abdominal wall. For endometriosis: maximum duration of therapy 6 mo. For prostate cancer, 10.8 mg S.C. q 12 wk into upper abdominal wall. *Palliative treatment of advanced breast cancer in pre- and perimenopausal women —* **Adults:** 3.6 mg S.C. q 28 days into upper abdominal wall.	• After cleaning area and injecting local anesthetic, stretch skin with one hand while grasping barrel of syringe with other. Insert needle into subcutaneous fat; then change needle direction so it parallels abdominal wall. Push needle in until hub touches skin; then withdraw needle about 1 cm before depressing plunger completely. • Don't aspirate after inserting needle. • Implant comes in preloaded syringe. If package damaged, don't use syringe. Make sure drug is visible.
granisetron hydrochloride Kytril *Selective 5-hydroxytryptamine receptor antagonist Antiemetic/antinauseant* Pregnancy Risk Category: B	*Prevention of nausea and vomiting associated with emetogenic cancer chemotherapy —* **Adults and children 2 to 16 yr:** 10 mcg/kg I.V. infused over 5 min. Begin infusion within 30 min before chemotherapy administration. Or, 1 mg P.O. up to 1 hr before chemotherapy, and repeated 12 hr later.	• *I.V. use:* Dilute with 0.9% NaCl solution or D₅W to volume of 20 to 50 ml. • Don't mix with other drugs. • Stress importance of taking 2nd dose of oral drug 12 hr later for maximum effectiveness. • Warn to report adverse reactions promptly.
grepafloxacin hydrochloride Raxar *Fluoroquinolone antibiotic Antibiotic* Pregnancy Risk Category: C	*Acute bacterial exacerbations of chronic bronchitis caused by susceptible strains of H. influenzae, S. pneumoniae, or M. catarrhalis —* **Adults:** 400 or 600 mg P.O. once daily for 10 days. *Community-acquired pneumonia caused by*	• May start therapy pending results of culture and sensitivity tests. • Use cautiously in patients with known or suspected CNS disorders that predispose to seizures. Drug isn't recommended for patients with proarrhythmic conditions.

- Serious, sometimes fatal, reactions possible. Stop drug at first sign of reaction.
- Mild to life-threatening pseudomembranous colitis has been reported.
- Achilles and other tendon ruptures that require surgical repair have been reported. Discontinue drug if patient experiences pain, inflammation, or rupture of a tendon.
- Patients exposed to direct sunlight or tanning booths may experience phototoxicity reactions.

susceptible strains of H. influenzae, S. pneumoniae, M. catarrhalis, or M. pneumoniae — **Adults:** 600 mg P.O. once daily for 10 days.
Uncomplicated gonorrhea (urethral in males and endocervical and rectal in females) caused by N. gonorrhoeae — **Adults:** 400 mg P.O. as single dose.
Nongonococcal urethritis and cervicitis caused by Chlamydia trachomatis — **Adults:** 400 mg P.O. once daily for 7 days.

- Advise patient to take drug after high-fat meal.
- Inform patient that prolonged treatment may be needed to control infection and prevent relapse, even if symptoms abate in first few days.
- Instruct patient to keep skin clean and dry and to maintain good hygiene.
- Caution patient to avoid intense sunlight and alcoholic beverages.

(continued)

griseofulvin microsize
Fulcin‡, Fulvicin-U/F, Grifulvin V, Grisactin, Grisovin‡, Grisovin 500‡, Grisovin-FP
griseofulvin ultramicrosize
Fulvicin P/G, Grisactin Ultra, Griseostatin‡, Gris-PEG
Penicillin antibiotic
Antifungal
Pregnancy Risk Category: C

Ringworm infections of skin, hair, nails — **Adults:** 500 mg (microsize) P.O. q.d. in single or divided doses. Severe infections may require up to 1 g q.d. Or, 330 to 375 mg (ultramicrosize) P.O. q.d. in single or divided doses. **Children > 2 yr:** 125 to 250 mg (microsize) P.O. q.d. or 7.3 mg/kg (ultramicrosize) P.O. q.d. for child 13.1 to 22.7 kg (29 to 50 lb); or 250 to 500 mg (microsize) P.O. q.d. for child > 22.7 kg.
Tinea pedis; tinea unguium — **Adults:** 0.75 to 1 g (microsize) P.O. q.d. Or, 660 to 750 mg (ultramicrosize) P.O. q.d. in divided doses. **Children ≥ age 2:** 125 to 250 mg (mi-

‡Canadian †Australian

DRUG/CLASS/ CATEGORY	INDICATIONS/ DOSAGES	KEY NURSING CONSIDERATIONS
griseofulvin (continued)	crosize) P.O. q.d. or 7.3 mg/kg (ultramicrosize) P.O. q.d. for child 13.1 to 22.7 kg; or 250 to 500 mg (microsize) P.O. q.d. for child >22.7 kg.	
guaifenesin (glyceryl guaiacolate) Anti-Tuss, Glytuss, Halotussin, Humibid L.A. Neo-Spect, Robitussin *Propanediol derivative Expectorant* Pregnancy Risk Category: C	*Expectorant —* **Adults and children ≥ 12 yr:** 100 to 400 mg P.O. q 4 hr, maximum 2.4 g/day; or 600 to 1,200 mg extended-release capsules q 12 hr. Maximum 2,400 mg daily. **Children 6 to 12 yr:** 100 to 200 mg P.O. q 4 hr, maximum 1,200 mg P.O. q.d. For extended-release capsules, 600 mg q 12 hr, not to exceed 1,200 mg in 24 hr. **Children 2 to 6 yr:** 50 to 100 mg P.O. q 4 hr. Maximum 600 mg q.d. For extended-release capsules, 300 mg q 12 hr, not to exceed 600 mg in 24 hr.	▪ Explain that persistent cough may signal serious condition; instruct patient to contact doctor if cough lasts > 1 wk, recurs frequently, or is associated with high fever, rash, or severe headache. ▪ Advise patient to take each dose with glass of water. ▪ Encourage deep-breathing exercises.
haloperidol Apo-Haloperidol†, Haldol, Novo-Peridol†, Peridol†, Serenace‡ **haloperidol decanoate** Haldol Decanoate, Haldol LA†	*Psychotic disorders —* **Adults and children ≥ 12 yr:** dosage varies. Initial range 0.5 to 5 mg P.O. b.i.d. or t.i.d.; or 2 to 5 mg I.M. q 4 to 8 hr. Maximum 100 mg P.O. t.i.d. **Children 3 to 12 yr:** 0.05 mg/kg to 0.15 mg/kg P.O. q.d. in 2 or 3 divided doses. *Chronic psychotic patients who require prolonged therapy —* **Adults:** 50 to 100 mg I.M. haloperidol decanoate q 4 wk.	▪ Don't give decanoate form I.V. ▪ Monitor for tardive dyskinesia, which may follow prolonged use. ▪ Warn patient to avoid activities that require alertness and psychomotor coordination until CNS effects known. ▪ Tell patient to avoid alcohol. ▪ Instruct patient to relieve dry mouth with sugarless gum or hard candy.

haloperidol lactate
Haldol
Butyrophenone
Antipsychotic
Pregnancy Risk Category: C

Nonpsychotic behavior disorders — **Children 3 to 12 yr:** 0.05 mg/kg P.O. q.d. Maximum 6 mg q.d.
Adjust-a-dose: In debilitated patients, give 0.5 to 2 mg P.O. b.i.d. or t.i.d; increase gradually, p.r.n.

heparin calcium
Calcilean, Calciparine
heparin sodium
Hepalean†, Liquaemin Sodium, Uniparin‡
Anticoagulant
Anticoagulant
Pregnancy Risk Category: C

Dosage highly individualized, depending on disease state, age, and renal and hepatic status.
Full-dose continuous I.V. infusion therapy for deep vein thrombosis (DVT), MI, pulmonary embolism — **Adults:** initially, 5,000 U by I.V. bolus, followed by 750 to 1,500 U/hr by I.V. infusion with pump. Adjust hourly rate 8 hr after bolus dose and according to PTT. **Children:** initially, 50 U/kg I.V., followed by 25 U/kg/hr or 20,000 U/m² daily by I.V. infusion pump. Adjust dose according to PTT.
Full-dose S.C. therapy for DVT, MI, pulmonary embolism — **Adults:** initially, 5,000 U I.V. bolus and 10,000 to 20,000 U in concentrated solution S.C., followed by 8,000 to 10,000 U S.C. q 8 hr or 15,000 to 20,000 U in concentrated solution q 12 hr.
Fixed low-dose therapy for venous thrombosis, pulmonary embolism, atrial fibrillation with embolism, postoperative DVT, embolism prevention— **Adults:** 5,000 U S.C. q 12 hr. In surgical patients, give first dose 2 hr

- Give low-dose injections sequentially between iliac crests in lower abdomen deep into S.C. fat. Inject slowly into fat pad. Leave needle in place for 10 sec after injection, then withdraw. Don't massage after S.C. injection. Watch for signs of bleeding at injection site. Alternate sites q 12 hr (right for morning, left for evening).
- **I.V. use:** Administer I.V. using infusion pump. Check constant infusions regularly.
- During intermittent I.V. therapy, always draw blood ½ hr before next scheduled dose to avoid falsely elevated PTT. May draw blood for PTT any time after 8 hr of initiation of continuous I.V. therapy. Never draw blood for PTT from I.V. tubing of infusion or from infused vein (falsely elevated PTT will result). Always draw blood from opposite arm.
- Never piggyback other drugs into infusion line while infusion running. Never mix with *(continued)*

DRUG/CLASS/ CATEGORY	INDICATIONS/ DOSAGES	KEY NURSING CONSIDERATIONS
heparin *(continued)*	before procedure, then 5,000 U.S.C. q 8 to 12 hr for 5 to 7 days or until patient can walk. *Consumptive coagulopathy (such as disseminated intravascular coagulation)* — **Adults:** 50 to 100 U/kg by I.V. bolus or continuous I.V. infusion q 4 hr. **Children:** 25 to 50 U/kg by I.V. bolus or continuous I.V. infusion q 4 hr. If no improvement within 4 to 8 hr, discontinue.	another drug in same syringe when giving bolus. • Measure PTT carefully and regularly. Anticoagulation present when PTT values 1.5 to 2 times control values. Monitor platelet count regularly. • Treat severe overdose with protamine sulfate, as ordered.
hydralazine hydrochloride Alphapress‡, Apresoline, Novo-Hylazin† *Peripheral vasodilator* *Antihypertensive* Pregnancy Risk Category: C	*Essential hypertension (orally); severe essential hypertension (parenterally)* — **Adults:** *P.O.:* 10 mg q.i.d.; increase gradually to 50 mg q.i.d. Maximum dosage 200 mg q.d., but some patients may require 300 to 400 mg q.d. *I.V.:* 10 to 20 mg repeated, p.r.n.; switch to P.O. as soon as possible. *I.M.:* 10 to 50 mg, repeated p.r.n.; switch to P.O. as soon as possible. **Children:** *P.O.:* 0.75 mg/kg/day divided into 4 doses; increase gradually over 3 to 4 wk to maximum 7.5 mg/kg or 200 mg q.d. *I.V. or I.M.:* 1.7 to 3.5 mg/kg q.d. or 50 to 100 mg/m² q.d. in 4 to 6 divided doses. Initial parenteral dose shouldn't exceed 20 mg.	• *I.V. use:* Give slowly and repeat as necessary, generally every 4 to 6 hr. Undergoes color changes in most infusion solutions; changes don't indicate potency loss. Check with pharmacist for compatibility information. • Monitor BP, pulse, and weight frequently. Elderly patients may be more sensitive to hypotensive effects. • Call doctor immediately if symptoms of lupus-like syndrome develop. • Instruct patient to take oral form with meals to increase absorption. • Advise patient to rise slowly and avoid sudden position changes to minimize orthostatic hypotension.

hydrochloro-thiazide Apo-Hydro†, Aquazide-H, Diaqua, Dichlotride‡, Esidrix, HydroDIURIL, Oretic *Thiazide diuretic* *Diuretic/antihypertensive* Pregnancy Risk Category: B	*Edema —* **Adults:** 25 to 100 mg P.O. q.d. or intermittently. **Children 2 to 12 yr:** 37.5 to 100 mg P.O. q.d. in 2 divided doses. **Children 6 mo to 2 yr:** 2 to 2.2 mg/kg P.O. or 60 mg/m² q.d. in 2 divided doses. **Infants < 6 mo:** up to 3 mg/kg P.O. q.d. in 2 divided doses. Maximum dose: from 12.5 to 37.5 mg q.d. *Hypertension —* **Adults:** 25 to 50 mg P.O. q.d. as single dose or divided b.i.d. Increase or decrease q.d. dose according to BP. Doses > 50 mg/day not required when combined with other antihypertensives.	• Monitor I&O, weight, BP, and serum electrolytes. • Monitor serum creatinine, BUN, and serum uric acid regularly. Cumulative drug effects may occur with impaired renal function. • Monitor elderly patients, who are especially susceptible to excessive diuresis. • Monitor blood glucose, especially in diabetic patients. • In hypertension, therapeutic response may be delayed several wk.
hydrocortisone (systemic) Cortef, Hydrocortone **hydrocortisone acetate** Cortifoam, Hydrocortone Acetate **hydrocortisone sodium phosphate** Hydrocortone Phosphate **hydrocortisone sodium succinate** A-hydroCort, Solu-Cortef *Glucocorticoid/mineralocorticoid* *Adrenocorticoid replacement* Pregnancy Risk Category: C	*Severe inflammation; adrenal insufficiency —* **Adults:** 5 to 30 mg P.O. b.i.d., t.i.d., or q.i.d. (up to 80 mg q.i.d. in acute situations); or initially, 100 to 500 mg succinate I.M. or I.V., and then 50 to 100 mg I.M., as indicated; or 15 to 240 mg phosphate I.M. or I.V. q.d. in divided doses q 12 hr; or 5 to 75 mg acetate I.V. into joints or soft tissue. Dosage varies with size of joint. Local anesthetics often injected with dose. *Shock —* **Adults:** initially, 50 mg/kg succinate I.V., repeated in 4 hr. Repeat q 24 hr, p.r.n. Or, 100 to 500 mg to 2 g q 2 to 6 hr; continue until patient stabilized (usually not longer than 48 to 72 hr). **Children:** phosphate (I.M.) or succinate (I.M. or I.V.) 0.16 to 1 mg/kg or succinate (I.M. or I.V.) 0.16 to 1 mg/kg or 6 to 30 mg/m² q.d. or b.i.d.	• May mask or exacerbate infections. • Watch for depression or psychotic episodes. • Diabetic patients may need increased insulin; monitor blood glucose. • Instruct patient to take oral form with milk or food. • Warn patient on long-term therapy about cushingoid symptoms. • Teach patient about symptoms of early adrenal insufficiency: fatigue, muscular weakness, joint pain, fever, anorexia, nausea, dyspnea, dizziness, and fainting. • Instruct patient to carry card identifying need for supplemental systemic glucocorticoids during stress. • Warn patient about easy bruising.

†Canadian ‡Australian

DRUG/CLASS/ CATEGORY	INDICATIONS/ DOSAGES	KEY NURSING CONSIDERATIONS
hydrocortisone (topical) Acticort, CaldeCort, Cortef, Cortizone 5, Squibb-HC‡ **hydrocortisone acetate** CortaGel, Cortaid, Cortamed†, Hydrocortisone Acetate **hydrocortisone butyrate** Locoid **hydrocortisone valerate** Westcort Cream *Glucocorticoid* *Topical adrenocorticoid* Pregnancy Risk Category: C	*Inflammation associated with corticosteroid-responsive dermatoses; adjunctive topical management of seborrheic dermatitis of scalp* — **Adults and children:** clean area; apply cream, gel, lotion, ointment, or topical solution sparingly q.d. to q.i.d. Spray aerosol onto affected area q.d. to q.i.d. until acute phase controlled; then reduce dosage to 1 to 3 times weekly, p.r.n. *Inflammation associated with proctitis —* **Adults:** 1 applicator of rectal foam P.R. q.d. or b.i.d. for 2 to 3 wk, then q.o.d., as necessary.	• Gently wash skin before applying. To prevent skin damage, rub in gently, leaving thin coat. When treating hairy sites, part hair and apply directly to lesions. Don't apply near eyes, mucous membranes, or in ear canal; may be safely used on face, groin, armpits, and under breasts. • Stop drug and tell doctor if skin infection, striae, atrophy, or fever develops. • When using aerosol around face, cover patient's eyes and warn against inhaling spray. Don't spray for > 3 sec or closer than 6" (15 cm). Apply to dry scalp after shampooing. No need to massage medication into scalp after spraying. • Know systemic absorption likely with use of occlusive dressings, prolonged treatment, or extensive body-surface treatment.
hydromorphone hydrochloride (dihydromorphinone hydrochloride) Dilaudid, Dilaudid-HP, Hydrostat *Opioid* *Analgesic/antitussive*	*Moderate to severe pain* — **Adults:** 2 to 10 mg P.O. q 3 to 6 hr, p.r.n. or around the clock; or 2 to 4 mg I.M., S.C., or I.V. (slowly over at least 3 to 5 min) q 4 to 6 hr, p.r.n. or around the clock; or 3 mg rectal suppository h.s., p.r.n. or around the clock. (Give 1 to 14 mg Dilaudid-HP S.C. or I.M. q 4 to 6 hr.)	• Respiratory depression and hypotension possible with I.V. use. Give very slowly and monitor constantly. Keep resuscitation equipment available. • Keep narcotic antagonist available. • Dilaudid-HP highly concentrated. • Tell patient to request drug or to take it before pain becomes intense.

Pregnancy Risk Category: C Controlled Substance Schedule: II	*Cough* — **Adults and children > 12 yr:** 1 mg P.O. q 3 to 4 hr, p.r.n. **Children 6 to 12 yr:** 0.5 mg P.O. q 3 to 4 hr, p.r.n.	• Warn outpatient to avoid hazardous activities until CNS effects known. • Tell patient to take drug with food if GI upset occurs.
hydroxyzine embonate‡ Atarax **hydroxyzine hydrochloride** Apo-Hydroxyzine†, Atarax, Hyzine-50, Multipax†, Vistaquel†, Vistaril, Vistazine 50 **hydroxyzine pamoate** Hy-Pam, Vamate, Vistaril *Antihistamine (piperazine derivative)* *Antianxiety agent/sedative/antipruritic/antiemetic/antispasmodic* Pregnancy Risk Category: C	*Anxiety; tension; hyperkinesia* — **Adults:** 50 to 100 mg P.O. q.i.d. **Children ≥ 6 yr:** 50 to 100 mg P.O. q.d. in divided doses. **Children < 6 yr:** 50 mg P.O. q.d. in divided doses. *Preoperative and postoperative adjunctive sedation; to control vomiting (excluding pregnancy); as adjunct to asthma treatment* — **Adults:** 25 to 100 mg I.M. q 4 to 6 hr. **Children:** 1.1 mg/kg I.M. q 4 to 6 hr. *Pruritus due to allergies* — **Adults:** 25 mg P.O. t.i.d. or q.i.d. **Children < 6 yr:** 50 mg P.O. q.d. in divided doses. **Children ≥ 6 yr:** 50 to 100 mg P.O. q.d. in divided doses.	• Parenteral form (hydroxyzine hydrochloride) for I.M. use only; Z-track method preferred. Never administer I.V. • Aspirate I.M. injection carefully to prevent inadvertent intravascular injection. Inject deeply into large muscle mass. • If patient receiving other CNS drugs, observe for oversedation. Warn patient to avoid hazardous activities that require alertness and psychomotor coordination until CNS effects known. • Tell patient to avoid alcohol. • To relieve dry mouth, suggest sugarless hard candy or gum.
hyoscyamine Cystospaz **hyoscyamine sulfate** Anaspaz, Bellaspaz, Levsin, Levsin S/L, Neoquess	*GI tract disorders caused by spasm; to diminish secretions and block cardiac vagal reflexes preoperatively; adjunctive therapy for peptic ulcerations* — **Adults and children ≥ 12 yr:** 0.125 to 0.25 mg P.O. or S.L. t.i.d. or q.i.d. before meals and h.s.; 0.375 mg to 0.75 mg P.O. (extended-release form)	• Give 30 min to 1 hr before meals and h.s. Bedtime dose can be larger; give at least 2 hr after last meal of day. • Monitor vital signs and urine output carefully. • Injection may cause allergic reaction in certain patients. *(continued)*

†Canadian ‡Australian

DRUG/CLASS/ CATEGORY	INDICATIONS/ DOSAGES	KEY NURSING CONSIDERATIONS
hyoscyamine *(continued)* *Belladonna alkaloid* Anticholinergic Pregnancy Risk Category: C	P.O. q 12 hr; or 0.25 to 0.5 mg (1 or 2 ml) I.M., I.V., or S.C. q 4 hr b.i.d. to q.i.d. Maximum 1.5 mg q.d. **Children < 12 yr:** dosage individualized according to weight.	• Tell patient to avoid hazardous activities if adverse CNS effects occur, to drink plenty of fluids, and to report rash or other skin eruption.
ibuprofen Aches-N-Pain, ACT-3‡, Advil, Children's Advil, Children's Motrin, Motrin, Motrin-IB Caplets, Motrin IB Tablets, Nuprin Caplets, Nuprin Tablets, Pedia Profen *NSAID* *Nonnarcotic analgesic/antipyretic/anti-inflammatory* Pregnancy Risk Category: B	*Rheumatoid arthritis; osteoarthritis; arthritis* — **Adults:** 300 to 800 mg P.O. t.i.d. or q.i.d., not to exceed 3.2 g/day. *Mild to moderate pain; dysmenorrhea* — **Adults:** 400 mg P.O. q 4 to 6 hr, p.r.n. *Fever* — **Adults:** 200 to 400 mg P.O. q 4 to 6 hr. Don't exceed 1.2 g q.d. or give > 3 days. **6 mo to 12 yr:** if fever < 102.5° F (39.2° C), 5 mg/kg P.O. q 6 to 8 hr. Treat higher fevers with 10 mg/kg q 6 to 8 hr. Maximum 40 mg/kg q.d. *Juvenile arthritis* — **Children:** 30 to 70 mg/kg/day in 3 or 4 divided doses.	• Check renal and hepatic function periodically with long-term therapy. • Changes in vision may occur. • Instruct parent not to give to children < 12 years; tell adult patient not to self-medicate for extended periods without consulting doctor. • Caution patient that using with aspirin, alcohol, or corticosteroids may increase risk of adverse GI reactions. • Teach patient about signs and symptoms of GI bleeding, and tell her to contact doctor immediately if these occur.
ibutilide fumarate Corvert *Ibutilide derivative* *Supraventricular antiarrhythmic* Pregnancy Risk Category: C	*Rapid conversion of fibrillation or atrial flutter of recent onset to sinus rhythm* — **Adults > 60 kg (132 lb):** 1 mg I.V. over 10 min. **Adults < 60 kg:** 0.01 mg/kg I.V. over 10 min. Stop infusion if arrhythmia ends or if ventricular tachycardia or marked prolongation of QT or QTc interval occurs. If ar-	• Only skilled personnel should give drug. • Before therapy, correct hypokalemia and hypomagnesemia. • Adequately anticoagulate patients with atrial fibrillation of > 2 to 3 days' duration (generally for at least 2 wk).

- Monitor ECG continuously during and at least 4 hr after administration or until QTc interval returns to baseline.
  - *I.V. use:* May give undiluted or diluted in 50 ml diluent.

- Cardiotoxicity is dose-limiting toxicity.
- Take preventive steps, such as adequate hydration, before treatment. Hyperuricemia may result from rapid lysis of leukemic cells; allopurinol may be ordered.
- Give over 10 to 15 min into free-flowing I.V. infusion of 0.9% NaCl or 5% dextrose solution running into large vein.
- Vesicant; tissue necrosis may result. If extravasation occurs, discontinue infusion immediately and notify doctor. Apply intermittent ice packs immediately for ½ hr, then for ½ hr q.i.d. for 4 days.
- Monitor hepatic and renal function tests and CBC frequently, as ordered.
- Notify doctor if signs or symptoms of heart failure occur.

- Adequate fluid intake (2 L/day) essential before and for 72 hr after therapy.
- Assess for mental status changes.
- Don't give at bedtime. If cystitis develops, discontinue and notify doctor.
- Monitor CBC and renal and liver function tests, as ordered.

---

rhythmia doesn't end 10 min after stopping infusion, may give second 10-min infusion of equal strength.

Dosage and indications vary. Check treatment protocol with doctor.

Acute myeloid leukemia, including French-American-British classifications M1 through M7, with other approved antileukemic agents — **Adults:** 12 mg/m²/day for 3 days by slow I.V. injection (over 10 to 15 min) with 100 mg/m²/day of cytarabine for 7 days by continuous I.V. infusion; or as 25 mg/m² bolus (cytarabine); then 200 mg/m²/day (cytarabine) for 5 days by continuous infusion. Second course may be given, p.r.n. **Adjust-a-dose:** If patient experiences severe mucositis, delay until recovery complete, and reduce dose by 25%. Also reduce dose in hepatic or renal impairment. Don't give if bilirubin > 5 mg/dl.

Testicular cancer — **Adults:** 1.2 g/m²/day I.V. for 5 consecutive days. Infuse each dose over ≥ 30 min. Repeat treatment q 3 wk or after patient recovers from hematologic toxicity. Administer with protecting agent (mesna) to prevent hemorrhagic cystitis.

---

idarubicin hydrochloride
Idamycin
*Antibiotic/antineoplastic
Antineoplastic*
Pregnancy Risk Category: D

ifosfamide
IFEX
*Alkylating agent (cell cycle–phase nonspecific)
Antineoplastic*
Pregnancy Risk Category: D

171

†Canadian ‡Australian

DRUG / CLASS / CATEGORY	INDICATIONS / DOSAGES	KEY NURSING CONSIDERATIONS
imipenem and cilastatin Primaxin IM, Primaxin IV *Carbapenem (thienamycin class) beta-lactam antibiotic* *Antibiotic* Pregnancy Risk Category: C	*Serious lower respiratory, urinary tract, intra-abdominal, gynecologic, bone and joint, skin and soft-tissue infections; bacterial septicemia and endocarditis* — **Adults and children > 40 kg (88 lb):** 250 mg to 1 g by I.V. infusion q 6 to 8 hr. Maximum 50 mg/kg/day or 4 g/day, whichever is less. Or, 500 to 750 mg I.M. q 12 hr. Maximum 1,500 mg/day. **Children < 40 kg:** 60 mg/kg I.V. q.d. in divided doses. **Premature infants < 36 weeks gestational age:** 20 mg/kg I.V. q 12 hr. *Adjust-a-dose:* Based on creatinine clearance. Refer to package insert.	▪ Obtain culture and sensitivity tests before 1st dose. ▪ *I.V. use:* Give each 250- or 500-mg dose by I.V. infusion over 20 to 30 min. Infuse each 1-g dose over 40 to 60 min. If nausea occurs, may slow infusion. ▪ If seizures develop and persist, notify doctor. Drug should be discontinued. ▪ Monitor for superinfections and resistant infections.
imipramine hydrochloride Apo-Imipramine†, Imprilt, Janimine, Melipramine†, Norfranil, Tipramine, Tofranil **imipramine pamoate** Tofranil-PM *Dibenzazepine tricyclic antidepressant* *Antidepressant* Pregnancy Risk Category: B	*Depression* — **Adults:** 75 to 100 mg P.O. or I.M. q.d. in divided doses, increased in 25- to 50-mg increments. Maximum for outpatients 200 mg q.d.; 300 mg q.d. may be used for hospital patients. Entire dose may be given h.s. **Elderly and adolescent patients:** initially, 30 to 40 mg q.d.; usually not necessary to exceed 100 mg q.d. *Childhood enuresis* — **Children ≥ 6 yr:** 25 mg P.O. 1 hr before bedtime. If no response within 1 wk, increase to 50 mg if child < 12 yr; 75 mg for children ≥ 12 yr. In either case, maximum 2.5 mg/kg/day.	▪ Reduce dosage in elderly, debilitated, or adolescent patients or in patient with aggravated psychotic symptoms. ▪ Don't withdraw abruptly. ▪ Discontinue gradually several days before surgery. ▪ Warn patient to avoid hazardous activities until CNS effects known. ▪ If signs of psychosis occur or increase, reduce dosage. Monitor for suicidal tendencies and allow only minimum drug supply.

indapamide
Lozide†, Lozol, Natrilix‡
Thiazide-like diuretic
Diuretic/antihypertensive
Pregnancy Risk Category: B

Edema — **Adults:** initially, 2.5 mg P.O. q.d. in morning. Increase to 5 mg q.d. after 1 wk, if needed.
Hypertension — **Adults:** initially, 1.25 mg P.O. q.d. in morning. Increase to 2.5 mg q.d. after 4 wk, if needed. Increase to 5 mg q.d. after 4 more wk, if needed.

- Monitor I&O, weight, BP, serum electrolytes, BUN, creatinine, uric acid, and glucose.
- Watch for signs of hypokalemia.
- May be used with potassium-sparing diuretic to prevent potassium loss.
- Monitor elderly patients closely.

indinavir sulfate
Crixivan
HIV protease inhibitor
Antiviral
Pregnancy Risk Category: C

Treatment of HIV infection when antiretroviral therapy warranted — **Adults:** 800 mg P.O. q 8 hr. Reduce to 600 mg P.O. q 8 hr in mild to moderate hepatic insufficiency due to cirrhosis.

- Maintain adequate hydration (≥ 1.5 L fluids q 24 hr while on indinavir).
- Inform patient that drug won't cure HIV infection and may not prevent complications of HIV. Hasn't been shown to reduce risk of HIV transmission.
- Advise women to avoid breast-feeding.

indomethacin
Apo-Indomethacin†, Indochron E-R, Indocid SR†, Indocin, Indocin SR, Novo-Methacin†, Rheumacin‡
indomethacin sodium trihydrate
Apo-Indomethacin†, Indocid P.D.A.†, Indocin I.V., Novo-Methacin†
NSAID

Moderate to severe rheumatoid arthritis or osteoarthritis; ankylosing spondylitis — **Adults:** 25 mg P.O. or P.R. b.i.d. or t.i.d. with food or antacids; increase daily dose 25 or 50 mg q 7 days, up to 200 mg q.d. Or, SR capsule (75 mg): 75 mg P.O. to start, in morning or h.s.; then, 75 mg b.i.d., p.r.n.
Acute gouty arthritis — **Adults:** 50 mg P.O. t.i.d. Reduce as soon as possible; then stop.
Acute painful shoulders (bursitis or tendinitis) — **Adults:** 75 to 150 mg P.O. q.d. in divided doses t.i.d. or q.i.d. for 7 to 14 days.
To close hemodynamically significant patent ductus arteriosus in premature infants (I.V.

- Monitor carefully for bleeding and for reduced urine output with I.V. use. Don't give second or third scheduled I.V. dose if anuria or marked oliguria evident; instead, notify doctor. Monitor for bleeding in coagulation defects, in patients receiving anticoagulants, and in neonates.
- If ductus arteriosus reopens, may give second course of 1 to 3 doses. If still ineffective, surgery may be necessary.
- May lead to reversible renal impairment; monitor patient closely.

(continued)

173

†Canadian ‡Australian

DRUG/CLASS/ CATEGORY	INDICATIONS/ DOSAGES	KEY NURSING CONSIDERATIONS
indomethacin *(continued)* *Nonnarcotic analgesic/antipyretic/anti-inflammatory* Pregnancy Risk Category: NR	*form only)* — **Neonates < 48 hr:** 0.2 mg/kg I.V., followed by 2 doses of 0.1 mg/kg at 12- to 24-hr intervals. **Neonates 2 to 7 days:** 0.2 mg/kg I.V., followed by 2 doses of 0.2 mg/kg I.V. at 12- to 24-hr intervals. **Neonates > 7 days:** 0.2 mg/kg I.V., followed by 2 doses of 0.25 mg/kg at 12- to 24-hr intervals.	• Causes sodium retention. Monitor for weight gain and increased BP. • May mask signs and symptoms of infection. • Give oral dosage with food, milk, or antacid if GI upset occurs.
infliximab Remicade *Tumor necrosis factor– alpha inhibitor Antibody* Pregnancy Risk Category: C	*Reduction of signs and symptoms in patients with moderately to severely active Crohn's disease with inadequate response to conventional therapy —* **Adults:** 5 mg/kg single I.V. infusion over not less than 2 hr. *Reduction in the number of draining enterocutaneous fistulas in patients with fistulizing Crohn's disease —* **Adults:** 5 mg/kg I.V. infused over not less than 2 hr. Give additional doses of 5 mg/kg at 2 and 6 wk after initial infusion.	• Monitor for infusion-related reactions. • Know that drug may affect normal immune responses. • *I.V. use:* Prepare only in glass infusion bottle or polyolefin or polyolefin infusion bag; administer through polyethylene-lined administration sets with an in-line, sterile, nonpyrogenic, low-protein-binding filter (pore size of ≤ 1.2 mm). • Use reconstituted dose promptly; don't infuse in same I.V. line with other agents.
insulin injection (regular insulin, crystalline zinc insulin) Humulin R, Novolin R, Regular (Conc.), Iletin II **insulin (lispro)**	*Diabetic ketoacidosis (use regular insulin only) —* **Adults:** 0.33 U/kg as I.V. bolus, followed by 0.1 U/kg/hr by continuous infusion. Continue infusion until blood glucose drops to 250 mg/dl, then begin S.C. insulin with dosage and intervals adjusted according to blood glucose level.	• Regular insulin used in circulatory collapse, diabetic ketoacidosis, or hyperkalemia. Don't use regular insulin (concentrated), 500 U/ml I.V. Don't use intermediate or long-acting insulins for emergencies requiring rapid drug action.

- Lispro is for S.C. use and has rapid onset of effect.
- *I.V. use:* Give regular insulin I.V. only. Inject directly, at ordered rate, into vein through intermittent infusion device or into port close to I.V. access site. Intermittent infusion not recommended.
- Dosage expressed in USP units. Use syringes calibrated for specific insulin concentration.
- U-500 insulin available for patients requiring large doses.
- Monitor pregnant patients closely.
- When mixing regular insulin with intermediate or long-acting, always draw up regular insulin into syringe first.
- May mix lispro insulin with Humulin N or Humulin U; give 15 min before meal.
- Rotate injection sites; chart to avoid overusing one area.
- Store in cool area.

I.V. and 50 to 100 U S.C. immediately; then additional doses q 2 to 6 hr based on blood glucose levels. To prepare infusion, add 100 U regular insulin and 1 g albumin to 100 ml 0.9% NaCl solution. Insulin concentration will be 1 U/ml. **Children:** 0.1 U/kg as I.V. bolus, then 0.1 U/kg/hr by continuous infusion until blood glucose drops to 250 mg/dl; then start S.C. insulin. Or, 1 to 2 U/kg in 2 divided doses, one I.V. and other S.C., followed by 0.5 to 1 U/kg I.V. q 1 to 2 hr based on blood glucose levels.

Type 1 diabetes mellitus: adjunct to type 2 diabetes mellitus — **Adults and children:** therapeutic regimen adjusted according to blood glucose levels.

Humalog
insulin zinc suspension, prompt (semilente)
Semilente‡
isophane insulin suspension (NPH)
Humulin N, Humulin NPH‡, Novolin N, NPH Insulin
isophane insulin suspension with insulin injection
Humulin 50/50, Humulin 70/30, Novolin 70/30
insulin zinc suspension (lente)
Humulin L, Lente Insulin, Novolin L
protamine zinc suspension (PZI)
insulin zinc suspension, extended (ultralente)
Humulin U, Ultralente Insulin
Pancreatic hormone
Antidiabetic
Pregnancy Risk Category: NR

DRUG / CLASS / CATEGORY	INDICATIONS / DOSAGES	KEY NURSING CONSIDERATIONS
interferon alfa-2a, recombinant (rIFN-A) Roferon-A *Biological response modifier* *Antineoplastic* Pregnancy Risk Category: C	*Hairy-cell leukemia* — **Adults:** for induction, 3 million IU S.C. or I.M. q.d. for 16 to 24 wk. For maintenance, 3 million IU S.C. or I.M. 3 times weekly. *AIDS-related Kaposi's sarcoma* — **Adults:** for induction, 36 million IU S.C. or I.M. q.d. for 10 to 12 wk. For maintenance, 36 million IU S.C. or I.M. 3 times/wk. *Philadelphia chromosome–positive chronic myelogenous leukemia* — **Adults:** initially, 3 million IU I.M. or S.C. q.d. for 3 days; then 6 million IU for 3 days, then 9 million IU for duration of treatment.	- Obtain allergy history. Contains phenol (preservative) and serum albumin (stabilizer). - Give by S.C. route if platelet count <50,000/mm³. - Administer h.s. to minimize daytime drowsiness. - Keep patient well hydrated, especially during initial treatment stage. - Monitor for CNS adverse reactions, such as decreased mental status and dizziness. - Different brands may not be equivalent and may require different dosage. - Neurotoxicity and cardiotoxicity more common in elderly patients, especially those with underlying CNS or cardiac impairment.
interferon alfa-2b, recombinant (IFN-alpha 2) Intron A *Biological response modifier* *Antineoplastic* Pregnancy Risk Category: C	*Hairy-cell leukemia* — **Adults:** 2 million IU/m² I.M. or S.C., 3 times/wk. *AIDS-related Kaposi's sarcoma* — **Adults:** 30 million IU/m² S.C. or I.M. 3 times/wk. *Chronic hepatitis B* — **Adults:** 30 to 35 million IU weekly I.M. or S.C., given either as 5 million IU q.d. or 10 million IU 3 times/wk for 16 wk.	- Give by S.C. route if platelet count <50,000/mm³. - Administer h.s. to minimize daytime drowsiness. - Keep patient well hydrated. - Monitor for adverse CNS reactions. - May increase bone marrow suppressant effects when used with blood dyscrasia–causing therapies.

interferon alfacon-1

Infergen

Biological response modifier

Antineoplastic

Pregnancy Risk Category: C

Treatment of chronic hepatitis C viral infection — **Adults:** 9 mcg S.C. three times weekly for 24 wk; for nonresponders or those who relapse, 15 mcg S.C. three times weekly for 6 mo.

Adjust-a-dose: In patients intolerant to higher doses, may reduce dose to 7.5 mcg. Don't give doses below 7.5 mcg; decreased efficacy may result.

- Obtain laboratory work before therapy, 2 wk after initiation, and periodically thereafter (CBC, platelets; serum creatinine, albumin, bilirubin, TSH, and thyroxine levels).
- Allow at least 48 hr to elapse between doses.
- Store drug in refrigerator at 36° to 46° F (2° to 8° C); don't freeze. May allow to reach room temperature just before use. Avoid vigorous shaking. Discard unused portion.

interferon beta-1a

Avonex

Biological response modifier

Antiviral immunoregulator

Pregnancy Risk Category: C

Treatment of relapsing forms of multiple sclerosis to slow progression of physical disability and decrease frequency of clinical exacerbation — **Adults:** 30 mcg I.M. q wk.

- Monitor closely for depression and suicidal ideation.
- Monitor WBCs, platelet counts and blood studies, including liver function tests.
- To reconstitute, inject 1.1 ml supplied diluent (sterile water for injection) into vial and gently swirl to dissolve drug. Don't shake.

interferon beta-1b, recombinant

Betaseron

Biological response modifier

Antiviral immunoregulator

Pregnancy Risk Category: C

To reduce frequency of exacerbations in relapsing-remitting multiple sclerosis — **Adults:** 8 million IU (0.25 mg) S.C. q.o.d.

- To reconstitute, inject 1.2 ml supplied diluent into vial and swirl to dissolve drug.
- Discard vials containing particulates or discolored solution.
- Inject immediately after preparation.
- Rotate injection sites.
- Monitor for mental depression.

†Canadian ‡Australian

DRUG / CLASS / CATEGORY	INDICATIONS / DOSAGES	KEY NURSING CONSIDERATIONS
interferon gamma-1b Actimmune *Biological response modifier* *Antineoplastic* Pregnancy Risk Category: C	*Chronic granulomatous disease* — **Adults with body surface area > 0.5 m²**: 50 mcg/m² (1.5 million U/m²) S.C. 3 times weekly, preferably at h.s. Preferred injection site deltoid or anterior thigh muscle. **Adults with body surface area ≤ 0.5 m²**: 1.5 mcg/kg 3 times weekly.	• Premedicate with acetaminophen to minimize symptoms at start of therapy. • Discard unused portion. • Refrigerate at once. Store vials at 36° to 46°F (2° to 8°C); don't freeze. Don't shake vial; avoid excessive agitation. Discard vials left at room temperature for > 12 hr.
ipecac syrup Ipecac syrup *Alkaloid emetic* *Emetic* Pregnancy Risk Category: C	*To induce vomiting in poisoning* — **Adults and children > 12 yr**: 30 ml P.O.; then 200 to 300 ml water. **Children 1 to 12 yr**: 15 ml P.O.; then 240 to 480 ml water. **Children 6 mo to 1 yr**: 5 to 10 ml P.O.; then 120 to 240 ml water. May repeat dose in patients > 1 yr if vomiting doesn't occur within 20 min. If no vomiting occurs within 30 to 35 min after second dose, perform gastric lavage.	• Usually induces vomiting within 20 to 30 min. • If 2 doses don't induce vomiting, be prepared to perform gastric lavage. • No systemic toxicity with doses of ≤ 30 ml (1 oz) or less. • In antiemetic toxicity, usually effective if < 1 hr has passed since antiemetic ingested.
ipratropium bromide Atrovent *Anticholinergic* *Bronchodilator* Pregnancy Risk Category: B	*Bronchospasm associated with COPD* — **Adults**: 1 to 2 inhalations q.i.d. More may be needed. Don't exceed 12 inhalations in 24 hr. Or, use inhalation solution. Give 500 mcg dissolved in 0.9% NaCl solution and administer by nebulizer q 6 to 8 hr. **Children 5 to 12 yr**: 125 to 250 mcg nebulizer solution dissolved in 0.9% NaCl solution given by nebulizer q 6 to 8 hr.	• If using face mask for nebulizer, avoid leakage around mask. • Warn patient that drug is ineffective for treating acute episodes of bronchospasm. • Teach patient to perform oral inhalation correctly: Clear nasal passages and throat. Breathe out as much as possible. Place mouthpiece well into mouth as dose is released, and then inhale deeply. Hold

breath for several seconds, and then exhale slowly. If > 1 exhalation ordered, wait at least 2 min before repeating.

- If patient also uses steroid inhaler, tell him to use ipratropium first, then wait 5 min before using steroid.

Perennial rhinitis — **Adults and children > 12 yr:** 2 sprays (42 mcg) of 0.03% nasal spray per nostril 2 to 3 times q.d.
Common cold-induced rhinorrhea — **Adults and children > 12 yr:** 2 sprays (84 mcg) 0.06% nasal spray/nostril 3 or 4 times q.d.

irbesartan
Avapro
Angiotensin II receptor antagonist
Antihypertensive
Pregnancy Risk Category: C (first trimester); D (second and third trimesters)

Hypertension — **Adults:** initially 150 mg P.O. q.d., increased to maximum of 300 mg q.d., if necessary.
Adjust-a-dose: In volume- and salt-depleted patients, initially 75 mg P.O. q.d.

- Symptomatic hypotension may occur in volume- or salt-depleted patients. Correct cause of volume depletion before administration or giving lower dose.
- May continue drug when blood pressure has stabilized after a transient hypotensive episode.

irinotecan hydrochloride
Camptosar
Topoisomerase inhibitor
Antineoplastic
Pregnancy Risk Category: D

Treatment of metastatic carcinoma of colon or rectum that has recurred or progressed after fluorouracil therapy — **Adults:** initially, 125 mg/m² I.V. infusion over 90 min. Recommended treatment 125 mg/m² I.V. q wk for 4 wk, followed by 2-wk rest period. Thereafter, may repeat additional treatment course q 6 wk (4 wk on therapy, followed by 2 wk off). May adjust subsequent doses to low of 50 mg/m² or to maximum 150 mg/m² in 25- to 50-mg/m² increments, depending on tolerance. Treatment with additional courses may continue indefinitely if patient

- Pretreat with effective antiemetic therapy 30 min before irinotecan therapy.
- Don't add other drugs to infusion.
- If extravasation occurs, flush site with sterile water, apply ice, and notify doctor.
- Can induce severe diarrhea. Diarrhea occurring ≤ 24 hr of use may be relieved by atropine I.V., unless contraindicated. Late diarrhea (occurring after 24 hr) may be prolonged and life-threatening. Treat late diarrhea with loperamide, as ordered. Monitor fluid status and serum electrolytes.

(continued)

179

DRUG/CLASS/CATEGORY	INDICATIONS/DOSAGES	KEY NURSING CONSIDERATIONS
irinotecan hydrochloride *(continued)*	responds favorably or if disease remains stable, unless intolerable toxicity occurs.	• Monitor WBC count with differential, Hgb, and platelet count before each dose. If low, doses may need to be reduced or held.
isoniazid (isonicotinic acid hydrazide, INH) Isotamine†, Laniazid, Nydrazid, PMS Isoniazid† *Isonicotinic acid hydrazine* *Antituberculotic* Pregnancy Risk Category: C	*Actively growing tubercle bacilli* — **Adults:** 5 to 10 mg/kg P.O. or I.M. q.d. in single dose, up to 300 mg/day for 9 mo to 2 yr. **Infants and children:** 10 to 20 mg/kg P.O. or I.M. q.d. in single dose, up to 300 mg/day, for 18 mo to 2 yr. Give with one other antituberculotic. *Prevention of tubercle bacilli in those exposed to TB or those with tests consistent with non-progressive TB* — **Adults:** 300 mg P.O. q.d. in single dose, continued for 6 mo. **Infants and children:** 10 mg/kg P.O. q.d. in single dose, up to 300 mg/day, continued for 6 mo.	• Always give with other antituberculotics to prevent development of resistant organisms. • Monitor hepatic function closely for changes. • Tell patient to avoid alcoholic beverages, fish, and tyramine-containing products such as aged cheese, beer, and chocolate. • Give pyridoxine, as ordered, to prevent peripheral neuropathy, especially in malnourished patients.
isoproterenol (isoprenaline) Dey-Dose Isoproterenol, Isuprel, Vapo-Iso **isoproterenol hydrochloride** Isuprel, Norisodrine Aerotrol	*Shock* — **Adults and children:** (hydrochloride) 0.5 to 5 mcg/min by continuous I.V. infusion titrated to response. Usual concentration 1 mg (5 ml) in 500 ml D₅W. *Bronchospasm during mild acute asthma attacks* — **Adults and children:** initially, 1 inhalation of sulfate form; repeat, if needed, after 2 to 5 min, with maximum 6 inhalations q.d. *Bronchospasm in COPD* — **Adults and**	• Correct volume deficit and hypotension before administering vasopressors. • If HR > 110 with I.V. infusion, notify doctor. Doses sufficient to increase HR > 130 may induce ventricular arrhythmias. • When giving I.V. to treat shock, monitor BP, CVP, ECG, ABGs, and urine output. Adjust infusion rate according to results. • May aggravate ventilation-perfusion abnormalities.

isoproterenol sulfate Medihaler-Iso **isoproterenol** Isuprel *Adrenergic* *Bronchodilator/cardiac* *stimulant* Pregnancy Risk Category: C	**children:** (hydrochloride) by handheld nebulizer; 5 to 15 deep inhalations of 0.5% solution. In adults requiring stronger solution, 3 to 7 deep inhalations of 1% solution no more frequently than q 3 to 4 hr. *Heart block; ventricular arrhythmias —* **Adults:** (hydrochloride) 0.02 to 0.06 mg I.V. Subsequent doses 0.01 to 0.2 mg I.V. or 5 mcg/min I.V. titrated to response; or 0.2 mg I.M., then 0.02 to 1 mg I.M., p.r.n. **Children:** (hydrochloride); I.V. infusion of 2.5 mcg/min to 0.1 mcg/kg/min. Dosage based on response.	▪ May cause slight rise in systolic BP and slight to marked drop in diastolic BP. ▪ *I.V. use:* Give by direct injection or infusion. For infusion, don't use with sodium bicarbonate injection. ▪ Don't use injection or inhalation solution if discolored or contains precipitate. ▪ If administering via inhalation with oxygen, make sure oxygen concentration won't suppress respiratory drive. ▪ Monitor for rebound bronchospasms when drug effects end.
isosorbide dinitrate Apo-ISDN†, Dilatrate-SR, Isonate, Isorbid, Isordil, Isordil Tembids, Isotrate, Sorbitrate **isosorbide mononitrate** Imdur, ISMO, Monoket *Nitrate* *Antianginal/vasodilator* Pregnancy Risk Category: C	*Acute anginal attacks (S.L. and chewable tablets isosorbide dinitrate only); prophylaxis in situations likely to cause anginal attacks —* **Adults:** *S.L. form:* 2.5 to 10 mg under tongue, repeated q 5 to 10 min (maximum 3 doses for each 30-min period). Prophylaxis, 2.5 to 10 mg q 2 to 3 hr. *Chewable form:* 5 to 10 mg, p.r.n. for acute attack or q 2 to 3 hr for prophylaxis, but only after initial test dose of 5 mg. *Oral form (dinitrate):* 5 to 30 mg P.O. t.i.d. or q.i.d. for prophylaxis (use smallest effective dose); 20 to 40 mg P.O. (SR form) q 6 to 12 hr. *Oral form (mononitrate, using Imdur):* 30 to 60 mg	▪ Monitor BP and intensity and duration of drug response. ▪ May cause headaches, especially when therapy begins. Dose may be reduced temporarily, but tolerance usually develops. Give aspirin or acetaminophen for headache, as ordered. ▪ Inform patient that abrupt discontinuation may cause coronary vasospasm with increased anginal symptoms and potential risk of MI. *(continued)*

†Canadian ‡Australian

DRUG/CLASS/ CATEGORY	INDICATIONS/ DOSAGES	KEY NURSING CONSIDERATIONS
isosorbide *(continued)*	P.O. q.d. on arising; increased to 120 mg q.d. after several days, p.r.n. *Oral form (mononitrate, using ISMO or Monoket)*: 20 mg P.O. b.i.d. with 2 doses given 7 hr apart.	• Tell patient to take S.L. tablet at first sign of attack. Warn him not to confuse S.L. with oral form. • To prevent development of tolerance, nitrate-free interval of 8 to 12 hr per day recommended.
isotretinoin Accutane, Roaccutane‡ *Retinoic acid derivative Antiacne agent/keratinization stabilizer* Pregnancy Risk Category: X	*Severe recalcitrant nodular acne unresponsive to conventional therapy* — **Adults and adolescents:** 0.5 to 2 mg/kg P.O. q.d. in 2 divided doses for 15 to 20 wk.	• Monitor liver function tests and serum lipids, glucose, and creatine kinase levels, before and during therapy. • Screen patients who experience headache, nausea and vomiting, or visual disturbances for papilledema.
isradipine DynaCirc *Calcium channel blocker Antihypertensive* Pregnancy Risk Category: C	*Hypertension* — **Adults:** initially, 2.5 mg P.O. b.i.d., alone or with thiazide diuretic. If response inadequate after first 2 to 4 wk, make dosage adjustments of 5 mg q.d. at 2- to 4-wk intervals to maximum 20 mg q.d.	• May cause symptomatic hypotension. • Monitor BP closely. • Before surgery, inform anesthesiologist that patient receiving calcium channel blocker.
itraconazole Sporanox *Synthetic triazole Antifungal* Pregnancy Risk Category: C	*Pulmonary, extrapulmonary blastomycosis; nonmeningeal histoplasmosis* — **Adults:** 200 mg P.O. q.d. Increase dose, p.r.n., in 100-mg increments. Maximum 400 mg q.d. Give doses > 200 mg q.d in 2 divided doses. *Aspergillosis* — **Adults:** 200 to 400 mg P.O. q.d.	• Perform baseline liver function tests, as ordered, and monitor periodically. • Teach patient to recognize and report signs and symptoms of liver disease (anorexia, dark urine, pale stools, unusual fatigue, or jaundice).

ketoconazole
Nizoral
Imidazole derivative
Antifungal
Pregnancy Risk Category: C

Oropharyngeal and esophageal candidiasis — **Adults:** 200 mg swished in mouth for several sec then swallowed, daily for 1 to 2 wk.

- Tell patient to take with food to ensure maximal absorption.
- Esophageal candidiasis requires minimum treatment of 3 wk.

Fungal infections caused by susceptible organisms — **Adults:** 400 mg P.O. q.d. in single dose. Maximum 400 mg q.d. **Children ≥ 2 yr:** 3.3 to 6.6 mg/kg P.O. q.d. as single dose.

- To minimize nausea, divide daily dosage into 2 doses or give with meals.
- Monitor for elevated liver enzymes, nausea that doesn't subside, unusual fatigue, jaundice, dark urine, or pale stools.

ketoconazole (topical)
Nizoral
Imidazole derivative
Antifungal
Pregnancy Risk Category: C

Tinea corporis, tinea cruris, tinea pedis, tinea versicolor caused by susceptible organisms; seborrheic dermatitis; cutaneous candidiasis — **Adults:** cover affected and surrounding area with 2% cream q.d. for ≥ 2 wk; for seborrheic dermatitis, apply b.i.d. for 4 wk. Shampoo twice weekly for 4 wk, with ≥ 3 days between shampoos, p.r.n.
Topical treatment of tinea infestations — **Adults and children:** Apply q.d. or b.i.d. for about 2 wk; for tinea pedis, apply for 4 wk.

- Most patients show improvement soon after treatment begins.
- Continue treatment of tinea cruris or tinea corporis for ≥ 2 wk.
- If condition worsens, may have to discontinue and redetermine diagnosis.
- For shampoo, wet hair, lather, and massage for 1 min. Rinse and repeat, but leave drug on scalp for 3 min before rinsing.

ketoprofen
Actron, Orudis, Oruvail
NSAID
Nonnarcotic analgesic/antipyretic/anti-inflammatory
Pregnancy Risk Category: B

Rheumatoid arthritis and osteoarthritis — **Adults:** 75 mg t.i.d. or 50 mg q.i.d. or 150 to 200 mg as extended-release q.d. Maximum 300 mg.
Mild to moderate pain; dysmenorrhea — **Adults:** 25 to 50 mg P.O. q 6 to 8 hrs, p.r.n.
Minor aches and pain or fever — **Adults:** 12.5 mg q 4 to 6 hr, up to 75 mg in 24 hr.

- May lead to reversible renal impairment. Check renal and hepatic function every 6 mo or p.r.n.
- May mask signs of infection.
- Full effect may be delayed for 2 to 4 wk.
- Warn patient to avoid hazardous activities until CNS effects known.

183

†Canadian ‡Australian

DRUG / CLASS / CATEGORY	INDICATIONS / DOSAGES	KEY NURSING CONSIDERATIONS
ketorolac tromethamine (ophthalmic) Acular *NSAID* *Ophthalmic anti-inflammatory* Pregnancy Risk Category: C	*Relief of ocular itching caused by seasonal allergic conjunctivitis* — **Adults:** 1 drop instilled into conjunctival sac of each eye q.i.d.	▪ Apply light finger pressure on lacrimal sac for 1 min after instillation. ▪ Store away from heat in dark, tightly closed container and protect from freezing.
ketorolac tromethamine (systemic) Toradol *NSAID* *Analgesic* Pregnancy Risk Category: C	*Short-term management of pain* — **Adults < 65 yr:** 60 mg I.M. or 30 mg I.V. as single dose, or multiple doses of 30 mg I.M. or I.V. q 6 hr; maximum 120 mg q.d. **Elderly > 65 yr:** 30 mg I.M. or 15 mg I.V. as single dose, or multiple doses of 15 mg I.M. or I.V. q 6 hr; maximum 60 mg q.d. *Adjust-a-dose:* In renally impaired patients or those weighing > 50 kg (110 lb), give 30 mg I.M. or 15 mg I.V. *Short-term management of moderately severe, acute pain when switching from parenteral to oral therapy* — **Adults < 65 yr:** 20 mg P.O. as single dose, then 10 mg P.O. q 4 to 6 hr, up to 40 mg/day. **Elderly ≥ 65 yr, renally impaired patients, or those < 50 kg:** 10 mg P.O. as single dose; then 10 mg P.O. q 4 to 6 hr, not to exceed 40 mg/day.	▪ Limit duration of therapy to 5 days. ▪ I.M. administration may cause pain at injection site. Apply pressure over site after injection. ▪ Don't mix with morphine sulfate, meperidine hydrochloride, promethazine hydrochloride, or hydroxyzine hydrochloride. ▪ Inhibits platelet aggregation and can prolong bleeding time; carefully observe patients with coagulopathies and those taking anticoagulants. Won't alter platelet count, PTT, or PT. ▪ May mask signs and symptoms of infection.

labetalol hydrochloride
Normodyne, Presolol‡, Trandate
Alpha- and beta-adrenergic blocker
Antihypertensive
Pregnancy Risk Category: C

Hypertension — **Adults:** 100 mg P.O. b.i.d. with or without diuretic. May increase by 100 mg b.i.d. q 2 or 4 days until optimum response reached. Usual maintenance 200 to 600 mg b.i.d., maximum 2,400 mg q.d.
Hypertensive emergencies — **Adults:** infuse 0.5 to 2 mg/min and titrate; usual cumulative dose 50 to 200 mg. Or, by repeated I.V. injection: initially, 20 mg I.V. slowly over 2 min. Then repeat injections of 40 to 80 mg q 10 min to maximum 300 mg.

- When given I.V. for hypertensive emergencies, produces rapid, predictable BP drop within 5 to 10 min.
- *I.V. use:* Give injection with infusion control device. Monitor BP q 5 min for 30 min, q 30 min for 2 hr, then hourly for 6 hr. Keep patient supine for 3 hr.
- Masks common signs of shock.
- I.V. form incompatible with sodium bicarbonate injection.
- May mask signs of hypoglycemia.

lactulose
Cephalac, Chronulac, Constulose, Duphalac, Enulose, Kristalose, Lactulax†
Disaccharide
Laxative
Pregnancy Risk Category: B

Constipation — **Adults:** 10 to 20 g (15 to 30 ml) P.O. q.d., increased to 40 g/day, if needed.
Hepatic encephalopathy — **Adults:** 20 to 30 g P.O. t.i.d. or q.i.d., until 2 or 3 soft stools q.d. Or, 300 ml diluted with 700 ml water or saline solution P.R. and retained for 40 to 60 min q 4 to 6 hr, p.r.n.

- To minimize sweet taste, dilute with water or fruit juice or give with food.
- Monitor serum sodium for possible hypernatremia, especially when giving to treat hepatic encephalopathy.
- Be prepared to replace fluid loss.

lamivudine
Epivir
Synthetic nucleoside analogue
Antiviral
Pregnancy Risk Category: C

Treatment of HIV infection with zidovudine — **Adults ≥ 50 kg (110 lb); children ≥ 12 yr:** 150 mg P.O. b.i.d. **Adults < 50 kg:** 2 mg/kg P.O. b.i.d. **Children 3 mo to 12 yr:** 4 mg/kg P.O. b.i.d. Maximum 150 mg b.i.d.
Adjust-a-dose: Reduce dosage in patients with creatinine clearance < 50 ml/min.

- Monitor CBC, platelet count, and liver function studies, as ordered.
- Stop treatment immediately and notify doctor if clinical signs, symptoms, or lab results suggest pancreatitis.

15

DRUG / CLASS / CATEGORY	INDICATIONS / DOSAGES	KEY NURSING CONSIDERATIONS
lamivudine/zidovudine Combivir *Synthetic nucleoside analogue* *Antiviral* Pregnancy Risk Category: C	*Treatment of HIV infection* — **Adults and children ≥ 12 yr weighing > 50 kg (110 lb):** 1 tablet P.O. b.i.d.	▪ Use combination cautiously in patients with bone marrow suppression. ▪ Notify doctor of signs of lactic acidosis or hepatotoxicity (abdominal pain, jaundice). ▪ Monitor for bone marrow toxicity. ▪ Assess fine motor skills and peripheral sensation for evidence of peripheral neuropathies.
lamotrigine Lamictal *Phenyltriazine* *Anticonvulsant* Pregnancy Risk Category: C	*Adjunct therapy in treatment of partial seizures caused by epilepsy* — **Adults:** 50 mg P.O. q.d. for 2 wk, then 100 mg q.d. in 2 divided doses for 2 wk. Usual maintenance dose 300 to 500 mg P.O. q.d. in 2 divided doses. For patients also taking valproic acid, 25 mg P.O. q.o.d. for 2 wk, then 25 mg P.O. q.d. for 2 wk. Maximum 150 mg P.O. q.d. in 2 divided doses. *Adjust-a-dose:* Give lower maintenance doses in patients with severe renal impairment.	▪ Don't discontinue abruptly. Instead, taper over at least 2 wk. Check adjunct anticonvulsant serum levels, as ordered. ▪ Warn patient not to engage in hazardous activities until CNS effects known.
lansoprazole Prevacid *Acid (proton) pump inhibitor* *Antiulcer agent* Pregnancy Risk Category: B	*Short-term treatment of active duodenal ulcer* — **Adults:** 15 mg P.O. q.d. before meals for 4 wk. *Short-term treatment of erosive esophagitis* — **Adults:** 30 mg P.O. q.d. before meals for up to 8 wk. If healing doesn't occur, may give for 8 more wk.	▪ Instruct patient to take before eating. ▪ May open capsules and sprinkle contents over applesauce. ▪ Breast-feeding may need to be discontinued during therapy. ▪ Don't use as maintenance therapy for treatment of duodenal ulcer or erosive

esophagitis.
- Monitor closely if also receiving ampicillin esters, digoxin, iron salts, or ketoconazole. May inhibit lansoprazole absorption.

Long-term treatment of pathologic hyper-secretory conditions, including Zollinger-Ellison syndrome — **Adults:** initially, 60 mg P.O. q.d. Increase dosage, p.r.n. Give daily doses of > 120 mg in divided doses.

latanoprost
Xalatan
Prostaglandin analogue
Antiglaucoma/ocular anti-hypertensive agent
Pregnancy Risk Category: C

Treatment of increased IOP in patients with ocular hypertension or open-angle glauco-ma who can't tolerate or who respond in-sufficiently to other IOP-lowering medica-tions — **Adults:** 1 drop in conjunctival sac of affected eye q.d. in evening.

- Don't administer while patient wears con-tact lenses.
- More frequent administration than recom-mended may decrease IOP-lowering effects.
- May gradually change eye color, increas-ing amount of brown pigment in iris.

leflunomide
Arava
Dihydroorotate dehydroge-nase inhibitor
Antiproliferative/anti-inflammatory
Pregnancy Risk Category: X

Treatment of active rheumatoid arthritis to reduce signs and symptoms and to retard structural damage (X-ray erosions and joint space narrowing) — **Adults:** 100 mg P.O. q 24 hr for 3 days, followed by 20 mg (maxi-mum daily dose) P.O. q 24 hours. Dose may be decreased to 10 mg q.d. if higher dose not well-tolerated.

- Use cautiously in patients with renal insuf-ficiency.
- Men planning to father a child should dis-continue therapy and follow recommended leflunomide removal protocol.
- Monitor liver enzymes before starting therapy and monthly thereafter until sta-ble.

letrozole
Femara
Aromatase inhibitor
Hormone/antineoplastic
Pregnancy Risk Category: D

Metastatic breast cancer in postmenopausal women with disease progression following antiestrogen therapy — **Adults:** 2.5 mg P.O. as single daily dose.

- No dosage adjustment needed in renally impaired patients with creatinine clearance ≥ 10 ml/min.
- Use cautiously in patients with severe liver impairment.
- May give without regard to meals.

187

†Canadian ‡Australian

DRUG/CLASS/ CATEGORY	INDICATIONS/ DOSAGES	KEY NURSING CONSIDERATIONS
leucovorin calcium (citrovorum factor, folinic acid) Wellcovorin *Formyl derivative (active re- duced form of folic acid)* *Vitamin/antidote* Pregnancy Risk Category: C	*Overdose of folic acid antagonist* — **Adults and children:** I.M. or I.V. dose equivalent to weight of antagonist given. *Leucovorin rescue after high methotrexate dose* — **Adults and children:** 10 mg/m² P.O., I.M., or I.V. q 6 hr until methotrexate levels < 5 × 10⁻⁸ M. *Megaloblastic anemia caused by congenital enzyme deficiency* — **Adults and children:** 3 to 6 mg I.M. q.d. *Folate-deficient megaloblastic anemia* — **Adults and children:** up to 1 mg I.M. q.d.	• *I.V. use:* When using powder for injection, reconstitute 50-mg vial with 5 ml, 100-mg vial with 10 ml, or 350-mg vial with 17 ml sterile or bacteriostatic water for injection. With doses > 10 mg/m², don't use dilu- ents containing benzyl alcohol. Don't exceed 160 mg/min when giving by direct injection. • Don't confuse folinic acid with folic acid. • Don't administer simultaneously with sys- temic methotrexate.
levalbuterol Xopenex *Beta blocker/mast cell mediator inhibitor* *Short-acting sympatho- mimetic bronchodilator* Pregnancy Risk Category: C	*For the treatment or prevention of broncho- spasm in patients with reversible obstructive airway disease* — **Adults and children ≥ 12 yr:** 0.63 mg administered t.i.d. q 6 to 8 hr, by nebulization. **Elderly:** Safety and efficacy of levalbuterol solution may be different in pa- tients < 65 yr and patients ≥ 65 yr. In general, start patients > 65 yr at dose of 0.63 mg. **Adjust-a-dose:** Patients with more severe asthma who do not respond adequately to dose of 0.63 mg may benefit from dose of 1.25 mg t.i.d.	• Can produce paradoxical bronchospasm, which may be life-threatening. If this oc- curs, discontinue immediately. • Can produce clinically significant cardio- vascular effects and ECG changes; use with caution in patients with cardiovascular disorders, especially coronary artery insuf- ficiency, arrhythmias, and hypertension. • Protect unit-dose vials from light and ex- cessive heat. • Keep unopened vials in foil pouch. After foil pouch is opened, use vials within 2 wk.

levobunolol hydrochloride Betagan *Beta blocker* *Antiglaucoma agent* Pregnancy Risk Category: C	*Chronic open-angle glaucoma and ocular hypertension* — **Adults:** 1 to 2 drops q.d. (0.5%) or b.i.d. (0.25%).	• Apply light finger pressure on lacrimal sac for 1 min after instilling. • Avoid letting dropper touch eye or surrounding tissue.
levodopa Dopar, Larodopa *Dopamine precursor* *Antiparkinsonian* Pregnancy Risk Category: C	*Parkinsonism* — **Adults:** initially, 0.5 to 1 g P.O. q.d., b.i.d., t.i.d., or q.i.d. with food; increase by no more than 0.75 g q.d. q 3 to 7 days, as tolerated; usual optimal dose 3 to 6 g q.d. divided into 3 doses. Don't exceed 8 g/day except for exceptional patients. Significant therapeutic response may not occur for 6 mo.	• Report muscle twitching. • With long-term therapy, test regularly for diabetes and acromegaly; periodically monitor renal, liver, and hematopoietic function. • Multivitamins, fortified cereals, and OTC medications may block drug effects.
levofloxacin Levaquin *Fluoroquinolone antibiotic* *Antibiotic* Pregnancy Risk Category: C	*Acute maxillary sinusitis due to susceptible organisms* — **Adults:** 500 mg P.O. or I.V. q.d. for 10 to 14 days. *Acute exacerbation of chronic bronchitis due to susceptible organisms* — **Adults:** 500 mg P.O. or I.V. q.d. for 7 days. *Community-acquired pneumonia due to susceptible organisms* — **Adults:** 500 mg P.O. or I.V. q.d. for 7 to 14 days. *Mild to moderate skin infections due to susceptible organisms* — **Adults:** 500 mg P.O. or I.V. q.d. for 7 to 10 days. *UTIs due to susceptible organisms* — **Adults:** 250 mg P.O. or I.V. q.d. for 10 days. *Acute pyelonephritis caused by E. coli* — **Adults:** 250 mg P.O. or I.V. q.d. for 10 days.	• Discontinue and notify doctor if symptoms of excessive CNS stimulation occur. Institute seizure precautions. Use cautiously in renal impairment. • Notify doctor if diarrhea occurs. • Monitor blood glucose and renal, hepatic, and hematopoietic blood studies. • *I.V. use:* Give injection by I.V. infusion only. Dilute drug in single-use vials according to manufacturer's instructions. Reconstituted solution should be clear and slightly yellow. Don't mix with other medications. Infuse over 60 min.

189

DRUG / CLASS / CATEGORY	INDICATIONS / DOSAGES	KEY NURSING CONSIDERATIONS
levonorgestrel Norplant System *Progestin* *Contraceptive* Pregnancy Risk Category: X	*Prevention of pregnancy* — **Women:** 6 capsules implanted subdermally in midportion of upper arm, about 8 cm above elbow crease, during first 7 days of onset of menses. Capsules placed in fanlike position, 15° apart (total of 75°). Contraceptive efficacy lasts for 5 yr.	• Irregular bleeding may mask symptoms of cervical or endometrial cancer. • Expect implant to be removed if patient develops active thrombophlebitis or thromboembolic disease, will be immobilized for significant time, or if jaundice develops.
levothyroxine sodium (T₄ or L-thyroxine sodium) Eltroxin†, Levo-T, Levothroid, Levoxine, Levoxyl, Synthroid *Thyroid hormone* *Thyroid hormone replacement therapy* Pregnancy Risk Category: A	*Myxedema coma* — **Adults:** 200 to 500 mcg I.V.; if no response in 24 hr, give 100 to 300 mcg I.V. Maintenance dose 50 to 200 mcg I.V. q.d. *Thyroid hormone replacement* — **Adults:** initially, 50 mcg P.O. q.d., increased by 25 to 50 mcg P.O. q.d. q 2 to 4 wk. May give I.V. or I.M. **Adults > 65 yr:** 12.5 to 50 mcg P.O. q.d. Increase by 12.5 to 25 mcg at 2- to 8-wk intervals, p.r.n. **Children >12 yr:** over 150 mcg or 2 to 3 mcg/kg/day. **Children 6 to 12 yr:** 100 to 150 mcg, or 4 to 5 mcg/kg/day. **Children 1 to 5 yr:** 75 to 100 mcg or 5 to 6 mcg/kg/day. **Children 6 to 12 mo:** 50 to 75 mcg/kg/day. **Children < 6 mo:** 25 to 50 mcg or 8 to 10 mcg/kg/day.	• Rapid replacement in arteriosclerotic patients may trigger angina, coronary occlusion, or CVA; use cautiously. • **I.V. use:** Prepare I.V. dose immediately before injection. Don't mix with other solutions. Inject into vein over 1 to 2 min. • Monitor BP and HR closely. Normal serum T₄ levels should occur within 24 hr; then threefold increase in serum liothyronine (T₃) in 3 days. • When switching *to* T₃: stop T₄ and begin T₃. Increase dose in small increments after residual effects of T₄ disappear. When switching *from* T₃, start T₄ several days before withdrawing T₃. • Discontinue 4 wk before radioactive iodine uptake studies.
lidocaine hydrochloride	*Ventricular arrhythmias resulting from MI,* cardiac manipulation, or cardiac glyco-	• **I.V. use:** Patient must be on cardiac monitor. Use infusion control device. Don't ex-

(lignocaine hydrochloride)
LidoPen Auto-Injector,
Xylocaine
Amide derivative
Ventricular antiarrhythmic/
local anesthetic
Pregnancy Risk Category: B

sides — **Adults:** 50 to 100 mg (1 to 1.5 mg/kg) by I.V. bolus at 25 to 50 mg/min. Repeat bolus dose q 5 to 10 min until arrhythmias subside or adverse reactions develop. Don't exceed 300-mg total bolus over 1-hr period. Simultaneously, begin constant infusion of 20 to 50 mcg/kg/min (1 to 4 mg/min). **Elderly:** reduce dose and rate of infusion by 50%. **Children:** 0.5 to 1 mg/kg by I.V. bolus, followed by infusion of 10 to 50 mcg/kg/min.

Adjust-a-dose: In patients with heart failure or renal or liver disease or in those weighing < 50 kg (110 lb), use reduced dosage.

ceed rate of 4 mg/min. Seizures may be first clinical sign of toxicity. Therapeutic levels 2 to 5 mcg/ml.

- If signs of toxicity occur, stop drug immediately and notify doctor. Keep oxygen and resuscitative equipment available.
- Discontinue infusion and notify doctor if arrhythmias worsen or ECG changes appear.
- Give I.M. injections in deltoid muscle only.
- Monitor patient response, especially BP, electrolytes, BUN, and creatinine levels.

lindane
GBH†, G-well, Kwelladat†,
Scabene
Chlorinated hydrocarbon
insecticide
Scabicide/pediculicide
Pregnancy Risk Category: B

Parasitic infestation (scabies, pediculosis) — **Adults and children:** CDC recommends avoiding bathing before skin application. If patient bathes, let skin dry and cool thoroughly before using. Apply thin layer of cream or lotion over entire skin surface (with special attention to folds, creases, interdigital spaces, and genital area) for scabies, or to hairy areas for pediculosis. After 8 to 12 hr, wash off drug. Repeat in 1 wk if mites appear or new lesions develop.

Apply shampoo undiluted to affected area and work into lather for 4 to 5 min.

- Apply topical corticosteroids or administer oral antihistamines for pruritus.
- Don't apply to face, eyes, or mucous membranes.
- Place hospitalized patient in isolation, with special linen-handling precautions.
- Modest amounts (6% to 13%) absorbed through intact skin.
- Wash off skin and notify doctor immediately if skin irritation or hypersensitivity develops.
- In case of accidental contact with eyes, flush with water and notify doctor.

DRUG/CLASS/ CATEGORY	INDICATIONS/ DOSAGES	KEY NURSING CONSIDERATIONS
liothyronine sodium (T₃) Cyronine, Cytomel, Tertroxin‡, Triostat *Thyroid hormone* *Thyroid hormone replacement agent* Pregnancy Risk Category: A	*Cretinism —* **Children:** 5 mcg P.O. q.d. with 5-mcg increase q 3 to 4 days, p.r.n. *Myxedema —* **Adults:** initially, 5 mcg P.O. q.d., increased by 5 to 10 mcg q 1 or 2 wk. Maintenance dose 50 to 100 mcg q.d. *Myxedema coma; premyxedema coma —* **Adults:** initially, 10 to 20 mcg I.V. for known or suspected CV disease; 25 to 50 mcg I.V. for patients without known CV disease. *Nontoxic goiter —* **Adults:** initially, 5 mcg P.O. q.d.; increase by 5 to 10 mcg q.d. q 1 to 2 wk. May increase by 12.5 or 25 mcg q.d. q 1 to 2 wk. Maintenance: 75 mcg q.d. *Thyroid hormone replacement —* **Adults:** initially, 25 mcg P.O. q.d., increased by 12.5 to 25 mcg q 1 to 2 wk. Maintenance: 25 to 75 mcg q.d. **Elderly:** 5 mcg q.d., increased in 5-mcg daily increments.	▪ Rapid replacement in patients with arteriosclerosis may trigger angina, coronary occlusion, or CVA; use cautiously. In patients with CAD, observe carefully for possible coronary insufficiency. ▪ Alters thyroid function tests. Monitor PT; decreased anticoagulant dosage usually required. ▪ When switching *from* levothyroxine (T₄), stop that drug and start T₃ at low dosage. Increase dosage in small increments after residual effects of T₄ disappear. When switching *to* T₄, start T₄ several days before withdrawing T₃ ▪ Discontinue 7 to 10 days before radioactive iodine uptake studies.
lisinopril Prinivil, Zestril *ACE inhibitor* *Antihypertensive* Pregnancy Risk Category: C (first trimester); D (second and third trimesters)	*Hypertension —* **Adults:** initially, 5 to 10 mg P.O. q.d. Most patients well controlled on 20 to 40 mg q.d. as single dose. **Adjust-a-dose:** In patients receiving a diuretic, give 5 mg P.O. q.d. *Treatment adjunct in heart failure (with diuretics and cardiac glycosides) —* **Adults:** initially, 5 mg P.O. q.d. Most patients well	▪ Monitor BP often. If drug doesn't adequately control BP, may add diuretic. ▪ Monitor WBC with differential before therapy, every 2 wk for first 3 mo, and periodically thereafter. ▪ When used in acute MI, patient should receive standard recommended treatment,

as appropriate (such as thrombolytics, aspirin, and beta blockers).
- Angioedema (including laryngeal edema) may occur, especially after 1st dose. Advise patient to report breathing difficulty or swelling of face, eyes, lips, or tongue.
- Light-headedness may occur, especially in first few days. Tell patient to rise slowly and report symptoms. Advise to stop drug and call doctor immediately if fainting occurs.

---

controlled on 5 to 20 mg q.d. as single dose.
Acute MI — **Adults:** initially, 5 mg P.O. followed by 5 mg in 24 hr, 10 mg in 48 hr, and then 10 mg q.d. for 6 wk. In patients with low systolic BP (≤ 120) when treatment starts or during first 3 days after MI, reduce to 2.5 mg P.O. If systolic BP ≤ 100, may reduce daily maintenance dose from 5 mg to 2.5 mg.

- Blood drug level measurements crucial to safe use. Monitor weekly to monthly during maintenance therapy.
- Monitor electrolyte levels and baseline ECG, thyroid, and renal studies, as ordered.
- May alter glucose tolerance in diabetics.
- Check fluid I&O. Weigh daily; check for edema or sudden weight gain.
- Warn ambulatory patient to avoid hazardous activities until CNS effects known.

---

lithium carbonate
Carbolith†, Eskalith CR, Lithane, Lithicarb‡, Lithobid, Lithonate, Lithotabs
lithium citrate
Cibalith-S
Alkali metal
Antimanic agent /antipsychotic
Pregnancy Risk Category: D

Prevention or control of mania — **Adults:** 300 to 600 mg P.O. up to q.i.d., or 900 mg (Eskalith CR tablets) P.O. q 12 hr; increase on basis of blood levels to achieve optimal dosage.

---

lomefloxacin hydrochloride
Maxaquin
Fluoroquinolone
Broad-spectrum antibiotic
Pregnancy Risk Category: C

Acute bacterial exacerbations of chronic bronchitis, uncomplicated UTI (cystitis), and complicated UTI caused by susceptible organisms — **Adults:** 400 mg P.O. q.d. for 10 to 14 days.
Adjust-a-dose: In patients with creatinine clearance of 10 to 40 ml/min, give loading

- Obtain culture and sensitivity tests before 1st dose. Begin therapy pending results.
- Photosensitization and phototoxicity may occur.
- Prolonged use may result in overgrowth of resistant organisms.

(continued)

†Canadian ‡Australian

DRUG / CLASS / CATEGORY	INDICATIONS / DOSAGES	KEY NURSING CONSIDERATIONS
lomefloxacin hydrochloride *(continued)*	dose of 400 mg P.O. on day 1, followed by 200 mg q.d. for duration of therapy. *Prophylaxis of UTI after transrectal prostate biopsy* — **Adults:** 400 mg P.O. as single dose 1 to 6 hr before procedure.	• Warn patient to avoid hazardous tasks until CNS effects known. • Drug interactions possible with antacids, sucralfate, cimetidine, probenecid, warfarin, or cyclosporine. Give these no less than 4 hr before or 2 hr after lomefloxacin.
lomustine (CCNU) CeeNU *Alkylating agent/nitrosourea (cell cycle-phase nonspecific)* *Antineoplastic* Pregnancy Risk Category: D	*Brain tumor; Hodgkin's disease* — **Adults and children:** 100 to 130 mg/m^2 P.O. as single dose q 6 wk. Reduce dosage according to degree of bone marrow suppression. Don't repeat doses until WBC count > 4,000/mm^3 and platelet count > 100,000/mm^3.	• Give 2 to 4 hr after meals for more complete absorption. • Monitor CBC weekly. Usually not given more often than q 6 wk; bone marrow toxicity cumulative and delayed, usually occurring 4 to 6 wk after administration. • Periodically monitor liver function tests.
loperamide Imodium A-D, Kaopectate II Caplets *Piperidine derivative* *Antidiarrheal* Pregnancy Risk Category: B	*Acute, nonspecific diarrhea* — **Adults and children > age 12:** initially, 4 mg P.O., then 2 mg after each unformed stool. Maximum 16 mg q.d. **Children 9 to 11 yr:** 2 mg t.i.d. on first day. **Children 6 to 8 yr:** 2 mg b.i.d. on first day. **Children 2 to 5 yr:** 1 mg t.i.d. on first day. Maintenance dose ⅓ to ½ of initial dose.	• In acute diarrhea, tell patient to discontinue and seek medical attention if no improvement within 48 hr; in chronic diarrhea, tell him to notify doctor and discontinue if no improvement after taking 16 mg q.d. for at least 10 days. • Advise patient with acute colitis to stop drug immediately.
loracarbef Lorabid *Synthetic beta-lactam anti-*	*Secondary bacterial infections of acute bronchitis* — **Adults:** 200 to 400 mg P.O. q 12 hr for 7 days.	• Obtain specimen for culture and sensitivity tests before 1st dose. • Monitor for superinfection.

biotic (carbacephem class)
Antibiotic
Pregnancy Risk Category: B

Acute bacterial exacerbations of chronic bronchitis — **Adults:** 400 mg P.O. q 12 hr for 7 days.
Pneumonia — **Adults:** 400 mg P.O. q 12 hr for 14 days.
Pharyngitis; sinusitis; tonsillitis — **Adults:** 200 mg P.O. q 12 hr for 10 days. **Children:** 15 mg/kg P.O. in divided doses q 12 hr for 10 days.
Acute otitis media — **Children:** 15 mg/kg (oral suspension) P.O. q 12 hr for 10 days.
Adjust-a-dose: In patients with creatinine clearance of 10 to 49 ml/min, give 50% usual dose at same interval; for creatinine clearance < 10 ml/min, give usual dose q 3 to 5 days.

- To reconstitute powder for oral suspension, add 30 ml water in 2 portions to 50-ml bottle or 60 ml water in 2 portions to 100-ml bottle; shake well after each addition. After reconstitution, store oral suspension for 14 days at room temperature (59° to 86° F [15° to 30° C]).
- Monitor for seizures. If seizures occur, discontinue and notify doctor. Give anticonvulsants, as ordered.

---

loratadine
Claratyne‡, Claritin
Tricyclic antihistamine
Antihistaminic
Pregnancy Risk Category: B

Symptomatic treatment of seasonal allergic rhinitis — **Adults and children 12 ≥ yr:** 10 mg P.O. q.d.
Adjust-a-dose: In patients with liver failure or glomerular filtration rate < 30 ml/min, initially give 10 mg q.o.d.

- May affect allergy skin tests results.
- Tell patient to stop drug 7 days before allergy skin tests to preserve test accuracy.

---

lorazepam
Alzapam, Apo-Lorazepam†, Ativan, Lorazepam Intensol, Novo-Lorazem†, Nu-Loraz†
Benzodiazepine
Antianxiety agent/sedative-hypnotic

Anxiety; agitation; irritability — **Adults:** 2 to 6 mg P.O. q.d. in divided doses. Maximum 10 mg q.d. Or, 0.05 mg/kg up to 4 mg I.M. q.d. in divided doses, or 0.044 to 0.05 mg/kg up to 4 mg I.V. q.d. in divided doses.
Insomnia due to anxiety — **Adults:** 2 to 4 mg P.O. h.s.

- Monitor respirations q 5 to 15 min and before each repeated I.V. dose. Have resuscitation equipment and oxygen available.
- *I.V. use:* Give slowly, at rate not > 2 mg/min. Dilute with equal volume of sterile water for injection, 0.9% NaCl for injec-
(continued)

195

†Canadian ‡Australian

DRUG/CLASS/ CATEGORY	INDICATIONS/ DOSAGES	KEY NURSING CONSIDERATIONS
lorazepam *(continued)* Pregnancy Risk Category: D Controlled Substance Schedule: IV	*Preoperative sedation —* **Adults:** 0.05 mg/kg I.M. 2 hr before procedure. Maximum 4 mg. Or, 0.044 mg/kg (maximum total dose 2 mg) I.V., 15 to 20 min before surgery. In adults <50 yr, may give 0.05 mg/kg (maximum 4 mg) if increased lack of recall of preoperative events desired.	tion, or dextrose 5% injection. ▪ Reduce dose in elderly or debilitated patients. ▪ Inject I.M. doses deeply into muscle mass. ▪ With repeated or prolonged therapy, monitor liver, renal, and hematopoietic function studies periodically, as ordered. ▪ Possibility of abuse and addiction exists. Don't withdraw abruptly after long-term use; withdrawal symptoms may occur.
losartan potassium Cozaar *Angiotensin II receptor antagonist* *Antihypertensive* Pregnancy Risk Category: C (first trimester), D (second and third trimesters)	*Hypertension —* **Adults:** initially, 25 to 50 mg P.O. q.d. Maximum 100 mg q.d., given q.d. or b.i.d. **Adjust-a-dose:** In patients with hepatic impairment and intravascular volume depletion, initially, give 25 mg.	▪ If pregnancy suspected, notify doctor. ▪ Monitor BP closely to evaluate effectiveness. ▪ Closely monitor patient with severe heart failure; acute renal failure possible. ▪ Tell patient to avoid sodium substitutes. ▪ Regularly assess renal function, as ordered.
lovastatin (mevinolin) Mevacor *Lactone* *Cholesterol-lowering agent* Pregnancy Risk Category: X	*Reduction of LDL and total cholesterol levels in primary hypercholesterolemia (types IIa and IIb) —* **Adults:** initially, 20 mg P.O. q.d. with evening meal. For patients with severely elevated cholesterol (>300 mg/dl), initial dose 40 mg. Recommended daily dosage 20 to 80 mg in single or divided doses.	▪ Initiate only after diet and other nonpharmacologic therapies prove ineffective. Patient should be on low-cholesterol diet. ▪ Obtain liver function test results at start of therapy and periodically thereafter. ▪ Inform women when that drug contraindicated during pregnancy. ▪ Advise patient to have periodic eye exams.

loxapine hydrochloride
Loxapac†, Loxitane C,
Loxitane IM
loxapine succinate
Loxapac†, Loxitane
Dibenzoxazepine
Antipsychotic
Pregnancy Risk Category: NR

Psychotic disorders — **Adults:** 10 mg P.O. b.i.d. to q.i.d., rapidly increased to 60 to 100 mg P.O. q.d. for most patients; dosage varies among individuals. If patient can't take oral dose, 12.5 to 50 mg I.M. q 4 to 6 hr or longer, both dose and interval depending on patient response. Doses > 250 mg/day not recommended.

- Obtain baseline BP before therapy and monitor regularly.
- Dilute liquid concentrate with orange or grapefruit juice just before giving.
- Monitor for tardive dyskinesia. May treat acute dystonic reactions with diphenhydramine.
- Monitor for neuroleptic malignant syndrome.
- Warn patient to avoid hazardous activities until CNS effects known.

Lyme disease vaccine (recombinant OspA)
LYMErix
Vaccine
Vaccine
Pregnancy Risk Category: C

Active immunization against Lyme disease — **Adults and children ≥15 yr:** 30 mcg I.M. repeat dose at 1 and 12 mo after first dose. Safety and efficacy based on administration of second and third doses several wk before *Borrelia burgdorferi* transmission season.

- Review history for vaccine adverse reactions. Have epinephrine available.
- Vaccine should be turbid white suspension; if not, discard. Discard any unused vaccine.
- Administer I.M. injection in deltoid region.

magaldrate (aluminum-magnesium complex)
Antiflux†, Iosopan, Lowsium, Riopan
Aluminum magnesium salt
Antacid
Pregnancy Risk Category: C

Antacid — **Adults:** 480 to 960 mg P.O. (or 5 to 10 ml P.O. of suspension) with water between meals and h.s.; or 1 to 2 chewable tablets (chewed before swallowing) between meals and h.s.

- Monitor serum magnesium in mild kidney impairment. Symptomatic hypermagnesemia usually occurs only in severe renal failure.
- Not typically used in renal failure to help control hypophosphatemia.
- Very low sodium content; good choice for patients on restricted sodium intake.

†Canadian ‡Australian

DRUG/CLASS/CATEGORY	INDICATIONS/DOSAGES	KEY NURSING CONSIDERATIONS
magnesium citrate (citrate of magnesia) Citroma, Citro-Magt, Citro-Nesia, Evac-Q-Mag **magnesium hydroxide (milk of magnesia)** Milk of Magnesia, Phillips' Milk of Magnesia **magnesium sulfate (epsom salts)** *Magnesium salt* Antacid/antiulcer agent/laxative Pregnancy Risk Category: NR	*Constipation; to evacuate bowel before surgery* — **Adults and children ≥ 12 yr:** 11 to 25 g magnesium citrate P.O. q.d.; 2.4 to 4.8 g (30 to 60 ml) magnesium hydroxide P.O. q.d.; 10 to 30 g magnesium sulfate P.O. q.d. **Children 6 to 12 yr:** 5.5 to 12.5 g magnesium citrate P.O. q.d.; 1.2 to 2.4 g (15 to 30 ml) magnesium hydroxide P.O. q.d.; 5 to 10 g magnesium sulfate P.O. q.d. **Children 2 to 6 yr:** 2.7 to 6.25 g magnesium citrate P.O. q.d.; 0.4 to 1.2 g (5 to 15 ml) magnesium hydroxide P.O. q.d.; 2.5 to 5 g magnesium sulfate P.O. q.d. *Note:* All doses may be single or divided. *Antacid* — **Adults:** 5 to 15 ml milk of magnesia P.O. t.i.d. or q.i.d.	• Produces watery stools in 3 to 6 hr. Time doses so drug won't interfere with scheduled activities or sleep. • Before giving for constipation, determine if patient has adequate fluid intake, exercise, and diet. • Chill magnesium citrate before use to make more palatable. • Shake suspension well; give with large amount of water when used as laxative. • May accumulate in renal insufficiency. Monitor serum electrolytes, as ordered, during prolonged use.
magnesium chloride Slow-Mag **magnesium sulfate** *Mineral/electrolyte* Anticonvulsant Pregnancy Risk Category: NR	*Mild hypomagnesemia* — **Adults:** 1 g I.V. by piggyback or I.M. q 6 hr for 4 doses, depending on serum magnesium level. Or, 3 g P.O. q 6 hr for 4 doses. *Severe hypomagnesemia (serum magnesium 0.8 mEq/L or less, with symptoms)* — **Adults:** 2 to 5 g I.V. in 1 L solution over 3 hr. Subsequent doses depend on serum magnesium levels. *Magnesium supplementation* — **Adults:**	• *I.V. use:* Inject I.V. bolus dose slowly, using infusion pump for continuous infusion. Maximum infusion rate 150 mg/min. • When giving I.V. for severe hypomagnesemia, watch for respiratory depression and signs of heart block. Respirations should be > 16 before giving dose. • Monitor I&O. • Test knee-jerk and patellar reflexes before each additional dose. If absent, notify doc-

	54 to 483 mg/day in divided doses.	tor and withhold drug until reflexes return. • Incompatible with alkalis.
magnesium oxide Mag-Ox 400, Maox 420, Uro-Mag *Magnesium salt* *Antacid/laxative* Pregnancy Risk Category: NR	*Antacid* — **Adults:** 140 mg P.O. with water or milk after meals and h.s. *Laxative* — **Adults:** 4 g P.O. with water or milk, usually h.s. *Oral replacement therapy in mild hypomagnesemia* — **Adults:** 400 to 840 mg P.O. q.d.	• Monitor serum magnesium. With prolonged use and renal impairment, watch for symptoms of hypermagnesemia (hypotension, nausea, vomiting, depressed reflexes, respiratory depression, and coma). • If diarrhea occurs, use another drug.
magnesium salicylate Doan's, Mobidin, Bayer Select Maximum Strength Backache Pain Relief Formula *Salicylate* *Nonnarcotic analgesic/antipyretic/anti-inflammatory* Pregnancy Risk Category: NR	*Arthritis* — **Adults:** 545 mg to 1.2 g P.O. t.i.d. or q.i.d. *Mild pain or fever* — **Adults and children >11 yr:** 300 to 600 mg P.O. q 4 hr, not to exceed 3.5 g/day.	• Don't give to children or teenagers with chickenpox or flulike illness. • Febrile, dehydrated children can develop toxicity rapidly. • Therapeutic level in arthritis 10 to 30 mg/100 ml. With chronic therapy, mild toxicity may occur at 20 mg/100 ml. • Monitor Hgb and PT in long-term, high-dose treatment.
magnesium sulfate *Mineral/electrolyte* *Anticonvulsant* Pregnancy Risk Category: A	*Prevention or control of seizures in pre-eclampsia or eclampsia* — **Adults:** 4 g I.V. in 250 ml D₅W and 4 to 5 g deep I.M. each buttock; then 4 g deep I.M. alternate buttock q 4 hr, p.r.n. Or, 4 g I.V. loading dose, then 1 to 2 g/hr as I.V. infusion. Maximum 40 g q.d. *Hypomagnesemia; seizures* — **Adults:** 1 to 2 g (as 10% solution) I.V. over 15 min, then 1 g I.M. q 4 to 6 hr, per response and drug levels.	• **I.V. use:** If necessary, dilute to maximum concentration of 20%. Infuse no faster than 150 mg/min (1.5 ml/min of 10% solution or 0.75 ml/min of 20% solution). Compatible with D₅W. • Monitor vital signs q 15 min when giving I.V. Watch for respiratory depression and signs of heart block. *(continued)*

†Canadian ‡Australian

DRUG/CLASS/CATEGORY	INDICATIONS/DOSAGES	KEY NURSING CONSIDERATIONS
magnesium sulfate (continued)	*Seizures, hypomagnesemia associated with acute nephritis in children* — **Children:** 0.2 ml/kg 50% solution I.M. q 4 to 6 hr, p.r.n., or 100 to 200 mg/kg 1% to 3% solution I.V. slowly. *Management of paroxysmal atrial tachycardia* — **Adults:** 3 to 4 g I.V. over 30 sec. *Management of life-threatening ventricular arrhythmias* — **Adults:** 1 to 6 g I.V. over several min, then I.V. infusion of 3 to 20 mg/min for 5 or 48 hr.	• Keep I.V. calcium gluconate at hand to reverse magnesium intoxication; however, use cautiously in patients undergoing digitalization. • Check blood magnesium after repeated doses. Absence of knee-jerk and patellar reflexes signals impending toxicity. • Observe neonates for signs of magnesium toxicity, including neuromuscular or respiratory depression, when I.V. form given to toxemic mothers within 24 hr before delivery.
mannitol Osmitrol *Osmotic diuretic* Diuretic/prevention and management of acute renal failure or oliguria/reduction of IIntracranial pressure or IOP/treatment of drug intoxication Pregnancy Risk Category: B	*Test dose for marked oliguria or suspected inadequate renal function* — **Adults and children > 12 yr:** 200 mg/kg or 12.5 g as 25% I.V. solution over 3 to 5 min. Response adequate if 30 to 50 ml urine/hr excreted over 2 to 3 hr; if inadequate, give 2nd test dose. If still inadequate, discontinue. *Oliguria* — **Adults and children > 12 yr:** 50 to 100 g I.V. as 5% to 25% solution over 1½ to several hr.	• To redissolve crystallized solution, warm bottle in hot water and shake vigorously. Cool to body temperature before giving. • **I.V. use:** Give as intermittent or continuous infusion, using in-line filter. Direct injection not recommended. • Monitor vital signs, CVP, and I&O hourly. Check weight, renal function, and serum and urine sodium and potassium q.d.
measles, mumps, and rubella virus vaccine, live	*Routine immunization* — **Adults:** 0.5 ml S.C. Give 2 doses ≥ 1 mo apart to patients born after 1957. Inject into outer aspect of upper	• Obtain history of allergies. • Keep epinephrine 1:1,000 available. • Use diluent supplied. Discard after 8 hr.

M-M-R II
Vaccine
Viral vaccine
Pregnancy Risk Category: C

arm. **Children:** 0.5 ml S.C. Two-dose schedule recommended, with 1st dose given at 15 mo (12 mo in high-risk areas) and 2nd given either at 4 to 6 yr or 11 to 12 yr.

- Refrigerate; protect from light. Solution may be red, pink, or yellow, but must be clear.
- Review vaccine schedule with parent.

measles and rubella virus vaccine, live attenuated
M-R-Vax II
Vaccine
Viral vaccine
Pregnancy Risk Category: C

Immunization — **Adults and children ≥ 15 mo:** 0.5 ml (1,000 U) S.C. Inject into outer upper arm. Don't administer I.V.

- Obtain history of allergies, especially anaphylactic reactions to antibiotics.
- Keep epinephrine 1:1,000 available to treat anaphylaxis.
- Use only diluent supplied. Discard 8 hr after reconstituting.
- Refrigerate; protect from light. May be red, pink, or yellow, but must be clear.

measles virus vaccine, live attenuated
Attenuvax
Vaccine
Viral vaccine
Pregnancy Risk Category: C

Immunization — **Adults and children ≥ 15 mo:** 0.5 ml (1,000 U) S.C. Two-dose schedule recommended, with 1st dose given at 15 mo and 2nd at 4 to 6 yr or 11 to 12 yr.
Measles outbreak control — **Adults:** School personnel or those in medical facility born in or after 1957 who lack proof of measles immunity should be revaccinated. **Children:** if cases occur in children < 1 yr, vaccinate as young as 6 mo. All students and siblings without documentation of measles immunity should be revaccinated.

- Obtain history of allergies. Defer immunization in patients with acute illness or after blood or plasma administration.
- Keep epinephrine 1:1,000 available to treat anaphylaxis.
- Use only diluent supplied. Discard 8 hr after reconstituting.
- Don't give I.V.
- Refrigerate and protect from light. Reconstituted solution is clear yellow with no precipitation. Don't use if discolored.

†Canadian ‡Australian

DRUG/CLASS/ CATEGORY	INDICATIONS/ DOSAGES	KEY NURSING CONSIDERATIONS
mebendazole Vermox *Benzimidazole* *Anthelmintic* Pregnancy Risk Category: C	*Pinworm* — **Adults and children > 2 yr:** 100 mg P.O. as single dose; repeat if infection persists 2 to 3 wk later. *Roundworm; whipworm; hookworm* — **Adults and children > 2 yr:** 100 mg P.O. b.i.d. for 3 days; repeat if infection persists 3 wk later.	• Tablets may be chewed, swallowed whole, or crushed and mixed with food. • Administer to all family members, as prescribed, to decrease risk of spreading infection.
mechlorethamine hydrochloride (nitrogen mustard) Mustargen *Alkylating agent (cell cycle–phase nonspecific)* *Antineoplastic* Pregnancy Risk Category: D	*Chronic lymphocytic leukemia; Hodgkin's disease; bronchogenic cancer* — **Adults:** 0.4 mg/kg I.V. as single dose or in divided doses of 0.1 to 0.2 mg/kg/day. Give through running I.V. infusion. Give subsequent courses when patient recovers hematologically from previous course (usually 3 to 6 wk).	• Prepare immediately before infusion. Very unstable solution. Inspect before using; use within 15 min. Discard unused solution. • If extravasation occurs, apply cold compresses and infiltrate area with isotonic sodium thiosulfate. • Neurotoxicity increases with dose and patient age. • Watch for signs of infection and bleeding.
meclizine hydrochloride Antivert, Bonamine†, D-Vert, Meni-D, Vergon *Piperazine-derivative antihistamine* *Antiemetic/antivertigo agent* Pregnancy Risk Category: B	*Vertigo* — **Adults:** 25 to 100 mg P.O. q.d. in divided doses. Dosage varies with response. *Motion sickness* — **Adults:** 25 to 50 mg P.O. 1 hr before travel, then q.d. for duration of trip.	• May mask symptoms of ototoxicity, brain tumor, or intestinal obstruction. • Advise patient to avoid hazardous activities that require alertness until CNS effects known.

**medroxyproges-
terone acetate**
Amen, Curretab, Cycrin,
Depo-Provera, Provera
Progestin
Progestin/antineoplastic
Pregnancy Risk Category: X

Abnormal uterine bleeding caused by hormonal imbalance — **Adults:** 5 to 10 mg P.O. q.d. for 5 to 10 days starting on 16th day of menstrual cycle. If patient also has received estrogen, 10 mg P.O. q.d. for 10 days starting on 16th day of cycle.
Secondary amenorrhea — **Adults:** 5 to 10 mg P.O. q.d. for 5 to 10 days.
Endometrial or renal cancer — **Adults:** 400 to 1,000 mg I.M. weekly.
Contraception in women — **Adults:** 150 mg I.M. q 3 mo; give first injection during first 5 days of menstrual cycle.

- Don't use as test for pregnancy; may cause birth defects and masculinization of female fetus.
- I.M. injection may be painful. Monitor sites for sterile abscess. Rotate injection sites.
- Tell patient to report unusual symptoms immediately and to stop drug and call doctor if visual disturbances or migraines occur.
- FDA regulations require that patient read package insert before 1st dose for information on possible side effects. Also give verbal information.

megestrol acetate
Megace, Megostat†
Progestin
Antineoplastic
Pregnancy Risk Category: D

Breast cancer — **Adults:** 40 mg P.O. q.i.d.
Endometrial cancer — **Adults:** 40 to 320 mg P.O. q.d. in divided doses.
Treatment of unexplained significant weight loss — **Adults:** 800 mg P.O. (oral suspension) q.d.

- Advise patient to discontinue breast-feeding during therapy; possible infant toxicity.
- Advise women of childbearing age to use effective contraception during therapy.
- Inform patient that therapeutic response isn't immediate.

**melphalan
(L-phenylalanine
mustard)**
Alkeran
*Alkylating agent (cell cycle–
phase nonspecific*
Antineoplastic
Pregnancy Risk Category: D

Multiple myeloma — **Adults:** initially, 6 mg P.O. q.d. for 2 to 3 wk; then stop drug for up to 4 wk, or until WBC and platelet counts begin to rise again; then maintenance of 2 mg q.d. Or, 16 mg/m² by I.V. infusion over 15 to 20 min at 2-wk intervals for 4 doses. After toxicity recovery, give at 4-wk intervals.
Adjust-a-dose: In patients with renal insuf-

- *I.V. use:* Immediately before administering, reconstitute with 10 ml of sterile diluent supplied by manufacturer. Shake vigorously until solution clear.
- Promptly dilute and administer; reconstituted product begins to degrade within 30 min. Administer within 60 min of reconstitution.
(continued)

†Canadian ‡Australian

DRUG / CLASS / CATEGORY	INDICATIONS / DOSAGES	KEY NURSING CONSIDERATIONS
melphalan *(continued)*	ficiency, reduce dose up to 50%. *Nonresectable advanced ovarian cancer —* **Adults:** 0.2 mg/kg P.O. q.d. for 5 days. Repeat q 4 to 5 wk.	▪ Don't refrigerate reconstituted product. ▪ Give oral form on empty stomach. ▪ Monitor serum uric acid and CBC, as ordered. ▪ To prevent bleeding, avoid all I.M. injections when platelet count <100,000/mm³.
meningococcal polysaccharide vaccine Menomune-A/C/Y/W-135 *Vaccine* *Bacterial vaccine* *Pregnancy Risk Category: C*	*Meningococcal meningitis prophylaxis —* **Adults and children ≥ 2 yr:** 0.5 ml S.C.	▪ Obtain history of allergies and reaction to immunization. ▪ Keep epinephrine 1:1,000 available to treat anaphylaxis. ▪ Stress importance of avoiding pregnancy for 3 mo after vaccination. Offer contraception information.
menotropins Pergonal *Gonadotropin* *Ovulation stimulant/spermatogenesis stimulant* *Pregnancy Risk Category: X*	*Production of follicular maturation —* **Women:** 75 IU each of follicle-stimulating hormone (FSH) and luteinizing hormone (LH) I.M. q.d. for 7 to 12 days, then 5,000 to 10,000 USP human chorionic gonadotropin (HCG) I.M. 1 day after last dose of menotropins; repeat for 2 more menstrual cycles. May increase to 150 IU each of FSH and LH I.M. q.d. for 7 to 12 days, then 5,000 to 10,000 USP units HCG I.M. 1 day after last dose of menotropins; repeat for two menstrual cycles.	▪ Monitor closely to ensure adequate ovarian stimulation without hyperstimulation. ▪ Reconstitute with 1 to 2 ml sterile 0.9% NaCl for injection. Use immediately. ▪ Rotate injection sites. ▪ Advise patient that multiple births possible. ▪ Initiate treatment for stimulation of spermatogenesis after 4 to 6 mo of treatment with HCG.

Stimulation of spermatogenesis — **Adults:** 75 IU I.M. 3 times weekly (with 2,000 USP units HCG twice weekly) for 4 mo. After 4 mo, may continue with 75 to 150 IU FSH/LH 3 times weekly.

meperidine hydrochloride (pethidine hydrochloride) Demerol *Opioid Analgesic/adjunct to anesthesia* Pregnancy Risk Category: C Controlled Substance Schedule: II	*Moderate to severe pain —* **Adults:** 50 to 150 mg P.O., I.M., I.V., or S.C. q 3 to 4 hr. **Children:** 1.1 to 1.8 mg/kg P.O., I.M., I.V., or S.C. q 3 to 4 hr, or 175 mg/m² q.d. in 6 divided doses. Maximum single dose not to exceed 100 mg. *Preoperatively —* **Adults:** 50 to 100 mg I.M., I.V., or S.C. 30 to 90 min before surgery. **Children:** 1 to 2.2 mg/kg I.M., I.V., or S.C. up to adult dose 30 to 90 min before surgery. Don't exceed adult dosage.	■ Monitor respiratory and CV status. Don't give if respirations < 12, if respiratory rate or depth decreases, or if pupil change occurs. ■ *I.V. use:* Give slowly by direct I.V. injection. May also give by slow infusion. ■ Keep narcotic antagonist (naloxone) available when giving I.V. ■ Watch for withdrawal symptoms if drug stopped abruptly after long-term use.
mercaptopurine (6-mercaptopurine, 6-MP) Purinethol *Antimetabolite (cell cycle-phase specific, S phase) Antineoplastic* Pregnancy Risk Category: D	*Acute myeloblastic leukemia; chronic myelocytic leukemia —* **Adults:** 80 to 100 mg/ m² P.O. q.d. as single dose up to 5 mg/kg/ day. **Children:** 70 mg/m² P.O. q.d. *Acute lymphoblastic leukemia —* **Children:** 70 mg/m² P.O. q.d. **Usual maintenance for adults and children:** 1.5 to 2.5 mg/kg/day. **Adjust-a-dose:** In renally impaired patients, dosage may be reduced to avoid increased accumulation.	■ Watch for hepatic dysfunction, which is reversible on discontinuation. If hepatic tenderness occurs, stop drug and notify doctor. ■ Watch for signs of bleeding or infection. ■ To prevent bleeding, avoid all I.M. injections when platelet count < 100,000/mm³.

DRUG / CLASS / CATEGORY	INDICATIONS / DOSAGES	KEY NURSING CONSIDERATIONS
meropenem Merrem IV *Carbapenem derivative* *Antibiotic* Pregnancy Risk Category: B	*Complicated appendicitis and peritonitis caused by susceptible organisms; bacterial meningitis (pediatric patients only) caused by susceptible organisms* — **Adults:** 1 g I.V. q 8 hr over 15 to 30 min as I.V. infusion or over about 3 to 5 min as I.V. bolus injection. Maximum 2 g I.V. q 8 hr. **Children ≥ 3 mo:** 20 to 40 mg/kg I.V. q 8 hr as I.V. infusion over 15 to 30 min as I.V. infusion or over about 3 to 5 min as I.V. bolus injection. Maximum 2 g I.V. q 8 hr. **Children > 110 lb (50 kg):** 2 g I.V. q 8 hr for meningitis.	▪ Obtain specimen for culture and sensitivity test before giving 1st dose. ▪ Monitor for superinfection. ▪ Serious and occasionally fatal hypersensitivity reactions reported. Determine if previous hypersensitivity reactions to antibiotics have occurred. ▪ If seizures occur, discontinue infusion and notify doctor. ▪ Assess organ system functions periodically during prolonged therapy.
mesalamine Rowasa *Salicylate* *Anti-inflammatory* Pregnancy Risk Category: B	*Active mild to moderate distal ulcerative colitis, proctitis, or proctosigmoiditis* — **Adults:** 500 mg P.R. (suppository) b.i.d. or 4 g (retention enema) q.d., preferably h.s. for 3 to 6 wk. Rectal form should be retained overnight (for about 8 hr).	▪ Monitor periodic renal function studies with long-term therapy, as ordered. ▪ May cause hypersensitivity reactions in patients sensitive to sulfites. ▪ Instruct to stop if fever or rash occurs. ▪ Advise patient to carefully follow instructions supplied with medication.
mesna Mesnex, Dromitexan *Thiol derivative* *Uroprotectant* Pregnancy Risk Category: B	*Prophylaxis of hemorrhagic cystitis in patients receiving ifosfamide* — **Adults:** dosage varies with amount of ifosfamide administered; calculated as 20% (w/w) of ifosfamide dose at time of ifosfamide administration. Usual dose 240 mg/m² as I.V. bolus with ifosfamide administration; repeat	▪ *I.V. use:* Prepare solution by diluting commercially available ampules with D₅W solution, dextrose 5% and 0.9% NaCl for injection, 0.9% NaCl for injection, or lactated Ringer's to obtain final solution of 20 mg mesna/ml.

- Monitor urine samples daily in patients receiving mesna for hematuria.

at 4 and 8 hr after ifosfamide given.

mesoridazine besylate

Serentil, Serentil Concentrate

Phenothiazine (piperidine derivative)

Antipsychotic

Pregnancy Risk Category: NR

Alcoholism — **Adults and children > 12 yr:** 25 mg P.O. b.i.d. Maximum 200 mg q.d.

Behavioral problems associated with chronic organic mental syndrome — **Adults and children > 12 yr:** 25 mg P.O. t.i.d. to maximum 300 mg q.d.

Psychoneurotic manifestations (anxiety) — **Adults and children > 12 yr:** 10 mg P.O. t.i.d. to maximum 150 mg q.d.

Schizophrenia — **Adults and children > 12 yr:** initially, 50 mg P.O. t.i.d. or 25 mg I.M., repeated in 30 to 60 min, p.r.n. Maximum oral dose 400 mg q.d.; maximum I.M. dose 200 mg.

- Obtain baseline BP before starting.
- Watch for tardive dyskinesia. Treat acute dystonic reactions with diphenhydramine.
- Assess for neuroleptic malignant syndrome.
- Withhold dose and notify doctor if patient develops jaundice, symptoms of blood dyscrasia, or persistent extrapyramidal reactions (> several hours).
- Arrange for weekly bilirubin tests during first month; periodic blood tests (CBC and liver function); and ophthalmic tests.
- Wear gloves when preparing solutions and avoid contact with skin and clothing.

metaproterenol sulfate

Alupent, Dey-Dose Metaproterenol, Dey-Lute Metaproterenol, Metaprel

Adrenergic

Bronchodilator

Pregnancy Risk Category: C

Acute episodes of bronchial asthma — **Adults and children ≥ 12 yr:** 2 to 3 inhalations. Don't repeat inhalation more often than q 3 to 4 hr. Maximum 12 inhalations/day.

Bronchial asthma and reversible bronchospasm — **Adults and children > 9 yr or > 27 kg (60 lb):** 20 mg P.O. q 6 to 8 hr. **Children 6 to 9 yr or < 27 kg:** 10 mg P.O. q 6 to 8 hr. Or, via IPPB or nebulizer: **Adults and children ≥ 12 yr:** 0.2 to 0.3 ml of 5% solution diluted in about 2.5 ml of 0.45% or

- May use tablets and aerosol together.
- Inhalant solution can be given by IPPB with drug diluted in 0.45% or 0.9% NaCl solution or with hand nebulizer at full strength.
- If patient also uses steroid inhaler, tell him to use bronchodilator first, then wait about 5 min before using steroid.
- Warn patient to discontinue immediately and notify doctor if paradoxical bronchospasm occurs.

(continued)

DRUG/CLASS/ CATEGORY	INDICATIONS/ DOSAGES	KEY NURSING CONSIDERATIONS
metaproterenol sulfate *(continued)*	0.9% NaCl solution, or 2.5 ml commercially available 0.4% or 0.6% solution q 4 hr, p.r.n. **Children 6 to 12 yr:** 0.1 to 0.2 ml of 5% solution diluted in 0.9% NaCl solution to final volume of 3 ml q 4 hr, p.r.n.	▪ Instruct patient to notify doctor if drug ineffective or to request dosage adjustment.
metformin hydrochloride *Glucophage* *Biguanide* *Antidiabetic* Pregnancy Risk Category: B	*Adjunct to diet to lower blood glucose in type 2 diabetes mellitus* — **Adults:** initially, 500 mg P.O. b.i.d. with morning and evening meals, or 850 mg P.O. q.d. with morning meal. With 500-mg form, increase dosage 500 mg weekly to maximum 2,500 mg P.O. q.d. in divided doses, p.r.n. With 850-mg form, increase dosage 850 mg every other wk to maximum 2,550 mg P.O. q.d. in divided doses, p.r.n. *Adjust-a-dose:* In elderly or debilitated patients, give lower dose.	▪ Monitor renal function. If renal impairment detected, expect to switch to different antidiabetic. ▪ Give with meals. ▪ Monitor blood glucose level regularly to evaluate effectiveness. ▪ Monitor blood glucose level closely during times of increased stress because patient may need insulin therapy.
methadone Dolophine, Methadose, Physeptone‡ *Opioid* *Analgesic/narcotic detoxification adjunct* Pregnancy Risk Category: C	*Severe pain* — **Adults:** 2.5 to 10 mg P.O., I.M., or S.C. q 3 to 4 hr, p.r.n. *Narcotic withdrawal syndrome* — **Adults:** 15 to 40 mg P.O. q.d. (highly individualized). Maintenance 20 to 120 mg P.O. q.d. Adjust dosage, p.r.n. Daily doses > 120 mg require special state and federal approval.	▪ Oral liquid form legally required in maintenance programs. Completely dissolve tablets in 120 ml orange juice or powdered citrus drink. ▪ For parenteral use; I.M. injection preferred. ▪ Around-the-clock regimen necessary to manage severe, chronic pain.

Controlled Substance Schedule: II

methamphetamine
Desoxyn
CNS stimulant/adjunctive anorexigenic/sympathomimetic amine
Pregnancy Risk Category: C
Controlled Substance
Schedule: I

Attention deficit disorder with hyperactivity — **Children ≥ 6 yr:** 2.5 to 5 mg P.O. q.d. or b.i.d.; increase in 5-mg increments weekly, p.r.n. Usual effective dose 20 to 25 mg q.d.
Short-term adjunct in exogenous obesity — **Adults:** 2.5 to 5 mg P.O. b.i.d. to t.i.d., 30 min before meals; or 10 to 15 mg long-acting tablets P.O. q.d. before breakfast.

- Not recommended for first-line treatment of obesity. Use as anorexigenic prohibited in some states.
- When used for obesity, be sure patient on weight-reduction program.
- If tolerance to anorexigenic effect develops, notify doctor.

methimazole
Tapazole
Thyroid hormone antagonist
Antihyperthyroid agent
Pregnancy Risk Category: D

Hyperthyroidism — **Adults:** if mild, 15 mg P.O. q.d.; if moderately severe, 30 to 45 mg q.d.; if severe, 60 mg q.d. All given in 3 equally divided doses q 8 hr. Maintenance 5 to 30 mg q.d. **Children:** 0.4 mg/kg/day P.O. divided q 8 hr. Maintenance 0.2 mg/kg/day divided q 8 hr.

- Monitor hepatic function and CBC.
- Doses > 30 mg/day increase risk of agranulocytosis.
- Watch for signs of hypothyroidism.
- Discontinue and notify doctor of severe rash or enlarged cervical lymph nodes.
- Advise patient not to take OTC cough medicines.

methocarbamol
Robaxin
Carbamate derivative of guaifenesin
Skeletal muscle relaxant
Pregnancy Risk Category: NR

Adjunct in acute, painful musculoskeletal conditions — **Adults:** 1.5 g P.O. q.i.d. for 2 to 3 days. Maintenance 4 to 4.5 g P.O. q.d. in 3 to 6 divided doses. Or, 1 g I.M. or I.V. Maximum 3 g q.d. I.M. or I.V. for 3 consecutive days.
Supportive therapy in tetanus management — **Adults:** 1 to 2 g I.V. push or 1 to 3 g as infusion q 6 hr. **Children:** 15 mg/kg I.V. q 6 hr.

- Irritates veins; may cause fainting or phlebitis or aggravate seizures if injected rapidly. Keep patient supine during infusion. Avoid infiltration.
- Give I.M. deeply, only into outer quadrant of each buttock, with maximum 5 ml in each buttock. Don't give S.C.
- Warn patient to avoid activities that require alertness until CNS effects known.

†Canadian ‡Australian

209

DRUG/CLASS/ CATEGORY	INDICATIONS/ DOSAGES	KEY NURSING CONSIDERATIONS
methotrexate (amethopterin, MTX) **methotrexate sodium** Folex PFS, Mexate-AQ, Rheumatrex *Antimetabolite (cell cycle–phase specific, S phase)* *Antineoplastic* Pregnancy Risk Category: X	*Trophoblastic tumors (choriocarcinoma, hydatidiform mole)* — **Adults:** 15 to 30 mg P.O. or I.M. q.d. for 5 days. Repeat after ≥ 1 wk, according to response or toxicity. *Acute lymphocytic leukemia* — **Adults and children:** 3.3 mg/m²/day P.O., I.M., or I.V. for 4 to 6 wk or until remission; then 20 to 30 mg/m² P.O. or I.M. weekly in 2 divided doses or 2.5 mg/kg I.V. q 14 days. *Meningeal leukemia* — **Adults and children:** 12 mg/m² or less (maximum 15 mg) intrathecally q 2 to 5 days until CSF normal, then 1 additional dose.	■ Reconstitute solutions without preservatives just before use; discard unused drug. ■ Leucovorin rescue necessary with high-dose (> 100 mg) protocols; start 24 hr after methotrexate treatment begins. ■ Rash, redness, or ulcerations in mouth or adverse pulmonary reactions may signal serious complications. ■ Monitor pulmonary function tests periodically, as ordered. ■ Monitor I&O daily. Encourage intake of 2 to 3 L daily. ■ Watch for infection or bleeding.
methylcellulose Citrucel, Cologel *Adsorbent* *Bulk-forming laxative* Pregnancy Risk Category: C	*Chronic constipation* — **Adults:** maximum 6 g q.d., divided into 0.45 to 3 g/dose. **Children 6 to 12 yr:** maximum 3 g q.d., divided into 0.45 to 1.5 g/dose.	■ Especially useful in debilitated patients and in those with postpartum constipation, irritable bowel syndrome, diverticulitis, and colostomies.
methyldopa Aldomet, Apo-Methyldopa†, Dopamet†, Novomedopa† **methyldopate hydrochloride** Aldomet, Aldomet Ester Injection‡	*Hypertension; hypertensive crisis* — **Adults:** initially, 250 mg P.O. b.i.d. to t.i.d. in 1st 48 hr. Then increase, p.r.n., q 2 days. Maintenance 500 mg to 3 g q.d. in 2 to 4 divided doses; maximum: 3 g q.d. Or, 250 to 500 mg I.V. q 6 hr, diluted in D₅W and given over 30 to 60 min; maximum dose 1 g q 6 hr.	■ *I.V. use:* Observe for and report involuntary choreoathetoid movements. ■ After dialysis, monitor for hypertension and notify doctor, if necessary. ■ Monitor Coombs' test results. ■ Monitor CBC with differential.

Centrally acting antiadrener-gic *Antihypertensive* Pregnancy Risk Category: B	**Children:** 10 mg/kg P.O. q.d. in 2 to 4 divid-ed doses; or 20 to 40 mg/kg I.V. q.d. in 4 di-vided doses. Dosage increased 65 mg/kg or 3 g. Maximum daily dose 65 mg/kg or 3 g.	• Caution patient not to stop taking suddenly but to contact doctor if unpleasant adverse reactions occur.
methylergonovine maleate Methergine *Ergot alkaloid* *Oxytocic* Pregnancy Risk Category: C	*Prevention and treatment of postpartum hemorrhage caused by uterine atony or subinvolution* — **Adults:** 0.2 mg I.M. q 2 to 4 hr; for excessive uterine bleeding or other emergencies, 0.2 mg I.V. over 1 min while BP and uterine contractions monitored. Af-ter initial I.M. or I.V. dose, 0.2 mg P.O. q 6 to 8 hr for 2 to 7 days. Decrease dosage if se-vere cramping occurs.	• **I.V. use:** Don't routinely give I.V. If neces-sary, administer slowly over 1 min with BP monitoring. May dilute 1 ml with 5 ml with 0.9% NaCl solution. Contractions be-gin immediately after I.V. use and continue for up to 45 min. • Monitor and record BP, pulse rate, and uterine response; report sudden changes.
methylphenidate hydrochloride PMS-Methylphenidate†, Ritalin, Ritalin-SR *Piperidine CNS stimulant* *CNS stimulant (analeptic)* Pregnancy Risk Category: NR Controlled Substance Schedule: II	*Attention deficit hyperactivity disorder* — **Children ≥ 6 yr:** initial dose, 5 to 10 mg P.O. q.d. before breakfast and lunch, increased in 5- to 10-mg increments weekly, p.r.n., up to 2 mg/kg or 60 mg q.d Usual effective dose 20 to 30 mg. *Narcolepsy* — **Adults:** 10 mg P.O. b.i.d. or t.i.d. 30 to 45 min before meals. Dose varies with patient needs; average 40 to 60 mg/day.	• May trigger Tourette syndrome in children. • Observe for signs of excessive stimula-tion. Monitor BP. • Monitor height and weight in children on long-term therapy. May delay growth spurt, but children will attain normal height when drug stopped. • Monitor for tolerance or psychological de-pendence.
methylpredniso-lone Medrol **methylpredniso-lone acetate**	*Multiple sclerosis* — **Adults:** 200 mg P.O. q.d. for 1 wk, followed by 80 mg q.o.d. for 1 mo. *Severe inflammation or immunosuppres-sion* — **Adults:** 2 to 60 mg P.O. q.d. in 4 di-	• Give oral dose with food when possible. Critically ill patients may require concomi-tant antacid or H_2-receptor antagonist. *(continued)*

DRUG/CLASS/ CATEGORY	INDICATIONS/ DOSAGES	KEY NURSING CONSIDERATIONS
methylpredniso- lone (continued) depMedalone 40, Depoject- 40, Depo-Medrol, Depopred- 40, Depo-Predate 40, Du- ralone-40, Medralone-40, **methylpredniso- lone sodium succi- nate** A-methaPred, Solu-Medrol *Glucocorticoid* *Anti-inflammatory/immuno- suppressant* Pregnancy Risk Category: C	vided doses; 10 to 80 mg acetate I.M. q.d., or 10 to 250 mg succinate I.M. or I.V. up to q 4 hr; or 4 to 40 mg acetate into smaller joints or 20 to 80 mg acetate into larger joints. **Children:** 0.03 to 0.2 mg/kg succi- nate or 1 to 6.25 mg/m² I.M. q.d. or b.i.d. *Shock* — **Adults:** 100 to 250 mg succinate I.V. at 2- to 6-hr intervals; or 30 mg/kg I.V. initially; repeated q 4 to 6 hr, p.r.n. Continue therapy for 2 to 3 days or until patient stable.	▪ *I.V. use:* Use only methylprednisolone sodium succinate; never give acetate form I.V. Reconstitute according to manufactur- er's directions. ▪ Give direct injection over at least 1 min. Give massive doses over at least 10 min. If used for continuous infusion, change solution q 24 hr. ▪ May mask or exacerbate infections. ▪ Watch for depression or psychotic episodes. ▪ Diabetic patients may need increased in- sulin.
methyltestosterone Android, Oreton Methyl, Testred *Androgen* *Androgen replacement* Pregnancy Risk Category: X Controlled Substance Schedule: III	*Breast cancer in women* — **Adults:** 50 to 200 mg P.O. q.d.; or 25 to 100 mg buccally q.d. *Male hypogonadism* — **Adults:** 10 to 50 mg P.O. q.d.; or 5 to 25 mg buccally q.d. Semen evaluation q 3 to 4 mo.	▪ In children, obtain wrist bone X-rays be- fore therapy to establish bone maturation level. ▪ Check Hgb, Hct, cholesterol, calcium, and cardiac and liver function. ▪ Stop therapy if disease progression oc- curs.
methysergide maleate	*Prevention of frequent, severe, uncontrol- lable, disabling migraine or vascular*	▪ Monitor laboratory studies of cardiac and renal function, and CBC.

Deserilt, Sansert
Ergot alkaloid
Vasoconstrictor
Pregnancy Risk Category: X

headaches — **Adults:** 4 to 8 mg P.O. q.d. with meals for up to 6 mo.

- Monitor heart sounds for signs of valve disorders.
- May withdraw gradually q 6 mo, then restart after at least 3 wk.

metoclopramide hydrochloride
Apo-Metoclop†, Clopra, Maxolon, Octamide, Reclomide, Reglan
Para-aminobenzoic acid derivative
Antiemetic/GI stimulant
Pregnancy Risk Category: B

Prevention or reduction of nausea and vomiting associated with cancer chemotherapy — **Adults:** 1 to 2 mg/kg I.V. 30 min before cancer chemotherapy, then repeated q 2 hr for 2 doses, then q 3 hr for 3 doses.
Prevention of postoperative nausea and vomiting — **Adults:** 10 to 20 mg I.M. near end of procedure; then q 4 to 6 hr, p.r.n.
To facilitate small-bowel intubation and to aid in radiologic exams — **Adults and children > 14 yr:** 10 mg I.V. as single dose over 1 to 2 min. **Children < 6 yr:** 0.1 mg/kg I.V.
Children 6 to 14 yr: 2.5 to 5 mg I.V.
Gastroesophageal reflux — **Adults:** 10 to 15 mg P.O. q.i.d., p.r.n., 30 min before meals and h.s.

- **I.V. use:** Give lower doses (≤ 10 mg) by direct injection over 1 to 2 min. Dilute doses > 10 mg in 50 ml compatible diluent; infuse over ≥ 15 min. Protection from light unnecessary if mixture given ≤ 24 hr.
- Compatible with D_5W, 0.9% NaCl for injection, D_5W in 0.45% NaCl, or lactated Ringer's injection.
- Use diphenhydramine 25 mg I.V., as ordered, to counteract extrapyramidal adverse effects associated with high doses.
- Advise patient to avoid activities requiring alertness for 2 hr after each dose.
- Monitor BP in patient receiving I.V. form.

metolazone
Mykrox (prompt-release), Zaroxolyn (extended-release)
Quinazoline derivative
(thiazide-like) diuretic
Diuretic/antihypertensive
Pregnancy Risk Category: B

Edema in heart failure or renal disease — **Adults:** 5 to 20 mg (extended-release) P.O. q.d.
Hypertension — **Adults:** 2.5 to 5 mg (extended-release) P.O. q.d. Maintenance based on BP. Or 0.5 mg (prompt-release) P.O. q.d. in morning; increased to 1 mg P.O. q.d.

- To prevent nocturia, give in morning.
- Monitor I&O, weight, BP, and electrolytes.
- Watch for signs of hypokalemia, such as muscle weakness and cramps.
- Advise patient to avoid sudden posture changes.

†Canadian ‡Australian

213

DRUG / CLASS / CATEGORY	INDICATIONS / DOSAGES	KEY NURSING CONSIDERATIONS
metoprolol succinate Toprol XL **metoprolol tartrate** Apo-Metoprolol†, Lopresor SR†, Lopressor, Minax‡ *Beta blocker* *Antihypertensive/adjunctive treatment of acute MI* Pregnancy Risk Category: C	*Hypertension* — **Adults:** 100 mg P.O. in single or divided doses; maintenance 100 to 450 mg q.d. in 2 or 3 divided doses. Or, 50 to 100 mg of extended-release tablets q.d. (maximum 400 mg q.d.). *Early intervention in acute MI* — **Adults:** three 5-mg (tartrate) I.V. boluses q 2 min. Then, 15 min after last dose, 25 to 50 mg P.O. q 6 hr for 48 hr. Maintenance 100 mg P.O. b.i.d. *Angina pectoris* — **Adults:** initially, 100 mg P.O. q.d. in 2 divided doses. Maintenance 100 to 400 mg q.d.	• Check apical pulse before giving. If < 60, withhold dose and call doctor immediately. • Masks common signs of hypoglycemia. Monitor blood glucose level closely in diabetic patients. • Masks common signs of shock. Monitor BP frequently. • May precipitate asthma attacks. Monitor for breathing difficulties.
metronidazole (systemic) Apo-Metronidazole†, Flagyl, Metrozine‡, Neo-Metric†, PMS Metronidazole†, Protostat, Trikacide† **metronidazole hydrochloride** Flagyl I.V. RTU, Metro I.V., Novonidazol† *Nitroimidazole* *Antibacterial/antiprotozoal/ amebicide*	*Intestinal amebiasis* — **Adults:** 750 mg P.O. t.i.d. for 5 to 10 days. **Children:** 30 to 50 mg/kg q.d. (in 3 doses) for 10 days. *Trichomoniasis* — **Adults:** 250 mg P.O. t.i.d. for 7 days or 2 g P.O. in single dose; 4 to 6 wk should elapse between courses of therapy. **Children:** 5 mg/kg dose P.O. t.i.d. for 7 days. *Refractory trichomoniasis* — **Adults:** 250 or 500 mg P.O. b.i.d. for 10 or 7 days, respectively. *Bacterial infections caused by anaerobic microorganisms* — **Adults:** loading dose 15 mg/kg I.V. infused over 1 hr. Maintenance	• Infuse over ≥ 1 hr. Don't give I.V. push. • Record number and character of stools when used to treat amebiasis. Should be used only after *T. vaginalis* confirmed by wet smear or culture or *E. histolytica* identified. Asymptomatic sexual partners of patients being treated for *T. vaginalis* should be treated simultaneously to avoid reinfection. • Instruct patient to take oral form with food. • Tell patient to avoid alcohol or alcohol-containing medications during therapy and for at least 48 hr afterward.

Pregnancy Risk Category: B

dose 7.5 mg/kg I.V. or P.O. q 6 hr. Give first maintenance dose 6 hr after loading dose. Maximum 4 g q.d.

Prevention of postoperative infection in contaminated or potentially contaminated colorectal surgery — **Adults:** 15 mg/kg I.V. infused over 30 to 60 min 1 hr before surgery. Then, 7.5 mg/kg I.V. infused over 30 to 60 min at 6 and 12 hr after initial dose.

- Inform patient that metallic taste and dark or reddish brown urine may occur.
- Don't refrigerate neutralized diluted solution; precipitation may occur. If Flagyl I.V. RTU refrigerated, crystals may form; these disappear after solution warms to room temperature.

---

metronidazole (topical)
MetroGel, MetroGel-Vaginal
Nitroimidazole
Antiprotozoal/antibacterial
Pregnancy Risk Category: B

Acne rosacea — **Adults:** apply thin film to affected area b.i.d., morning and evening. Frequency and duration of therapy adjusted after response evaluated.
Bacterial vaginosis — **Adults:** 1 applicatorful b.i.d., morning and evening, for 5 days.

- Avoid using topical gel around eyes. Clean area before use and wait 15 to 20 min before applying drug. Cosmetics may be used after applying drug.
- If local reactions occur, tell patient to apply less frequently or to stop and contact doctor.

---

mexiletine hydrochloride
Mexitil
Lidocaine analogue/sodium channel antagonist
Ventricular antiarrhythmic
Pregnancy Risk Category: C

Refractory life-threatening ventricular arrhythmias, including ventricular tachycardia and PVCs — **Adults:** 200 mg P.O. q 8 hr. May increase dose in increments of 50 to 100 mg q 8 hr. Or, loading dose of 400 mg with maintenance dose of 200 mg q 8 hr. Maximum no more than 1,200 mg q.d.

- When switching from lidocaine, stop infusion when first mexiletine dose given. Keep infusion line open until arrhythmia controlled.
- Tremor early toxicity sign; progresses to dizziness and later to ataxia and nystagmus.
- Monitor BP and heart rate and rhythm often.

---

mezlocillin sodium
Mezlin
Extended-spectrum penicillin, acylaminopenicillin
Antibiotic

Systemic infections caused by susceptible strains of gram-positive and especially gram-negative organisms — **Adults:** 200 to 300 mg/kg q.d. I.V. or I.M. in 4 to 6 divided doses. Usual dose 3 g q 4 hr or 4 g q 6 hr.

- Before giving, ask about previous allergic reactions to penicillin.
- Obtain specimen for culture and sensitivity tests before 1st dose.

(continued)

†Canadian ‡Australian

DRUG / CLASS / CATEGORY	INDICATIONS / DOSAGES	KEY NURSING CONSIDERATIONS
mezlocillin sodium (continued) Pregnancy Risk Category: B	For serious infections, may give up to 24 g q.d. **Children ≤12 yr:** 200 to 300 mg/kg/day I.M. or I.V. in divided doses q 4 to 6 hr.	• With I.M., don't give > 2 g per injection. • May cause thrombocytopenia. Check CBC and platelet counts frequently, as ordered. • Monitor serum potassium.
miconazole nitrate Micatin, Monistat-Derm Cream and Lotion, Monistat 3 Vaginal Suppository, Monistat 7 *Imidazole derivative* *Antifungal* Pregnancy Risk Category: C	*Tinea pedis; tinea cruris; tinea corporis* — **Adults and children:** apply or spray sparingly b.i.d. for 2 to 4 wk. *Vulvovaginal candidiasis* — **Adults:** 1 applicatorful or 100 mg suppository (Monistat 7) inserted intravaginally h.s. for 7 days; repeat course, if necessary. Or, 200 mg suppository (Monistat 3) intravaginally h.s. for 3 days.	• Concurrent use of intravaginal forms and certain latex products, such as vaginal contraceptive diaphragms, not recommended. • Instruct patient to avoid sexual intercourse during vaginal treatment. • Caution patient to discontinue if sensitivity or chemical irritation occurs.
midazolam hydrochloride Hypnovel†, Versed *Benzodiazepine* *Preoperative sedative/agent for conscious sedation/adjunct for induction of general anesthesia/amnesic agent* Pregnancy Risk Category: D Controlled Substance Schedule: IV	*Preoperative sedation* — **Adults:** 0.07 mg to 0.08 mg/kg I.M. 1 hr before surgery. *Conscious sedation before short diagnostic procedures* — **Adults:** 1 to 2 mg by slow I.V. injection before procedure. *Induction of general anesthesia* — **Adults:** 0.15 to 0.35 mg/kg over 20 to 30 sec. Additional increments of 25% initial dose may be needed. Maximum: 0.6 mg/kg. **Unpremedicated adults ≥55 yr:** initially, 0.3 mg/kg. **Adjust-a-dose:** In debilitated patients, initial dose 0.2 to 0.25 mg/kg.	• Monitor BP, heart rate and rhythm, respirations, airway integrity, and SaO₂. • Have oxygen and resuscitation equipment available. • May mix in same syringe with morphine sulfate, meperidine, atropine sulfate, or scopolamine. • **I.V. use:** Administer slowly over at least 2 min, and wait at least 2 min when titrating. • I.V. dose may cause respiratory depression and respiratory arrest.

midodrine hydrochloride

ProAmatine

Peripheral alpha-adrenergic agonist

Vasopressor/antihypertensive

Pregnancy Risk Category: C

Treatment of symptomatic orthostatic hypotension unresponsive to standard clinical care — **Adults:** 10 mg P.O. t.i.d. Suggested dosing schedule: 1st dose shortly before or on arising in morning; 2nd dose at midday; 3rd dose in late afternoon (no later than 6 p.m.). Use cautiously in abnormal renal function; initially, 2.5-mg doses recommended.

- Monitor supine and sitting BP; notify doctor if supine BP increases excessively.
- Tell patient to take during day when he can be upright and doing daily activities. Space doses ≥ 3 hr apart. Tell him not to take after evening meal or within 4 hr before bedtime.
- Perform renal and hepatic function tests before and during therapy, as ordered.
- Instruct patient to consult doctor before taking OTC medications.

milrinone lactate

Primacor

Bipyridine phosphodiesterase inhibitor

Inotropic vasodilator

Pregnancy Risk Category: C

Short-term treatment of heart failure — **Adults:** initial loading dose 50 mcg/kg I.V., given slowly over 10 min, followed by continuous I.V. infusion of 0.375 to 0.75 mcg/kg/min. Adjust infusion dose according to clinical and hemodynamic responses, as ordered. **Adjust-a-dose:** With creatinine clearance ≤ 50 ml/min, titrate dose to maximum clinical effect, not to exceed 1.13 mg/kg/day.

- Improved cardiac output may enhance urine output. Potassium loss may predispose patient to digitalis toxicity.
- Monitor fluid and electrolyte status, BP, HR, and renal function. Excessive BP decrease requires discontinuing or slowing rate of infusion.

minocycline hydrochloride

Apo-Minocycline†, Dynacin, Minocin

Tetracycline

Antibiotic

Pregnancy Risk Category: NR

Infections caused by susceptible gram-negative and gram-positive organisms — **Adults:** initially, 200 mg I.V.; then 100 mg I.V. q 12 hr. No > 400 mg/day. Or, 200 mg P.O. initially; then 100 mg P.O. q 12 hr. Can use 100 or 200 mg P.O. initially, followed by 50 mg q.i.d. **Children > 8 yr:** initially, 4 mg/kg P.O. or I.V.; then 2 mg/kg q 12 hr. Given I.V. in 500-

- Obtain specimen for culture and sensitivity tests before first dose. May begin therapy pending test results.
- With large doses or prolonged therapy, monitor for superinfection, especially in high-risk patients.
- Check tongue for signs of candidal infection. Stress good oral hygiene.

(continued)

217

†Canadian ‡Australian

DRUG/CLASS/CATEGORY	INDICATIONS/DOSAGES	KEY NURSING CONSIDERATIONS
minocycline hydrochloride *(continued)*	to 1,000-ml solution without calcium over 6 hr. *Gonorrhea in patients allergic to penicillin* — **Adults:** initially, 200 mg P.O.; then 100 mg q 12 hr for at least 4 days. *Syphilis in patients allergic to penicillin* — **Adults:** initially, 200 mg P.O.; then 100 mg q 12 hr for 10 to 15 days. *Meningococcal carrier state* — **Adults:** 100 mg P.O. q 12 hr for 5 days. *Uncomplicated urethral, endocervical, rectal infection caused by C. trachomatis* — 100 mg P.O. b.i.d. for at least 7 days.	• May cause tooth discoloration in children < 8 yr. Observe for brown pigmentation; inform doctor if present. • Don't expose to heat or light. Keep cap tightly closed. • Thrombophlebitis may occur with I.V. administration. Avoid extravasation. Switch to oral therapy as soon as possible. • Tell patient to take oral form with full glass of water. May be taken with food. • Instruct patient not to take within 1 hr of bedtime.
minoxidil (oral) Loniten *Peripheral vasodilator* *Antihypertensive* Pregnancy Risk Category: C	*Severe hypertension* — **Adults:** initially, 5 mg P.O. as single dose. Effective dosage range usually 10 to 40 mg q.d. Maximum 100 mg q.d. **Children < 12 yr:** 0.2 mg/kg P.O. (maximum 5 mg) as single daily dose. Effective dosage range usually 0.25 to 1 mg/kg q.d. Maximum 50 mg q.d.	• Closely monitor BP and HR at start of therapy. Elderly patients may be more sensitive to hypotensive effects. • Removed by hemodialysis. Be sure to administer dose after dialysis. • Monitor fluid I&O. Check for weight gain and edema.
minoxidil (topical) Rogaine *Direct-acting vasodilator* *Hair-growth stimulant* Pregnancy Risk Category: C	*Androgenic alopecia* — **Adults:** 1 ml of 2% solution applied to affected area b.i.d. Maximum 2 ml q.d.	• Ensure that hair and scalp thoroughly dry; don't apply to other body areas. Advise not to use on irritated or sunburned scalp or with other medication on scalp. Instruct to wash hands thoroughly after application.

mirtazapine
Remeron
Piperazinoazepine
Tetracyclic antidepressant
Pregnancy Risk Category: C

Depression — **Adults:** initially, 15 mg P.O. h.s. Maintenance range 15 to 45 mg q.d. Dosage adjustments at intervals of at least 1 to 2 wk.

- Caution patient not to perform hazardous activities if somnolence occurs.
- Instruct patient not to use alcohol or other CNS depressants.
- Monitor closely for signs of dependence; not known if drug causes physical or psychological dependence.

misoprostol
Cytotec
Prostaglandin E₁ analogue
Antiulcer agent/gastric mucosal protectant
Pregnancy Risk Category: X

Prevention of NSAID-induced gastric ulcer in elderly or debilitated patients at high risk for complications from gastric ulcer and in patients with history of NSAID-induced ulcer — **Adults:** 200 mcg P.O. q.i.d. with food; if not tolerated, may decrease to 100 mcg P.O. q.i.d. Give last dose h.s. Give for duration of NSAID therapy.

- Provide oral and written warnings about dangers to fetus. Ensure that patient can comply with contraception and has negative serum pregnancy test within 2 wk of starting drug.
- Advise patient not to begin therapy until second or third day of next menstrual period.

**mitomycin
(mitomycin-C)**
Mutamycin
Antineoplastic antibiotic (cell cycle–phase nonspecific)
Antineoplastic
Pregnancy Risk Category: NR

Dosage and indications vary. Check treatment protocol with doctor.
Disseminated adenocarcinoma of stomach or pancreas — **Adults:** 20 mg/m² as I.V. single dose. Cycle repeated after 6 to 8 wk when WBC and platelet counts return to normal.

- Stop infusion immediately and notify doctor if extravasation occurs. Extravasation may cause necrosis.
- Monitor for dyspnea with cough.
- Watch for signs of infection and bleeding.

modafinil
Provigil
Racemic compound

Improvement of wakefulness in patients with excessive daytime sleepiness associated with narcolepsy — **Adults:** 200 mg P.O.

- May increase risk of unintended pregnancy when using steroidal contraceptives, including *(continued)*

DRUG / CLASS / CATEGORY	INDICATIONS / DOSAGES	KEY NURSING CONSIDERATIONS
modafinil *(continued)* *Wakefulness-promoting agent* Pregnancy Risk Category: C	q.d., given as single dose in morning. Although doses of 400 mg q.d. as single dose have been well tolerated, may be no additional benefit with doses > 200 mg. **Elderly:** Lower dose may be needed because of reduced elimination of drug and its metabolites. *Adjust-a-dose:* In patients with severe hepatic impairment, reduce dose by 50%.	ing depot or implantable contraceptives, during and for 1 mo after stopping therapy. ▪ Advise to inform doctor if taking or planning to take any prescription or OTC drugs. ▪ Advise patients to report rash, hives, or related allergic phenomenon.
moexipril hydrochloride Univasc *ACE inhibitor* *Antihypertensive* Pregnancy Risk Category: C (first trimester); D (second and third trimesters)	*Hypertension —* **Adults:** initially, 7.5 mg (3.75 mg if patient receiving diuretic) P.O. q.d. 1 hr before meal. If control inadequate, may increase or divide dose. Recommended maintenance dose 7.5 to 30 mg q.d., in 1 or 2 divided doses 1 hr before meals. Subsequent dosage depends on response. *Adjust-a-dose:* In patients with creatinine clearance < 40 ml/min, initially, give 3.75 mg/day; adjust to maximum of 15 mg/day.	▪ Monitor CBC with differential before therapy. ▪ Assess renal function before and during therapy. Monitor serum potassium level. ▪ Monitor for excessive hypotension. Measure BP at trough (just before dose) to verify BP control. ▪ Angioedema can cause fatal airway obstruction. Be prepared with S.C. epinephrine 1:1,000 (0.3 to 0.5 ml) and equipment to ensure patent airway.
molindone hydrochloride Moban *Dihydroindolone* *Antipsychotic* Pregnancy Risk Category: NR	*Psychotic disorders —* **Adults:** initially, 50 to 75 mg P.O. q.d., increased to 100 to 225 mg/day in 3 or 4 days. Maintenance doses as follows: mild severity, 5 to 15 mg P.O. t.i.d. to q.i.d.; moderate severity, 10 to 25 mg P.O. t.i.d. or q.i.d.; extreme severity, 225	▪ Monitor for tardive dyskinesia. ▪ Assess for neuroleptic malignant syndrome. ▪ May treat acute dystonic reactions with diphenhydramine. ▪ Warn patient to avoid hazardous activities until CNS effects known. Drowsiness and dizziness usually subside after first few wk.

mg/day P.O. **Elderly:** Initiate therapy with lowest recommended dose.

- Do not abruptly substitute drug for inhaled or oral corticosteroids.
- Drug isn't indicated for use in patients with acute asthmatic attacks or status asthmaticus or as monotherapy for management of exercise-induced bronchospasm. Patient should continue appropriate rescue medication for acute exacerbations.

---

montelukast sodium
Singulair
Leukotriene receptor antagonist
Antiasthmatic
Pregnancy Risk Category: B

For prophylaxis and chronic treatment of asthma — **Adults and children ≥ 15 yr:** 10 mg (film-coated tablet) P.O. once daily in evening. **Children 6 to 14 yr:** 5 mg (chewable tablet) P.O. once daily in evening.

---

moricizine hydrochloride
Ethmozine
Sodium channel blocker
Antiarrhythmic
Pregnancy Risk Category: B

Life-threatening ventricular arrhythmias — **Adults:** dosages individualized. Therapy should begin in hospital. Most patients respond to 600 to 900 mg P.O. q.d. in divided doses q 8 hr. Daily dose increased q 3 days by 150 mg.

- Determine electrolyte status and correct imbalances before therapy, as ordered.
- Notify doctor if chest pain or discomfort or fever occurs.

---

morphine hydrochloride
Morphitec, M.O.S.,†
morphine sulfate
Astramorph PF, Duramorph, Epimorph†, Infumorph 200, Morphine H.P.†, MS Contin, Roxanol
morphine tartrate†
Opioid
Narcotic analgesic

Severe pain — **Adults:** 5 to 20 mg S.C. or I.M., or 2.5 to 15 mg I.V. q 4 hr, p.r.n.; or 10 to 30 mg P.O. or 10 to 20 mg P.R. q 4 hr, p.r.n. When given by continuous I.V., loading dose of 15 mg I.V. may be followed by continuous infusion of 0.8 to 10 mg/hr. May also give 15 to 30 mg controlled-release tablets P.O. q 8 to 12 hr. As epidural injection, 5 mg; then, if adequate pain relief not obtained within 1 hr, additional doses of 1 to 2 mg. Maximum total epidural dose

- Keep narcotic antagonist (naloxone) and resuscitation equipment available.
- When given epidurally, monitor for respiratory depression up to 24 hr after injection.
- Monitor circulatory, respiratory, bowel, and bladder functions carefully. May cause transient BP decrease. May worsen or mask gallbladder pain.
- May cause CNS depression, hypotension, urine retention, nausea, vomiting, or ileus. *(continued)*

†Canadian †Australian

DRUG/CLASS/ CATEGORY	INDICATIONS/ DOSAGES	KEY NURSING CONSIDERATIONS
morphine (continued) Pregnancy Risk Category: C Controlled Substance Schedule: II	shouldn't exceed 10 mg/24 hr. **Children:** 0.1 to 0.2 mg/kg S.C. or I.M. q 4 hr. Maximum single dose 15 mg.	• Withhold dose and notify doctor if respirations < 12. • Tell patient not to crush, break, or chew controlled-release tablets.
mumps virus vaccine, live Mumpsvax Vaccine Viral vaccine Pregnancy Risk Category: C	*Immunization* — **Adults and children ≥ 1 yr:** 0.5 ml (20,000 U) S.C.	• Obtain history of allergies, especially anaphylactic reactions to antibiotics, and reaction to immunization. • Keep epinephrine 1:1,000 available to treat anaphylaxis. • Use only diluent supplied. Discard 8 hr after reconstituting.
mupirocin Bactroban Antibiotic Topical antibacterial Pregnancy Risk Category: B	*Impetigo* — **Adults and children:** apply to affected areas t.i.d. for 1 to 2 wk.	• Wash and dry affected area thoroughly. Apply thin film, rubbing in gently. • If no improvement in 3 to 5 days, tell patient to notify doctor immediately. • Warn patient about local adverse reactions.
mycophenolate mofetil CellCept **mycophenolate mofetil hydrochloride**	*Prophylaxis of organ rejection in patients receiving allogenic cardiac and renal transplants* — **Adults:** 1 g P.O. or I.V. b.i.d. (renal transplant) or 1.5 g P.O. or I.V. b.i.d. (cardiac transplant) within 72 hr after transplantation, together with corticosteroids and	• Potential teratogenic effects. Don't open or crush capsule. Avoid inhaling powder in capsule or letting it contact skin or mucous membranes. If contact occurs, wash with soap and water and rinse eyes with plain water.

CellCept Intravenous
Mycophenolic acid derivative
Immunosuppressant
Pregnancy Risk Category: C

cyclosporine.
Adjust-a-dose: In patients with severe chronic renal impairment outside of immediate transplant period, avoid doses > 1 g b.i.d. If neutropenia occurs, interrupt or reduce dose.

- Stress importance of not stopping therapy without consulting doctor.
- Monitor CBC regularly, as ordered.
- Tell woman to use contraception during therapy and for 6 wk after discontinuation. Dilute infusion to 6 mg/dl in D_5W and infuse over ≥ 2 hr.

---

nabumetone
Relafen
NSAID
Antarthritic
Pregnancy Risk Category: C

Rheumatoid arthritis; osteoarthritis —
Adults: initially, 1,000 mg P.O. q.d. as single dose or in divided doses b.i.d. Maximum 2,000 mg q.d.

- May lead to reversible renal impairment.
- May cause serious GI toxicity. Teach patient about signs and symptoms of GI bleeding.
- With long-term therapy, monitor renal and liver function, CBC, and Hct.

---

nadolol
Corgard
Beta blocker
Antihypertensive/anti-anginal
Pregnancy Risk Category: C

Long-standing angina pectoris — **Adults:** 40 mg P.O. q.d. Increased in 40- to 80-mg increments until optimum response occurs. Usual maintenance dose 40 to 80 mg q.d. *Hypertension —* **Adults:** 40 mg P.O. q.d. Increased in 40- to 80-mg increments until optimum response occurs. Usual maintenance dose 40 to 80 mg q.d. Doses of 320 mg may be needed.
Adjust-a-dose: In renally impaired patients, dosage interval adjusted according to creatinine clearance.

- Check apical pulse before giving. If < 60, withhold dose and call doctor. Monitor BP frequently. If severe hypotension occurs, give vasopressor, as prescribed.
- Masks signs of shock and hyperthyroidism.
- Abrupt discontinuation can exacerbate angina and trigger MI. Reduce dosage gradually over 1 to 2 wk.

---

nafcillin sodium
Nallpen, Unipen

Systemic infections caused by penicillinase-producing staphylococci — **Adults:** 2 to 4 g P.O. q.d. in divided doses q 6 hr; or 2 to

- Ask about allergic reactions to penicillin. Obtain specimen for culture and sensitivity tests before 1st dose.

(continued)

DRUG/CLASS/ CATEGORY	INDICATIONS/ DOSAGES	KEY NURSING CONSIDERATIONS
nafcillin sodium *(continued)* *Penicillinase-resistant penicillin* *Antibiotic* Pregnancy Risk Category: B	12 g I.M. or I.V. q.d. in divided doses q 4 to 6 hr. **Children:** 25 to 50 mg/kg P.O. q.d. in divided doses q 6 hr. **Neonates:** 25 mg/kg I.V. b.i.d.	• Give P.O. 1 to 2 hr before or 2 to 3 hr after meals. • Give > 1 hr before bacteriostatic antibiotics.
nalbuphine hydrochloride Nubain *Narcotic agonist-antagonist/opioid partial agonist* *Analgesic/adjunct to anesthesia* Pregnancy Risk Category: NR	*Moderate to severe pain* — **Adults:** For typical (70-kg [154 lb]) person, give 10 to 20 mg S.C., I.M., or I.V. q 3 to 6 hr, p.r.n. Maximum 160 mg q.d. *Adjunct to balanced anesthesia* — **Adults:** 0.3 to 3 mg/kg I.V. over 10 to 15 min, then maintenance doses of 0.25 to 0.50 mg/kg in single I.V. dose, p.r.n.	• Causes respiratory depression, which can be reversed with naloxone. Monitor circulatory and respiratory status and bladder and bowel function. • Acts as narcotic antagonist; may trigger withdrawal syndrome. • *I.V. use:* Inject slowly over at least 2 to 3 min into vein or into I.V. line containing compatible, free-flowing I.V. solution.
naloxone hydrochloride Narcan *Narcotic (opioid) antagonist* *Narcotic antagonist* Pregnancy Risk Category: B	*Known or suspected narcotic-induced respiratory depression* — **Adults:** 0.4 to 2 mg I.V., S.C., or I.M. repeated q 2 to 3 min, p.r.n. If no response after 10 mg given, reconsider diagnosis of narcotic-induced toxicity. **Children:** 0.01 mg/kg I.V., followed by 2nd dose of 0.1 mg/kg I.V., if needed. If I.V. route not available, may give I.M. or S.C. in divided doses. **Neonates:** 0.01 mg/kg I.V., I.M., or	• Abrupt reversal of opiate-induced CNS depression may result in nausea, vomiting, diaphoresis, tachycardia, tachypnea, CNS excitement, and increased BP. • Monitor respiratory depth and rate. Be prepared to provide oxygen, ventilation, and other resuscitation measures. • *I.V. use:* Be prepared to administer continuous I.V. infusion. If 0.02 mg/ml not

available, may dilute adult concentration (0.4 mg) by mixing 0.5 ml with 9.5 sterile water or 0.9% NaCl for injection to make neonatal concentration (0.02 mg/ml).

S.C. May repeat dose q 2 to 3 min, p.r.n.

Postoperative narcotic depression —
Adults: 0.1 to 0.2 mg I.V. q 2 to 3 min, p.r.n. May repeat dosage within 1 to 2 hr, if needed. **Children:** 0.005 to 0.01 mg I.V. Repeat q 2 to 3 min, p.r.n. **Neonates (asphyxia neonatorum):** 0.01 mg/kg I.V. into umbilical vein. May repeat q 2 to 3 min.

---

naltrexone hydrochloride
ReVia
Narcotic (opioid) antagonist
Narcotic detoxification adjunct
Pregnancy Risk Category: C

Adjunct for maintenance of opioid-free state in detoxified individuals — **Adults:** 25 mg P.O. If no withdrawal signs < 1 hr, give additional 25 mg. When patient on 50 mg q 24 hr, may use flexible maintenance schedule. *Treatment of alcohol dependence —* **Adults:** 50 mg P.O. q.d.

- Treatment for opioid dependency should not begin until patient receives naloxone challenge. If signs of withdrawal persist, don't give naltrexone.
- Patient must be completely opioid-free before taking, or severe withdrawal symptoms may occur.

---

naphazoline hydrochloride (ophthalmic)
Allerest, Clear Eyes, Optazine†, VasoClear
Sympathomimetic
Decongestant/vasoconstrictor
Pregnancy Risk Category: C

Ocular congestion, irritation, itching —
Adults: 1 drop 0.1% solution instilled q 3 to 4 hr, or 1 drop 0.012% to 0.03% solution up to q.i.d.

- Wash hands before and after instilling. Apply light finger pressure on lacrimal sac. Don't touch dropper tip to eye or surrounding tissue.
- Notify doctor if photophobia, blurred vision, pain, or lid edema develops.
- Instruct patient not to use OTC preparations > 72 hr without consulting doctor.

---

naphazoline hydrochloride (nasal)
Privine
Sympathomimetic

Nasal congestion — **Adults and children ≥ 12 yr:** 2 drops or sprays instilled in each nostril q 3 to 4 hr (drops) or 3 to 6 hr (spray). **Children 6 to 12 yr:** 1 to 2 drops or

- For drops, instruct patient to tilt head back, instill drops, then lean head forward while inhaling, and then repeat procedure *(continued)*

DRUG/CLASS/ CATEGORY	INDICATIONS/ DOSAGES	KEY NURSING CONSIDERATIONS
naphazoline hydro-chloride (nasal) *(continued)* *Decongestant/vasoconstrictor* Pregnancy Risk Category: NR	sprays instilled in each nostril q 3 to 6 hr, p.r.n. Don't use > 3 to 5 days.	for other nostril. For spray, instruct patient to hold spray container and head upright. Tell him not to shake spray.
naproxen Inza 250‡, Naprosyn, Naprosyn SR†‡, Novo-Naprox† **naproxen sodium** Aleve, Anaprox, Apo-Napro-Na†, Naprelan, Napro-gesic‡, Synflex† *NSAID* *Nonnarcotic analgesic/antipyretic/anti-inflammatory* Pregnancy Risk Category: B	*Rheumatoid arthritis; osteoarthritis; ankylosing spondylitis; pain; dysmenorrhea; tendinitis; bursitis* — **Adults:** 250 to 500 mg (naproxen) b.i.d., maximum 1.5 g/day. Or, 375 to 500 mg delayed-release (EC-Naprosyn) b.i.d.; or 750 to 1,000 mg controlled-release (Naprelan) b.i.d.; or 275 to 550 mg naproxen sodium b.i.d. *Juvenile arthritis* — **Children:** 10 mg/kg P.O. in 2 divided doses. *Acute gout* — **Adults:** 750 mg (naproxen) P.O., then 250 mg q 8 hr until attack subsides. Or, 825 mg naproxen sodium, then 275 mg q 8 hr until attack subsides; or 1,000 to 1,500 mg/day controlled-release (Naprelan) on 1st day, then 1,000 mg q.d. *Mild to moderate pain* — **Adults:** 500 mg (naproxen) P.O., then 250 mg q 6 to 8 hr, up to 1.25 g/day. Or, 550 mg naproxen sodium, then 275 mg q 6 to 8 hr, up to 1.375 g/day; or 1,000 mg controlled-release (Naprelan) q.d.	• May lead to reversible renal impairment, especially in preexisting renal failure, liver dysfunction, or heart failure, and in elderly patients and patients taking diuretics. • Serious GI toxicity, including peptic ulcers and bleeding, can occur despite absence of GI symptoms. Teach patient about signs and symptoms of GI bleeding, and tell him to contact doctor immediately if they occur. • Caution that use with aspirin, alcohol, or corticosteroids may increase risk of adverse GI reactions. • May mask signs and symptoms of infection. • Warn against activities that require mental alertness until CNS effects known. • Advise patient to take with food or milk to minimize GI upset. Instruct to take each dose with full glass of water or other fluid. • If patient taking for arthritis, inform him that full therapeutic effect may be delayed 2 to 4 wk.

naratriptan hydrochloride
Amerge
Selective 5-hydroxy-tryptamine₁ receptor–subtype agonist
Antimigraine
Pregnancy Risk Category: C

Acute migraine headache attacks with or without aura — **Adults:** 1 or 2.5 mg P.O. as single dose. If headache returns or if only partial response occurs, may repeat dose after 4 hr; maximum 5 mg within 24 hr.
Adjust-a-dose: In patients with renal or hepatic impairment, use lower initial dose. Maximum dose 2.5 mg/24 hr.

- Use cautiously in patients with risk factors for CAD unless CV evaluation shows patient doesn't have cardiac disease.
- Can cause coronary artery vasospasm and increase risk of cerebrovascular events.
- Don't use for prophylactic therapy in managing hemiplegic or basilar migraine.

---

nedocromil sodium
Tilade
Pyranoquinoline
Anti-inflammatory respiratory inhalant
Pregnancy Risk Category: B

Maintenance in mild to moderate bronchial asthma — **Adults and children ≥ 12 yr:** 2 inhalations q.i.d. at regular intervals.

- Slow onset. Shouldn't be used during acute bronchospasm; isn't therapeutic in aborting acute attack.
- Must use regularly, even during symptom-free periods.

---

nefazodone hydrochloride
Serzone
Phenylpiperazine
Antidepressant
Pregnancy Risk Category: C

Depression — **Adults:** initially, 200 mg/day P.O. in 2 divided doses. Increase in increments of 100 to 200 mg/day at intervals of no less than 1 wk, p.r.n. Usual range 300 to 600 mg/day. Several wk may be required for full effect. **Elderly:** 50 mg P.O. b.i.d.
Adjust-a-dose: In debilitated patients, initially, 50 mg.

- At least 1 wk should elapse between stopping nefazodone and starting MAO inhibitor; at least 2 wk before starting nefazodone after MAO inhibitor therapy ends.
- Monitor for suicidal tendencies.
- Warn patient not to engage in hazardous activity until CNS effects known.

---

nelfinavir mesylate
Viracept
HIV protease inhibitor
Antiviral
Pregnancy Risk Category: B

HIV infection when antiretroviral therapy is warranted — **Adults:** 750 mg P.O. t.i.d. **Children 2 to 13 yr:** 20 to 30 mg/kg/dose P.O. t.i.d. Maximum 750 mg t.i.d.

- Monitor liver function test results.
- Administer oral powder to children unable to take tablets. Know that mixing with acidic foods or juice creates a bitter taste.
- Give with meals or a light snack.

227

†Canadian ‡Australian

DRUG/CLASS/ CATEGORY	INDICATIONS/ DOSAGES	KEY NURSING CONSIDERATIONS
neomycin sulfate (oral) Mycifradin, Neo-fradin, Neosulf†, Neo-Tabs *Aminoglycoside* *Antibiotic* Pregnancy Risk Category: NR	*Infectious diarrhea caused by* E. coli — **Adults:** 50 mg/kg P.O. in 4 divided doses for 2 to 3 days; maximum 3 g q.d. **Children:** 50 to 100 mg/kg q.d. P.O. divided q 4 to 6 hr for 2 to 3 days. *Suppression of intestinal bacteria preoperatively* — **Adults:** 1 g P.O. q hr for 4 doses, then 1 g q 4 hr for balance of 24 hr. Saline cathartic should precede therapy. **Children:** 50 to 100 mg/kg q.d. P.O. divided q 4 to 6 hr. First dose should follow saline cathartic.	• Monitor renal function (output, specific gravity, urinalysis, BUN, creatinine level, and creatinine clearance). Notify doctor of signs of decreasing renal function. • Evaluate hearing before, during, and after prolonged therapy. • For preoperative disinfection, provide low-residue diet and cathartic immediately before oral administration, as ordered.
neomycin sulfate (topical) Mycifradin†, Myciguent *Aminoglycoside* *Antibiotic* Pregnancy Risk Category: C	*Prevention or treatment of superficial bacterial infections* — **Adults and children:** rub into affected area q.d. to t.i.d.	• More absorption occurs on abraded areas. • Watch for signs of hypersensitivity and ototoxicity. • If no improvement or if condition worsens, tell patient to stop using and notify doctor.
neostigmine bromide/neostigmine methylsulfate Prostigmin *Cholinesterase inhibitor* *Muscle stimulant* Pregnancy Risk Category: C	*Symptomatic control of myasthenia gravis* — **Adults:** 0.5 mg S.C. or I.M. dose from 15 to 375 mg/day. Later dosages individualized. **Children:** 7.5 to 15 mg P.O. t.i.d. to q.i.d. *Diagnosis of myasthenia gravis* — **Adults:** 0.022 mg/kg I.M. 30 min after atropine I.M. **Children:** 0.025 to 0.04 mg/kg I.M. after atropine S.C.	• In myasthenia gravis, schedule doses between periods of fatigue. • *I.V. use:* Give at slow, controlled rate, not exceeding 1 mg/min in adults and 0.5 mg/min in children. • Monitor vital signs frequently, especially respirations. Have atropine injection available to give, as ordered;

	Postoperative abdominal distention and bladder atony — **Adults:** 0.5 to 1 mg I.M. or S.C. q 3 hr for 5 doses after bladder has emptied. *Antidote for nondepolarizing neuromuscular blocking agents* — **Adults:** 0.5 to 2 mg I.V. slowly. Repeat, p.r.n. to total of 5 mg. Before antidote dose, give atropine I.V.	provide respiratory support, as needed. • Monitor and document response after each dose. Optimum dosage hard to judge. Observe closely for improvement in strength, vision, and ptosis 45 to 60 min after each dose. • Resistance to drug may occur.
nevirapine Viramune *Nonnucleoside reverse transcriptase inhibitor* *Antiviral* Pregnancy Risk Category: C	*Adjunctive treatment in patients with HIV-1 infection who have experienced clinical or immunologic deterioration* —**Adults:** 200 mg P.O. q.d. for first 14 days, then 200 mg P.O. b.i.d. Used in combination with nucleoside analogue antiretroviral agents.	• Monitor liver function tests. • If therapy interrupted for > 7 days, restart as if administering for first time. • Advise women not to use hormonal birth control methods. • Notify doctor if severe rash occurs.
niacin (vitamin B₃, nicotinic acid) Niac, Niacor, Nico-400, Nicobid, Nicolar **niacinamide (nicotinamide)** *B-complex vitamin* *Vitamin B₃/antilipemic/ peripheral vasodilator* Pregnancy Risk Category: C	*Pellagra* — **Adults:** 300 to 500 mg P.O., S.C., I.M., or I.V. q.d. in divided doses, depending on severity of deficiency. **Children:** up to 300 mg P.O. q.d. in divided doses, depending on severity of niacin deficiency. *Hyperlipidemias, especially with hypercholesterolemia (niacin only)* — **Adults:** 1 to 2 g P.O. t.i.d. with or after meals, increased at intervals to 6 g q.d.	• *I.V. use:* Give no faster than 2 mg/min. • If needed, administer aspirin to possibly reduce flushing response. • Stress that niacin is potent medication, not just vitamin, and may cause serious adverse effects. Explain importance of adhering to therapeutic regimen. • Monitor hepatic function and blood glucose level early in therapy. • Give with meals.
nicardipine Cardene, Cardene IV, Cardene SR	*Chronic stable angina, hypertension* — **Adults:** initially, 20 mg P.O. t.i.d. (immediate-release only). Adjust to response q 3	• *I.V. use:* When switching to P.O. therapy other than nicardipine, initiate when infu- *(continued)*

†Canadian ‡Australian

DRUG/CLASS/ CATEGORY	INDICATIONS/ DOSAGES	KEY NURSING CONSIDERATIONS
nicardipine *(continued)* *Calcium channel blocker* *Antianginal/antihypertensive* Pregnancy Risk Category: C	days. Usual range 20 to 40 mg t.i.d. Usual range 30 to 60 mg (SR) b.i.d. *Short-term management of hypertension —* **Adults:** if unable to take oral nicardipine, give 5 mg/hr I.V. infusion, titrated to 2.5 mg/hr q 15 min to maximum 15 mg/hr.	sion stopped. If P.O. nicardipine to be used, give first dose of t.i.d. regimen 1 hr before infusion stopped. ▪ Measure BP frequently during initial therapy. Check for orthostatic hypotension. Adjust rate if hypotension or tachycardia occurs. ▪ Tell patient to report chest pain immediately.
nicotine polacrilex (nicotine resin complex) Nicorette, Nicorette DS *Nicotinic agonist* *Smoking cessation aid* Pregnancy Risk Category: X	*Relief of nicotine withdrawal symptoms in patients undergoing smoking cessation —* **Adults:** initially, one 2-mg square; highly dependent patients should start with 4-mg. Patients should chew 1 piece of gum slowly and intermittently for 30 min whenever urge occurs. Most require 9 to 12 pieces daily during first mo. For patients using 4-mg squares, maximum 20 pieces daily. For patients using 2-mg squares, maximum 30 pieces daily.	▪ Instruct patient to chew gum slowly and intermittently (chew several times; then place between cheek and gum) for about 30 min. Fast chewing tends to produce more adverse reactions. ▪ Most likely to benefit smokers with high physical nicotine dependence.
nicotine transdermal system Habitrol, Nicoderm, Nicotrol, ProStep *Nicotinic cholinergic agonist* *Smoking cessation aid* Pregnancy Risk Category: D	*Relief of nicotine withdrawal symptoms in patients undergoing smoking cessation —* **Adults:** initially, 1 transdermal system, delivering largest available nicotine dose in series, applied q.d. to nonhairy body part. For Habitrol, Nicoderm, and ProStep, patch should be kept on 24 hr, then removed and new system applied to alternate skin site. For Nicotrol,	▪ To reduce exposure to nicotine, avoid unnecessary contact with system. Wash hands with water alone; soap may enhance absorption. ▪ Teach patient proper disposal to prevent accidental poisoning of children or pets. ▪ Warn patient not to smoke.

patch should be applied on awakening and removed h.s. After 4 to 12 wk, taper to next lowest dose in series, followed in 2 to 4 wk by lowest system in series being used. Drug then stopped in 2 to 4 wk.		▪ Advise patient to apply patch promptly. Patch should not be altered in any way (folded or cut) before application.
nifedipine Adalat, Adalat CC, Adapinet, Apo-Nifedt, Nu-Nifedt, Procardia, Procardia XL *Calcium channel blocker* *Antianginal* Pregnancy Risk Category: C	*Prinzmetal's (variant) angina* — **Adults:** starting dose 10 mg P.O. t.i.d. Usual effective range 10 to 20 mg t.i.d. Maximum 180 mg q.d. *Hypertension* — **Adults:** 30 or 60 mg P.O. q.d. Adjust over 7 to 14 days. Doses > 90 mg (for Adalat CC) and 120 mg (for Procardia XL) aren't recommended.	▪ When rapid response to drug desired, have patient bite and swallow capsule. Continuous BP and ECG monitoring recommended. ▪ Patient may briefly develop anginal exacerbation.
nilutamide Anandron, Nilandron *Hormone* *Antiandrogen* Pregnancy Risk Category: C	*Adjunct therapy with surgical castration for treatment of metastatic prostate cancer* — **Adults:** 6 tablets (50 mg each) P.O. for total of 300 mg/day for 30 days; then 3 tablets q.d. for total of 150 mg/day thereafter.	▪ Used with surgical castration; should begin on same day or day after surgery for maximum benefit. ▪ Tell patient to report dyspnea or aggravation of preexisting dyspnea immediately.
nisoldipine Sular *Calcium channel blocker* *Antihypertensive* Pregnancy Risk Category: C	*Hypertension* — **Adults:** 20 mg (10 mg if patient > 65 or has liver dysfunction) P.O. q.d.; increased by 10 mg/wk or at longer intervals, p.r.n. Usual maintenance dosage 20 to 40 mg/day. Doses > 60 mg/day not recommended.	▪ Monitor carefully. Some patients experience increased frequency, duration, or severity of angina or even acute MI after starting drug or when dosage increased. ▪ Monitor BP regularly.
nitrofurantoin macrocrystals Macrobid, Macrodantin **nitrofurantoin microcrystals** Macrodantin	*UTIs caused by susceptible organisms* — **Adults and children > 12 yr:** 50 to 100 mg P.O. q.i.d. with meals and h.s. **Children 1 mo to 12 yr:** 5 to 7 mg/kg P.O. q.d. divided q.i.d. *Long-term suppression therapy* — **Adults:**	▪ Obtain urine specimen for culture and sensitivity tests before therapy. ▪ May cause growth of nonsusceptible organisms.

(continued)

†Canadian ‡Australian

DRUG/CLASS/ CATEGORY	INDICATIONS/ DOSAGES	KEY NURSING CONSIDERATIONS
nitrofurantoin *(continued)* Furadantin, Macrodantin *Nitrofuran* Urinary tract anti-infective Pregnancy Risk Category: B	50 to 100 mg P.O. q.d. h.s. **Children:** 1 mg/kg P.O. q.d. in single dose h.s. or divided into 2 doses.	▪ Give with food or milk to minimize GI distress and improve absorption. ▪ Monitor fluid I&O carefully. May turn urine brown or darker.
nitrofurazone Furacin *Synthetic antibacterial nitrofuran derivative* Topical antibacterial Pregnancy Risk Category: C	*Adjunctive treatment of second- and third-degree burns; prevention of skin allograft rejection —* **Adults and children:** Apply directly to lesion daily or q few days, depending on burn severity. May also apply to dressings used to cover affected area.	▪ Clean wound, as indicated by doctor, before reapplying dressings. ▪ When using wet dressing, protect skin around wound with zinc oxide ointment. ▪ Report irritation, sensitization, or infection.
nitroglycerin (glyceryl trinitrate) Anginine‡, Nitro-Bid, Nitrocine, Nitrodisc, Nitro-Dur, Nitrogard, Nitroglyn, Nitrol, Nitrolingual, Nitrostat, Transderm-Nitro, Transiderm-Nitro‡, Tridil *Nitrate* Antianginal/vasodilator Pregnancy Risk Category: C	*Prophylaxis against chronic anginal attacks —* **Adults:** 2.5 mg or 2.6 mg sustained-release capsule q 8 to 12 hr. Or, use 2% ointment range ½" to 5". Or, transdermal disc or pad 0.2 to 0.4 mg/hr q.d. *Acute angina pectoris; prophylaxis to prevent or minimize anginal attacks —* **Adults:** 1 S.L. tablet. Repeat q 5 min, p.r.n., for 15 min. Or, using Nitrolingual, 1 or 2 sprays into mouth. Repeat q 3 to 5 min, p.r.n., to maximum 3 doses in 15-min period. Or, 1 to 3 mg transmucosally q 3 to 5 hr during waking hours. *Hypertension; heart failure; acute angina*	▪ Advise patient that abrupt drug discontinuation can cause coronary vasospasms. ▪ Closely monitor vital signs during infusion. Excessive hypotension may worsen MI. ▪ Measure prescribed amount on application paper; then place on nonhairy area. Don't rub in. Cover with plastic film. If using Tape-Surrounded Appli-Ruler (TSAR) system, keep TSAR on skin to protect clothing. ▪ Remove transdermal patch before defibrillation.

	pectoris; to produce controlled hypotension during surgery (by I.V. infusion) — **Adults:** 5 mcg/min, increased p.r.n. by 5 mcg/min q 3 to 5 min until response.	▪ Keep S.L. tablets capped in original container. Protect from heat and moisture.
nitroprusside sodium Nitropress *Vasodilator Antihypertensive* Pregnancy Risk Category: C	*Hypertensive emergencies* — **Adults and children:** 50-mg vial diluted with 2 to 3 ml of D₅W and added to 250, 500, or 1,000 ml of D₅W; solution titrated at 0.3 to 10 mcg/min titrated to BP. Maximum rate 10 mcg/kg/min. *Acute heart failure* — **Adults and children:** I.V. infusion titrated to cardiac output and systemic BP. Same dosage range as for hypertensive emergencies.	▪ Obtain vital signs and parameters before giving. Check BP q 5 min at start and then q 15 min. If severe hypotension occurs, stop infusion and notify doctor. Check serum thiocyanate levels q 72 hr. Levels > 100 mcg/ml associated with toxicity. ▪ Sensitive to light; wrap I.V. solution in foil. Fresh solution should have faint brownish tint. Don't piggyback with other drugs.
nizatidine Axid, Axid AR, Tazac‡ *H₂-receptor antagonist Antiulcer agent* Pregnancy Risk Category: C	*Active duodenal ulcer* — **Adults:** 300 mg P.O. q.d. h.s. Or, 150 mg P.O. b.i.d. *Maintenance therapy for duodenal ulcer* — **Adults:** 150 mg P.O. q.d. h.s. *Benign gastric ulcer* — **Adults:** 150 mg P.O. b.i.d. or 300 mg h.s. for 8 wk. *Gastroesophageal reflux disease* — **Adults:** 150 mg P.O. b.i.d.	▪ Tell patient with trouble swallowing capsules that contents may be mixed with apple juice but not with tomato-based juices. ▪ Encourage patient to avoid cigarette smoking; may increase gastric acid secretion and worsen disease. ▪ Increases serum salicylate levels when used with high doses of aspirin.
norepinephrine bitartrate Levophed *Adrenergic Vasopressor* Pregnancy Risk Category: C	*To maintain BP in acute hypotensive states* — **Adults:** initially, 8 to 12 mcg/min I.V. infusion, then adjust to maintain normal BP. Average maintenance dose 2 to 4 mcg/min. **Children:** 2 mcg/m²/min I.V. infusion. Adjust dose per response.	▪ Check BP q 2 min until stabilized; then q 5 min. Frequently monitor ECG, cardiac output, CVP, PAWP, pulse rate, urine output, and color and temperature of extremities. Phentolamine is antidote for extravasation. ▪ When stopping, gradually slow rate.

233

DRUG / CLASS / CATEGORY	INDICATIONS / DOSAGES	KEY NURSING CONSIDERATIONS
norethindrone Micronor, Nor-Q.D. **norethindrone acetate** Aygestin, Norlutate *Progestin* *Contraceptive* Pregnancy Risk Category: X	*Amenorrhea; abnormal uterine bleeding* — **Adults:** 2.5 to 20 mg P.O. q.d. on days 5 to 25 of menstrual cycle. *Endometriosis* — **Adults:** 5 to 10 mg P.O. q.d. for 14 days; then increase by 2.5 to 5 mg q.d. q 2 wk up to 15 mg q.d. *Contraception in women* — **Adults:** initially, 0.35 mg norethindrone P.O. on 1st day of menstruation; then 0.35 mg q.d.	▪ Norethindrone acetate twice as potent as norethindrone. Acetate shouldn't be used for contraception. ▪ Watch carefully for signs of edema. ▪ Tell patient to report unusual symptoms immediately and to stop drug and call doctor if visual disturbances or migraine occurs.
norfloxacin Noroxin *Fluoroquinolone* *Broad-spectrum antibiotic* Pregnancy Risk Category: C	*UTIs caused by susceptible organisms* — **Adults:** for uncomplicated infections, 400 mg P.O. q 12 hr for 7 to 10 days. For complicated infections, 400 mg P.O. q 12 hr for 10 to 21 days. *Acute uncomplicated urethral, cervical gonorrhea* — **Adults:** 800 mg P.O. as single dose.	▪ Advise patient to take 1 hr before or 2 hr after meals. ▪ Tell patient to drink several glasses of water throughout day. ▪ Caution patient to avoid hazardous tasks that require alertness until CNS effects known.
norgestrel Ovrette *Progestin* *Contraceptive* Pregnancy Risk Category: X	*Contraception in women* — **Adults:** 0.075 mg P.O. q.d.	▪ Instruct patient to take q day at same time, even if menstruating.
nortriptyline hydrochloride Allegron‡, Aventyl, Pamelor *TCA*	*Depression* — **Adults:** 25 mg P.O. t.i.d. or q.i.d., gradually increased to maximum 150 mg q.d. Entire dosage may be given h.s. Monitor plasma levels when giving doses >	▪ Adverse anticholinergic effects can occur rapidly. ▪ Warn patient to avoid activities that require alertness until CNS effects known.

Antidepressant Pregnancy Risk Category: NR	100 mg/day. **Elderly:** 30 to 50 mg P.O. q.d. given once or in divided doses.		▪ Tell patient to consult doctor before taking other prescription or OTC drugs.
nystatin Mycostatin, Nadostine†, Nilstat, Nystex *Polyene macrolide* *Antifungal* Pregnancy Risk Category: C	*Intestinal candidiasis* — **Adults:** 500,000 to 1 million U as oral tablets t.i.d. *Oral infections* — **Adults and children:** 400,000 to 600,000 U oral suspension q.i.d. **Infants:** 200,000 U oral suspension q.i.d. **Neonates and premature infants:** 100,000 U oral suspension q.i.d. *Vaginal infections* — **Adults:** 100,000 U (tablets) high into vagina q.d. for 14 days.		▪ Not effective against systemic infections. ▪ Pregnant patients can use vaginal tablets up to 6 wk before term. ▪ For treatment of oral candidiasis (thrush): After mouth cleaned of food debris, instruct patient to hold suspension in mouth for several min before swallowing. When treating infants, swab medication on oral mucosa.
octreotide acetate Sandostatin, Sandostatin LAR *Synthetic octapeptide* *Somatotropic hormone* *Somatostatin hormone* Pregnancy Risk Category: B	*Flushing and diarrhea associated with carcinoid tumors* — **Adults:** 100 to 600 mcg q.d. S.C. in 2 to 4 divided doses for 1st 2 wk of therapy, then dose per response. *Watery diarrhea associated with vasoactive intestinal polypeptide secreting tumors* — **Adults:** 200 to 300 mcg q.d. S.C. in 2 to 4 divided doses for 1st 2 wk of therapy. *Acromegaly* — **Adults:** initially, 50 mcg S.C. t.i.d. then adjusted according to somatomedin C levels q 2 wk. May switch patients currently receiving Sandostatin injection directly to depot. Give 20 mg I.M. intragluteally q 4 wk for 3 mo, then adjust dose according to growth hormone levels.		▪ LAR preparation for intragluteal use only. ▪ Monitor somatomedin C levels q 2 wk, as ordered. ▪ Monitor thyroid function tests, urine 5-hydroxin-doleacetic acid, plasma serotonin, and substance P. ▪ May be linked to development of cholelithiasis. ▪ Monitor closely for symptoms of glucose imbalance.

DRUG/CLASS/ CATEGORY	INDICATIONS/ DOSAGES	KEY NURSING CONSIDERATIONS
ofloxacin Floxin, Floxin I.V. *Fluoroquinolone* *Antibiotic* Pregnancy Risk Category: C	*Lower respiratory tract infections* — **Adults:** 400 mg I.V. or P.O. q 12 hr for 10 days. *Cervicitis; urethritis* — **Adults:** 300 mg I.V. or P.O. q 12 hr for 7 days. *Acute, uncomplicated gonorrhea* — **Adults:** 400 mg I.V. or P.O. as single dose with doxycycline. *Mild to moderate skin infections* — **Adults:** 400 mg I.V. or P.O. q 12 hr for 10 days. *Cystitis; UTI* — **Adults:** 200 mg I.V. or P.O. q 12 hr for 3 to 7 days. *Prostatitis* — **Adults:** 300 mg I.V. or P.O. q 12 hr for 6 wk. *Pelvic inflammatory disease (outpatient)* — **Adults:** 400 mg P.O. q 12 hr for 14 days. *Adjust-a-dose:* Dose or interval decrease necessary in patients with renal failure.	▪ Use cautiously and with dosage adjustment in renal failure, as prescribed. ▪ Give serologic test for syphilis to patient treated for gonorrhea. Drug not effective against syphilis; gonorrhea treatment may mask or delay symptoms of syphilis. ▪ Advise patient to take with plenty of fluids but not with meals. ▪ Instruct patient to stop drug and notify doctor if rash or other hypersensitivity signs occur. ▪ Advise patient to use sunscreen and wear protective clothing.
olanzapine Zyprexa *Dibenzepine* *Antipsychotic* Pregnancy Risk Category: C	*Psychotic disorders* — **Adults:** initially, 5 to 10 mg P.O. q.d. Dose adjustments in 5-mg daily increments should occur at intervals of not less than 1 wk. Most patients respond to 10 mg/day. Don't exceed 20 mg/day.	▪ Monitor for signs of neuroleptic malignant syndrome. Stop drug immediately. ▪ Monitor for tardive dyskinesia. ▪ Obtain baseline and periodic liver function tests.
olsalazine sodium Dipentum *Salicylate*	*Maintenance of remission of ulcerative colitis in patients intolerant of sulfasalazine* — **Adults:** 500 mg P.O. b.i.d. with meals.	▪ Regularly monitor BUN, creatinine, and urinalysis in preexisting renal disease. ▪ Administer in divided doses and with food

Anti-inflammatory
Pregnancy Risk Category: C

omeprazole
Losec‡, Prilosec
Substituted benzimidazole
Gastric acid suppressant
Pregnancy Risk Category: C

Severe erosive esophagitis; gastroesophageal reflux disease — **Adults:** 20 mg P.O. q.d. for 4 to 8 wk.

Hypersecretory conditions — **Adults:** 60 mg P.O. q.d.; adjust to response. If dose > 80 mg, give in divided doses.

Duodenal ulcer — **Adults:** 20 mg P.O. q.d. for 4 to 8 wk.

Active benign gastric ulcer — **Adults:** 40 mg P.O. q.d. for 4 to 8 wk.

Treatment of H. pylori — **Adults:** 40 mg P.O. q morning with clarithromycin for 14 days, then 20 mg q.d. for 14 days.

to minimize adverse GI reactions.

- Increases its own bioavailability with repeated doses.
- Caution patient not to perform hazardous activities if dizziness occurs.
- Instruct patient to swallow tablets whole.
- Advise patient to report signs and symptoms of overdose: confusion, drowsiness, blurred vision, tachycardia, nausea and vomiting, diaphoresis, dry mouth, and headache.

ondansetron hydrochloride
Zofran
Serotonin (5-HT₃) receptor antagonist
Antiemetic
Pregnancy Risk Category: B

Prevention of nausea and vomiting associated with chemotherapy — **Adults and children ≥ 12 yr:** 8 mg P.O. 30 min before chemotherapy. Then 8 mg P.O. 8 hr after 1st dose, then 8 mg q 12 hr for 1 to 2 days. Or, single dose of 32 mg by I.V. infusion over 15 min, given 30 min before chemotherapy; or 3 divided doses of 0.15 mg/kg I.V. given over 15 min, 4 and 8 hr after 1st dose (30 min before chemotherapy). **Children 4 to 12 yr:** 4 mg P.O. 30 min before chemotherapy. Then 4 mg P.O. 4 and 8 hr after 1st dose, then 4 mg q 8 hr for 1 to 2 days. Or, 3 doses of 0.15

- Instruct patient to alert nurse immediately if difficulty breathing occurs after dose taken.
- Dilute I.V. form in 50 ml 5% dextrose or 0.9% NaCl solution before administering.
- Tell patient receiving I.V. form to report discomfort at insertion site promptly.
- Generally well tolerated. Common adverse reactions include headache, malaise, dizziness, sedation, diarrhea or constipation, and musculoskeletal pain.

(continued)

†Canadian ‡Australian

DRUG / CLASS / CATEGORY	INDICATIONS / DOSAGES	KEY NURSING CONSIDERATIONS
ondansetron hydrochloride *(continued)*	mg/kg I.V., given as for adults. *Prevention of nausea and vomiting associated with radiotherapy —* **Adults:** 8 mg P.O. t.i.d.	• Mix with sufficient water to ensure passage to stomach. • For overdose, use narcotic antagonist naloxone to reverse respiratory depression. • Opium content of tincture 25 times greater than that of camphorated tincture. Do not confuse the two. • Risk of physical dependence; don't use > 2 days.
opium tincture; opium tincture, camphorated (paregoric) Opiate *Antidiarrheal* Pregnancy Risk Category: NR Controlled Substance Schedule: II (tincture) or III (camphorated)	*Acute diarrhea —* **tincture — Adults:** 0.6 ml (range 0.3 to 1 ml) P.O. q.i.d. Maximum 6 ml q.d. **camphorated tincture — Adults:** 5 to 10 ml P.O. q.d., b.i.d., t.i.d., or q.i.d. until diarrhea subsides. **Children:** 0.25 to 0.5 ml/kg camphorated tincture P.O. q.d., b.i.d., t.i.d., or q.i.d. until diarrhea subsides.	
oprelvekin Neumega *Human thrombopoietic growth factor* *Platelet production stimulator* Pregnancy Risk Category: C	*Prevention of severe thrombocytopenia and reduction of need for platelet transfusions following myelosuppressive chemotherapy with nonmyeloid malignancies —* **Adults:** 50 mcg/kg S.C. q.d.	• Begin 6 to 24 hr after completion of chemotherapy and stop at least 2 days before starting the next planned cycle. • Use reconstituted drug within 3 hr. • Refrigerate drug and diluent. • Monitor fluid and electrolyte status in patients receiving diuretics.
orlistat Xenical *Lipase inhibitor* *Antihyperlipidemic*	*Obesity management when used with reduced-calorie diet; risk reduction for regaining weight after weight loss; for obese patients with initial body mass index ≥ 30 kg*	• Patient should take vitamin supplement q day at least 2 hr before or after taking drug. • Advise patient to distribute fat, carbohydrate, and protein intake over three main meals.

		• If patient occasionally misses meal or eats meal without fat, dose can be omitted.
Pregnancy Risk Category: B	*(66 lb)/m² or ≥ 27 kg (60 lb)/m² in presence of other risk factors* — **Adult:** 120 mg P.O. t.i.d. with each main meal containing fat.	
oxacillin sodium Bactocill *Penicillinase-resistant penicillin* *Antibiotic* Pregnancy Risk Category: B	*Infections due to penicillinase-producing staphylococci* — **Adults and children > 40 kg (88 lb):** 500 mg to 1 g P.O. q 4 to 6 hr; or 2 to 12 g I.V. or I.M. q.d. in divided doses q 4 to 6 hr. **Children ≤ 40 kg:** 50 to 100 mg/kg P.O. q.d. in divided doses q 6 hr; or 50 to 200 mg/ kg I.M. or I.V. q.d. in divided doses q 4 to 6 hr.	• Obtain specimen for culture and sensitivity tests before 1st dose. • Watch for superinfection. • When given orally, give 1 to 2 hr before or 2 to 3 hr after meals. • Give at least 1 hr before bacteriostatic antibiotics.
oxaprozin Daypro *NSAID* *Anti-inflammatory* Pregnancy Risk Category: C	*Osteoarthritis; rheumatoid arthritis* — **Adults:** initially, 600 to 1,200 mg P.O. q.d. Then individualized to smallest effective dose. Maximum 1,800 mg or 26 mg/kg.	• May cause renal toxicity in susceptible patients. Closely monitor renal function. • Elevated liver function tests can occur after chronic use. • May mask signs of infection.
oxazepam Alepam†, Serax, Zapex† *Benzodiazepine* *Antianxiety agent/sedative-hypnotic* Pregnancy Risk Category: NR Controlled Substance Schedule: IV	*Alcohol withdrawal; severe anxiety* — **Adults:** 15 to 30 mg P.O. t.i.d. or q.i.d. *Mild to moderate anxiety* — **Adults:** 10 to 15 mg P.O. t.i.d. or q.i.d. **Elderly:** initially, 10 mg t.i.d., increased to 15 mg t.i.d. to q.i.d., p.r.n.	• Use cautiously in elderly patients or in those with history of drug abuse. • Monitor liver, renal, and hematopoietic function studies periodically. • Possibility of abuse and addiction exists. Don't stop drug abruptly; withdrawal symptoms may occur.
oxycodone hydrochloride	*Moderate to severe pain* — **Adults:** 5 mg P.O. q 6 hr, p.r.n. Or, 1 to 3 suppositories P.R. q.d., p.r.n.	• For full analgesic effect, administer before intense pain occurs. *(continued)*

†Canadian ‡Australian

DRUG/CLASS/ CATEGORY	INDICATIONS/ DOSAGES	KEY NURSING CONSIDERATIONS
oxycodone hydrochloride *(continued)* OxyContin, Oxy IR, Roxicodone, Roxicodone Intensol, Supeudol† **oxycodone pectinate** *Opioid* *Analgesic* Pregnancy Risk Category: C Controlled Substance Schedule: II		- To minimize GI upset, give after meals or with milk. - Single-agent solution or tablets especially good for patients who shouldn't take aspirin or acetaminophen. - Monitor circulatory and respiratory status. Withhold dose and notify doctor if respirations are shallow or if rate < 12. - Monitor bladder and bowel patterns.
oxymetazoline hydrochloride (nasal) Afrin, Allerest 12 Hr Nasal Spray, Neo-Synephrine 12 Hr Nasal Spray *Sympathomimetic* *Decongestant/vasoconstrictor* Pregnancy Risk Category: NR	*Nasal congestion* — **Adults and children ≥ 6 yr:** 2 to 3 drops or sprays of 0.05% solution in each nostril b.i.d. **Children 2 to 6 yr:** 2 to 3 drops of 0.025% solution in each nostril b.i.d. Don't use > 3 to 5 days.	- Tell patient to hold head upright to minimize swallowing of drug, and then sniff spray briskly. - Caution patient not to exceed recommended dosage and to use only when needed. - Excessive use may cause bradycardia, hypotension, dizziness, and weakness. - Should be used by only 1 person.
oxymetazoline hydrochloride (ophthalmic)	*Relief of eye redness due to minor eye irritations* — **Adults and children ≥ 6 yr:** 1 to 2 drops in conjunctival sac 2 to 4 times q.d.	- Wash hands before and after instilling. Don't touch dropper to eye.

OcuClear, Visine L.R. *Sympathomimetic Decongestant/vasoconstrictor* Pregnancy Risk Category: C	- Apply light finger pressure on lacrimal sac for 1 min after instillation. - Tell patient to stop using and see doctor if eye pain occurs, vision changes, or redness or irritation continues, worsens, or lasts > 72 hr.
oxytocin, synthetic injection Pitocin *Exogenous hormone Oxytocic/lactation stimulant* Pregnancy Risk Category: NR	*Induction, stimulation of labor* — **Adults:** 1-ml (10 U) ampule in 1,000 ml dextrose 5% injection or 0.9% NaCl I.V. infused at 1 to 2 milliunits/min. Increase in increments of not > 1 to 2 milliunits/min q 15 to 30 min. *Reduction of postpartum bleeding after placenta expulsion* — **Adults:** 10 to 40 U added to 1 L D_5W or 0.9% NaCl infused at 20 to 40 milliunits/min. Also, 1 ml (10 U) can be given I.M. after placenta delivery. *Incomplete or inevitable abortion* — **Adults:** 10 U I.V. in 500 ml 0.9% NaCl or dextrose 5% in 0.9% NaCl at 10 to 20 milliunits/min.	- *I.V. use:* Don't give by bolus injection. Administer by infusion only; give piggyback so drug may be discontinued without interrupting I.V. line. Use infusion pump. - Monitor I&O. Antidiuretic effect may lead to fluid overload, seizures, and coma. - Monitor and record uterine contractions, HR, BP, intrauterine pressure, fetal HR, and character of blood loss q 15 min. - If contractions occur < 2 min apart and if contractions > 50 mm Hg recorded, or if contractions last ≥ 90 sec, stop infusion, turn patient on side, and notify doctor.
paclitaxel Taxol *Antimicrotubule Antineoplastic* Pregnancy Risk Category: D	*Metastatic ovarian cancer* — **Adults:** 135 or 175 mg/m² I.V. over 3 hr q 3 wk. *Breast cancer* — **Adults:** 175 mg/m² I.V. over 3 hr q 3 wk.	- Closely monitor patient throughout infusion. - Monitor blood counts during therapy. - Watch for signs of infection and bleeding.
pamidronate disodium Aredia *Bisphosphonate/pyro-*	*Moderate to severe hypercalcemia associated with cancer* — **Patients with albumin corrected serum calcium (CCa) levels 12 to 13.5 mg/dl:* 60 to 90 mg by I.V. infusion over	- Use after patient hydrated. - Monitor serum electrolytes, especially calcium, phosphate, and magnesium. Also *(continued)*

†Canadian ‡Australian

241

DRUG/CLASS/ CATEGORY	INDICATIONS/ DOSAGES	KEY NURSING CONSIDERATIONS
pamidronate disodium *(continued)* phosphate analogue *Antihypercalcemic* Pregnancy Risk Category: C	4 hr for 60-mg dose and over 24 hr for 90-mg dose. **Patients with CCa levels > 13.5 mg/dl:** 90 mg by I.V. infusion over 24 hr. Minimum of 7 days before retreatment. *Moderate to severe Paget's disease —* **Adults:** 30 mg I.V. as 4-hr infusion on 3 days for total dose of 90 mg. Repeat, p.r.n. *Osteolytic bone lesions of multiple myeloma —* **Adults:** 90 mg I.V. as 4-hr infusion q 4 wk.	monitor creatinine, CBC and differential, Hct, and Hgb. ▪ Carefully monitor patients with preexisting anemia, leukopenia, or thrombocytopenia during first 2 wk of therapy. ▪ *I.V. use:* Reconstitute vial with 10 ml sterile water for injection. After completely dissolved, add to 1,000 ml 0.45% or 0.9% NaCl for injection or D₅W. Don't mix with infusion solutions that contain calcium.
paricalcitol Zemplar *Synthetic vitamin D analogue* *Antihyperparathyroid agent* Pregnancy Risk Category: C	*Prevention and treatment of secondary hyperparathyroidism associated with chronic renal failure —* **Adults:** 0.04 to 0.1 mcg/kg (2.8 to 7 mcg) I.V. q.o.d. during dialysis. Doses as high as 0.24 mcg/kg (16.8 mcg) may be used. Dose may be increased by 2 to 4 mcg at 2- to 4-wk intervals.	▪ Patients taking digoxin are at greater risk for digitalis toxicity because of potential for hypercalcemia. ▪ Monitor serum calcium and phosphorus twice/wk when dose adjusted, then q mo. Check parathyroid hormone level q 3 mo. ▪ Administer as I.V. bolus only.
paroxetine hydrochloride Paxil, Paxil CR *Selective serotonin reuptake inhibitor* *Antidepressant* Pregnancy Risk Category: B	*Depression —* **Adults:** 20 mg P.O. q morning. If no response, increase by 10 mg/day to maximum 50 mg q.d. Give 25 mg/day (extended-release), initially; then increase to maximum of 62.5 mg/day. **Elderly or debilitated patients, patients with severe hepatic or renal disease:** 10 mg P.O. q morning. If no response, increase by 10 mg/day to	▪ If psychosis occurs or increases, expect to reduce dosage. ▪ Warn patient to avoid hazardous activities until CNS effects known. ▪ Inform patient that orthostatic hypotension may occur. Supervise walking. Advise getting out of bed slowly.

- Tell patient not to crush or chew Paxil CR tablet.

pegaspargase (PEG-L-asparaginase) Oncaspar *Modified version of enzyme L-asparaginase* *Antineoplastic* Pregnancy Risk Category: C	maximum 40 mg q.d. *Panic disorder* — **Adults:** 10 mg/day. Increase by 10 mg/wk, p.r.n. Maximum dose ≤ 60 mg/day.	

pegaspargase (PEG-L-asparaginase) Oncaspar *Modified version of enzyme L-asparaginase* *Antineoplastic* Pregnancy Risk Category: C	*Acute lymphoblastic leukemia in patients who require L-asparaginase but have developed hypersensitivity to native forms* — **Adults and children with body surface area (BSA) ≥ 0.6 m²:** 2,500 IU/m² I.M. or I.V. q 14 days. **Children with BSA < 0.6 m²:** 82.5 IU/kg I.M. or I.V. q 14 days.	- When giving I.M., limit volume administered at single injection site to 2 ml. - When giving I.V., administer over 1 to 2 hr in 100 ml 0.9% NaCl or dextrose 5% injection through infusion already running. - Handle with care. Gloves recommended. Avoid vapor inhalation and contact with skin or mucous membranes.

pemoline Cylert, Cylert Chewable *Oxazolidinedione derivative/CNS stimulant* *Analeptic* Pregnancy Risk Category: B Controlled Substance Schedule: IV	*Attention deficit hyperactivity disorder* — **Children ≥ 6 yr:** initially, 37.5 mg P.O. in morning with daily dose raised by 18.75 mg weekly, p.r.n. Effective dose range 56.25 to 75 mg q.d.; maximum 112.5 mg q.d.	- Perform liver function tests before and during therapy. Give drug only to patients without liver dysfunction and with normal baseline liver function tests. - May induce Tourette syndrome in children. - Advise patient to take at least 6 hr before bedtime to avoid sleep interference.

penicillamine Cuprimine, Depen, D-Penamine‡ *Chelating agent* *Anti-inflammatory* Pregnancy Risk Category: NR	*Wilson's disease* — **Adults and children:** 250 mg P.O. q.i.d. 30 to 60 min before meals. Adjust dosage to achieve urinary copper excretion of 0.5 to 1 mg q.d. *Cystinuria* — **Adults:** 250 mg to 1 g P.O. q.i.d. before meals. Adjust dosage to urinary cystine excretion < 100 mg q.d. with calculi	- Give dose on empty stomach, preferably 1 hr before or 3 hr after meals. - If patient has skin reaction, give antihistamines, as prescribed. - Report rash and fever to doctor immediately. - Monitor CBC and renal and hepatic function. *(continued)*

‡Canadian †Australian

DRUG/CLASS/ CATEGORY	INDICATIONS/ DOSAGES	KEY NURSING CONSIDERATIONS
penicillamine *(continued)*	present or 100 to 200 mg q.d. when no calculi present. Maximum 4 g q.d. before meals. **Children:** 30 mg/kg P.O. q.d., divided q.i.d. before meals. Dose adjusted to achieve urinary cystine excretion < 100 mg q.d. when renal calculi present, or 100 to 200 mg q.d. with no calculi. *Rheumatoid arthritis —* **Adults:** initially, 125 to 250 mg P.O. q.d., with increases of 125 to 250 mg q 1 to 3 mo, if necessary. Maximum 1.5 g q.d.	tion q 2 wk for first 6 mo, then q mo, as ordered. Monitor urinalysis regularly for protein loss. ■ Withhold drug and notify doctor if WBC count < 3,500/mm³ or platelet count < 100,000/mm³. Progressive decline in platelet or WBC count in three successive blood tests may necessitate temporary discontinuation. ■ Give supplemental pyridoxine daily.
penicillin G benzathine (benzylpenicillin benzathine) Bicillin L-A, Permapen *Natural penicillin* *Antibiotic* Pregnancy Risk Category: B	*Congenital syphilis —* **Children < 2 yr:** 50,000 U/kg I.M. once. *Group A streptococcal upper respiratory infections —* **Adults:** 1.2 million U I.M. once. **Children > 27 kg (60 lb):** 900,000 U I.M. once. **Children < 27 kg:** 300,000 to 600,000 U I.M. once. *Prophylaxis of poststreptococcal rheumatic fever —* **Adults and children:** 1.2 million U I.M. q mo or 600,000 U I.M. twice monthly. *Syphilis —* **Adults:** 2.4 million U I.M. once (<1-yr duration); or, q wk for 3 wk (> 1-yr duration).	■ Obtain specimen for culture and sensitivity tests before first dose. ■ Never give I.V. Inject deeply into upper outer quadrant of buttocks in adults; in midlateral thigh in infants and small children. Avoid injection into or near major nerves or blood vessels. ■ With large doses and prolonged therapy, superinfection may occur.
penicillin G potassium	*Moderate to severe systemic infection —* **Adults and children ≥ 12 yr:** individualized;	■ Obtain specimen for culture and sensitivity tests before 1st dose.

(benzylpenicillin potassium) Megacillin†, Pfizerpen *Natural penicillin* *Antibiotic* Pregnancy Risk Category: B	1.6 to 3.2 million U P.O. q.d. in divided doses q 6 hr; 1.2 to 24 million U I.M. or I.V. q.d. in divided doses q 4 hr. **Children <12 yr:** 25,000 to 100,000 U/kg P.O. q.d. in divided doses q 6 hr, or 25,000 to 400,000 U/kg I.M. or I.V. q.d. in divided doses q 4 hr.	▪ Monitor renal function closely. ▪ Give 1 to 2 hr before or 2 to 3 hr after meals. Food may interfere with absorption. ▪ Give at least 1 hr before bacteriostatic antibiotics.
penicillin G procaine (benzylpenicillin procaine) Ayercillin†, Crysticillin 300 A.S., Wycillin *Natural penicillin* *Antibiotic* Pregnancy Risk Category: B	*Moderate to severe systemic infection* — **Adults:** 600,000 to 1.2 million U.I.M. q.d. in single dose. **Children >1 mo:** 25,000 to 50,000 U/kg I.M. q.d. in single dose. *Uncomplicated gonorrhea* — **Adults and children >12 yr:** 4.8 million U I.M.; after 30 min, 4.8 million U I.M., divided between 2 sites. *Pneumococcal pneumonia* — **Adults and children >12 yr:** 600,000 to 1.2 million U I.M. q.d. for 7 to 10 days.	▪ Obtain specimen for culture and sensitivity tests before first dose. ▪ Never give I.V. ▪ Give deep I.M. in upper outer quadrant of buttocks in adults; in midlateral thigh in small children. Don't give S.C. Don't massage injection site. Avoid injection near major nerves or blood vessels.
penicillin G sodium (benzylpenicillin sodium) Crystapen† *Natural penicillin* *Antibiotic* Pregnancy Risk Category: B	*Moderate to severe systemic infection* — **Adults and children ≥12 yr:** 1.2 to 24 million U q.d. I.M. or I.V. in divided doses q 4 to 6 hr. **Children <12 yr:** 25,000 to 400,000 U/kg q.d. I.M. or I.V. in divided doses q 4 to 6 hr.	▪ For patients receiving ≥ 10 million U q.d., dilute in 1 to 2 L of compatible solution and give over 24 hr. Otherwise, give by intermittent I.V. infusion: Dilute drug in 50 to 100 ml, and give over 1 to 2 hr. ▪ Give at least 1 hr before bacteriostatic antibiotics.
pentamidine isethionate NebuPent, Pentacarinat,	P. carinii *pneumonia* — **Adults and children:** 3 to 4 mg/kg I.V. or I.M. for 14 to 21 days.	▪ Administer aerosol form only by Respirgard II nebulizer.

(continued)

†Canadian ‡Australian

DRUG/CLASS/ CATEGORY	INDICATIONS/ DOSAGES	KEY NURSING CONSIDERATIONS
pentamidine isethionate *(continued)* Pentam 300 *Diamidine derivative* *Antiprotozoal* Pregnancy Risk Category: C	*Prevention of* P. carinii *pneumonia in high-risk individuals* — **Adults:** 300 mg by inhalation q 4 wk.	• Don't mix with other drugs. • Monitor blood glucose, serum calcium, serum creatinine, and BUN daily.
pentazocine hydrochloride Fortral‡, Talwin† **pentazocine hydrochloride and naloxone hydrochloride** Talwin-Nx **pentazocine lactate** Fortral‡, Talwin *Narcotic agonist-antagonist/ opioid partial agonist* *Analgesic/adjunct to anesthesia* Pregnancy Risk Category: C Controlled Substance Schedule: IV	*Moderate to severe pain* — **Adults:** 50 to 100 mg P.O. q 3 to 4 hr, p.r.n. Maximum P.O. dose 600 mg/day. Or, 30 mg I.M., I.V., or S.C. q 3 to 4 hr, p.r.n. Maximum parenteral dose 360 mg/day. Single doses > 30 mg I.V. or 60 mg I.M. or S.C. not recommended. *Labor* — **Adults:** 30 mg I.M. or 20 mg I.V. q 2 to 3 hr with regular contractions.	• Have naloxone available. • May trigger withdrawal syndrome in narcotic-dependent patients. • Psychological and physical dependence may occur with prolonged use. • Talwin-Nx contains naloxone. This prevents illicit I.V. use.

pentobarbital Nembutal **pentobarbital sodium** Nembutal Sodium, Nova Rectal† *Barbiturate* *Anticonvulsant/sedative-hypnotic* Pregnancy Risk Category: D (suppositories C) Controlled Substance Schedule: II (suppositories III)	*Sedation* — **Adults:** 20 to 40 mg P.O. b.i.d., t.i.d., or q.i.d. **Children:** 2 to 6 mg/kg/day P.O. in 3 divided doses. Maximum 100 mg/day. *Insomnia* — **Adults:** 100 to 200 mg P.O. h.s. or 150 to 200 mg deep I.M.; 100 mg I.V., then doses ≤ 500 mg; 120 or 200 mg P.R. **Children:** 2 to 6 mg/kg or 125 mg/m² I.M. Maximum 100 mg. **Children 2 mo to 1 yr:** 30 mg P.R. **Children 1 to 4 yr:** 30 or 60 mg P.R. **Children 5 to 11 yr:** 60 mg P.R. **Children 12 to 14 yr:** 60 or 120 mg P.R. *Preoperative sedation* — **Adults:** 150 to 200 mg I.M. **Children:** 5 mg/kg P.O. or I.M. ≥ 10 yr; 5 mg/kg I.M. or P.R. if < 10 yr.	▪ *I.V. use:* May cause severe respiratory depression, laryngospasm, or hypotension. Have emergency resuscitation equipment available. ▪ Watch for signs of barbiturate toxicity. ▪ Assess mental status before starting therapy. Elderly patients more sensitive to adverse CNS effects. ▪ Inspect skin. Discontinue if skin reactions occur and call doctor. In some patients, high fever, stomatitis, headache, or rhinitis may precede skin reactions.
pentoxifylline Trental *Xanthine derivative* *Hemorheologic agent* Pregnancy Risk Category: C	*Intermittent claudication caused by chronic occlusive vascular disease* — **Adults:** 400 mg P.O. t.i.d. with meals. May decrease to 400 mg b.i.d. if adverse GI and CNS effects occur.	▪ Elderly patients may be more sensitive to effects. ▪ Instruct patient to swallow medication whole.
pergolide mesylate Permax *Dopaminergic agonist* *Antiparkinsonian* Pregnancy Risk Category: B	*Adjunctive treatment of Parkinson's disease* — **Adults:** 0.05 mg P.O. q.d. for first 2 days, then increase to 0.1 to 0.15 mg q 3rd day over 12 days. Then increase by 0.25 mg q 3rd day, p.r.n., until best response seen. Usually given in divided doses t.i.d.	▪ Monitor BP. Symptomatic orthostatic or sustained hypotension may occur. ▪ Advise patient of potential adverse reactions, especially hallucinations and confusion.
perphenazine Apo-Perphenazine†, PMS	*Psychosis in nonhospitalized patients* — **Adults:** 4 to 8 mg P.O. t.i.d., reduced as	▪ Obtain baseline BP before therapy and monitor regularly. Watch for orthostatic *(continued)* 247

†Canadian ‡Australian

DRUG / CLASS / CATEGORY	INDICATIONS / DOSAGES	KEY NURSING CONSIDERATIONS
perphenazine *(continued)* Perphenazinet, Trilafon, Trilafon Concentrate *Phenothiazine (piperazine derivative)* *Antipsychotic/antiemetic* Pregnancy Risk Category: NR	soon as possible to minimum effective dosage. **Children > 12 yr:** lowest adult dose. *Psychosis in hospitalized patients —* **Adults:** 8 to 16 mg P.O. b.i.d., t.i.d., or q.i.d., increased to 64 mg/day, p.r.n. Or, 5 to 10 mg I.M. q 6 hr, p.r.n. Maximum 30 mg. **Children > 12 yr:** lowest adult dose. *Severe nausea and vomiting —* **Adults:** 8 to 16 mg P.O. in divided doses to maximum 24 mg. Or, 5 to 10 mg I.M. p.r.n. May give I.V., diluted to 0.5 mg/ml with 0.9% NaCl solution. Maximum 5 mg.	hypotension. Keep patient supine for 1 hr after administration; tell him to change positions slowly. • Monitor for tardive dyskinesia. • Assess for neuroleptic malignant syndrome. • Monitor weekly bilirubin tests during 1st mo; periodic CBC, liver function, and ophthalmic tests (long-term use), as ordered. • Wear gloves to prepare liquid forms.
phenazopyridine hydrochloride **(phenylazo diamino pyridine hydrochloride)** Azo-Standard, Baridium, Phenazo†, Prodium, Pyridium *Azo dye* *Urinary analgesic* Pregnancy Risk Category: B	*Pain with urinary tract irritation or infection —* **Adults:** 200 mg P.O. t.i.d. after meals for 2 days. **Children:** 12 mg/kg P.O. q.d. in 3 equal doses after meals for 2 days.	• Caution patient to stop taking drug and notify doctor if skin or sclerae yellow-tinged. • When used with antibacterial agent, therapy shouldn't last > 2 days. • Advise patient to take with meals. • Tell diabetic patient to use Clinitest for accurate urine glucose results. Also inform him that drug may interfere with Acetest or Ketostix. • Tell patient that drug turns urine red or orange; may stain fabrics or contact lenses.
phenobarbital (phenobarbitone)	*All forms of epilepsy, febrile seizures —* **Adults:** 60 to 200 mg P.O. q.d. in divided	• *I.V. use:* I.V. injection for emergencies only. Give slowly under close supervision.

Ancalixirt, Barbita, Solfoton

phenobarbital sodium (phenobarbitone sodium)
Luminal Sodium
Barbiturate
Anticonvulsant/sedative-hypnotic
Pregnancy Risk Category: D
Controlled Substance
Schedule: IV

doses t.i.d. or as single dose h.s. **Children:** 3 to 6 mg/kg P.O. q.d., divided q 12 hr.
Status epilepticus — **Adults:** 200 to 600 mg I.V. **Children:** 100 to 400 mg I.V.
Sedation — **Adults:** 30 to 120 mg P.O. q.d. in 2 or 3 divided doses. **Children:** 3 to 5 mg/kg P.O. q.d. in divided doses t.i.d.
Preoperative sedation — **Adults:** 100 to 200 mg I.M. 60 to 90 min before surgery. **Children:** 16 to 100 mg I.M. or 1 to 3 mg/kg I.V., I.M., or P.O. 60 to 90 min before surgery.

- Monitor respirations closely. Don't give > 60 mg/min. Have resuscitation equipment available.
- Watch for signs of barbiturate toxicity; overdose can be fatal.
- Don't stop abruptly; seizures may worsen. Call doctor if adverse reactions develop.
- Therapeutic blood levels 10 to 25 mcg/ml.

phentermine hydrochloride
Fastin, Panshape M, Phentercot, Phentride
Amphetamine congener
Short-term adjunctive anorexigenic/indirect acting sympathomimetic amine
Pregnancy Risk Category: X
Controlled Substance
Schedule: IV

Short-term adjunct in exogenous obesity — **Adults:** 8 mg P.O. t.i.d. ½ hr before meals. Or, 15 to 30 mg (resin complex) or 15 to 37.5 mg (hydrochloride) P.O. q.d. as single dose in morning.

- Use in conjunction with weight-reduction program.
- Monitor for tolerance or dependence.
- Tell patient to take at least 6 hr before bedtime to avoid sleep interference.

phentolamine mesylate
Regitine, Rogitine†
Alpha-adrenergic blocker

To aid pheochromocytoma diagnosis; to control or prevent hypertension before or during pheochromocytomectomy — **Adults:** I.V. diagnostic dose 2.5 mg. Before tumor

- When given to diagnose pheochromocytoma, take BP first; monitor BP frequently during administration. Positive for
(continued)

†Canadian ‡Australian

DRUG/CLASS/ CATEGORY	INDICATIONS/ DOSAGES	KEY NURSING CONSIDERATIONS
phentolamine mesylate *(continued)* *Antihypertensive for pheochromocytoma/cutaneous vasodilator* Pregnancy Risk Category: C	removal, 5 mg I.M. or I.V. During surgery, may give 5 mg I.V. **Children:** I.V. diagnostic dose 1 mg. Before tumor removal, 1 mg I.V. or I.M. During surgery, may give 1 mg I.V. *Dermal necrosis and sloughing after I.V. extravasation of norepinephrine* — **Adults and children:** infiltrate with 5 to 10 mg in 10 ml 0.9% NaCl solution, or half through infiltrated I.V. and other half around site.	pheochromocytoma if I.V. test dose causes severe hypotension. ▪ Don't administer epinephrine to treat phentolamine-induced hypotension. Use norepinephrine instead. ▪ Tell patient to report adverse reactions. ▪ Must perform treatment for infiltration within 12 hr.
phenylephrine hydrochloride (systemic) Neo-Synephrine *Adrenergic* *Vasoconstrictor* Pregnancy Risk Category: C	*Mild to moderate hypotension* — **Adults:** 2 to 5 mg S.C. or I.M.; repeat in 1 to 2 hr, p.r.n. Or, 0.1 to 0.5 mg by slow I.V.; repeat 10 to 15 min. **Children:** 0.1 mg/kg I.M. or S.C.; repeat in 1 to 2 hr, p.r.n. *Severe hypotension and shock* — **Adults:** 10 mg in 250 to 500 ml D₅W or 0.9% NaCl. Start infusion at 100 to 180 mcg/min; decrease to 40 to 60 mcg/min when BP stable.	▪ Use CV catheter or large vein to minimize extravasation. Use continuous infusion pump to regulate infusion flow rate. ▪ Frequently monitor ECG, BP, HR, cardiac output, CVP, PAWP, urine output, and color and temperature of extremities. ▪ To treat extravasation, infiltrate site promptly with phentolamine.
phenylephrine hydrochloride (ophthalmic) AK-Dilate, AK-Nefrin Ophthalmic, Isopto Frin, Mydfrin, Neo-Synephrine *Adrenergic*	*Mydriasis without cycloplegia* — **Adults and children:** 1 drop of 2.5% or 10% solution instilled before examination. May repeat in 1 hr. *Mydriasis and vasoconstriction* — **Adults and adolescents:** 1 drop 2.5% or 10% solution. **Children:** 1 drop 2.5% solution. *Chronic mydriasis* — **Adults and adoles-**	▪ Wash hands before and after instilling. Apply light finger pressure on lacrimal sac for 1 min after drops instilled. ▪ Tell patient not to use brown solutions or solutions that contain precipitate. ▪ Monitor BP and pulse rate.

Vasoconstrictor Pregnancy Risk Category: C	**cents:** 1 drop 2.5% or 10% solution b.i.d. or t.i.d. **Children:** 1 drop 2.5% solution b.i.d. or t.i.d.	▪ Advise patient to contact doctor if condition persists > 12 hr after drug stopped.
phenylephrine hydrochloride (nasal) Alconefrin, Neo-Synephrine, Sinex *Adrenergic* *Vasoconstrictor* Pregnancy Risk Category: NR	*Nasal congestion* — **Adults and children ≥ 12 yr:** 1 to 2 sprays in nostril or small amount of jelly to nasal mucosa q 4 hr. Don't use > 3 to 5 days. **Children 6 to 12 yr:** 1 to 2 sprays of 0.25% solution in nostril q 4 hr. **Children < 6 yr:** 2 to 3 drops of 0.125% solution q 4 hr.	▪ Tell patient to hold head upright to minimize swallowing of medication, then sniff spray briskly. After use, rinse tip of spray with hot water and air. ▪ Tell patient not to exceed recommended dosage.
phenytoin (diphenylhydantoin) Dilantin, Dilantin Infatabs **phenytoin sodium** Dilantin, Phenytex **phenytoin sodium (extended)** Dilantin Kapseals *Hydantoin derivative* *Anticonvulsant* Pregnancy Risk Category: NR	*Control of tonic-clonic and complex partial seizures* — **Adults:** 100 mg P.O. t.i.d. increased in increments of 100 mg P.O. q 2 to 4 wk until desired response. **Children:** 5 mg/kg or 250 mg/m² P.O. divided b.i.d. or t.i.d. Maximum 300 mg q.d. *For patients requiring loading dose —* **Adults:** 1 g P.O. divided into 3 doses given at 2-hr intervals. Or, 10 to 15 mg/kg I.V. at rate not > 50 mg/min. **Children:** 5 mg/kg/day P.O. in 2 or 3 equally divided doses with later dose individualized to maximum 300 mg q.d. *Status epilepticus* — **Adults:** loading dose 10 to 15 mg/kg I.V. at rate not > 50 mg/min, then maintenance doses of 100 mg P.O. or I.V. q 6 to 8 hr. **Children:** loading dose 15 to 20 mg/kg I.V. at rate not > 1 to 3 mg/	▪ Extravasation has caused severe local tissue damage. Avoid administering by I.V. push into veins on back of hand. Inject into larger veins or central venous catheter, if available. ▪ Check vital signs, BP, and ECG during I.V. administration. Monitor blood levels. Therapeutic level 10 to 20 mcg/ml. Monitor CBC and serum calcium level q 6 mo, and periodically monitor hepatic function. ▪ Advise patient to avoid hazardous activities until CNS effects known. ▪ Inform patient that drug may color urine pink, red, or reddish brown. ▪ After loading dose, start normal maintenance dose in 24 hr. *(continued)*

251

†Canadian ‡Australian

DRUG/CLASS/ CATEGORY	INDICATIONS/ DOSAGES	KEY NURSING CONSIDERATIONS
phenytoin *(continued)*	kg/min, then individualized maintenance doses.	
phytonadione (vitamin K₁) AquaMEPHYTON, Mephyton *Vitamin K* *Blood coagulation modifier* Pregnancy Risk Category: C	*Hypoprothrombinemia secondary to vitamin K malabsorption, drug therapy, excessive vitamin A dosage* — **Adults:** 2.5 to 10 mg P.O., S.C., or I.M.; repeat and increase up to 50 mg P.O., I.M., or S.C. **Infants:** 2 mg P.O., I.M., or S.C. **Children:** 5 to 10 mg P.O., I.M., or S.C. *Hypoprothrombinemia secondary to effect of oral anticoagulants* — **Adults:** 2.5 to 10 mg P.O., S.C. or I.M. based on PT and INR. In emergency, 10 to 50 mg slow I.V., rate ≤ 1 mg/min, repeated q 4 hr, p.r.n.	■ *I.V. use:* Give I.V. by slow infusion over 2 to 3 hr. Rate ≤ 1 mg/min in adults. ■ For I.M. use in adults and older children, inject in upper outer quadrant of buttocks; for infants, inject in anterolateral aspect of thigh or deltoid region. ■ Monitor PT and INR. ■ Watch for flushing, weakness, tachycardia, and hypotension. ■ Protect parenteral products from light.
pilocarpine Ocusert Pilo **pilocarpine hydrochloride** Adsorbocarpine, Isopto Carpine, Miocarpine†, Pilocar, Pilopt‡ **pilocarpine nitrate** Pilagan, P.V. Carpine Liquifilm *Cholinergic agonist* *Miotic*	*Primary open-angle glaucoma* — **Adults and children:** 1 to 2 drops up to q.i.d., or 1-cm ribbon of 4% gel q.h.s. Or, 1 Ocusert Pilo system (20 or 40 mcg/hr) q 7 days. *Emergency treatment of acute angle-closure glaucoma* — **Adults and children:** 1 drop 2% solution q 5 to 10 min for 3 to 6 doses, then 1 drop q 1 to 3 hr until pressure controlled. *Mydriasis caused by mydriatic or cyclo-plegic agents* — **Adults and children:** 1 drop 1% solution.	■ Instruct patient to apply gel h.s. Warn him to avoid hazardous activities until temporary blurring subsides. ■ Apply light finger pressure on lacrimal sac for 1 min afterward. ■ If Ocusert Pilo system falls out of eye during sleep, tell patient to wash hands, rinse insert in cool tap water, and reposition in eye. ■ Inform patient that transient brow pain and myopia usually subside within 2 wk.

pimozide
Orap
Diphenylbutylpiperidine
Antipsychotic
Pregnancy Risk Category: C

Suppression of motor and phonic tics in Tourette syndrome — **Adults and children > 12 yr:** 1 to 2 mg P.O. q.d. in divided doses; increase q.o.d., p.r.n. Maintenance dose < 0.2 mg/kg/day or 10 mg/day, whichever less. Maximum 10 mg q.d.

- Monitor for prolonged QT interval before and during treatment.
- Monitor for tardive dyskinesia. May treat acute dystonic reactions with diphenhydramine.
- May lower seizure threshold.

pindolol
Apo-Pindol†, Visken
Beta blocker
Antihypertensive
Pregnancy Risk Category: B

Hypertension — **Adults:** initially, 5 mg P.O. b.i.d. Increase, as needed and tolerated, to maximum 60 mg q.d.

- Check apical pulse before giving. If extreme, withhold dose and call doctor.
- Monitor BP frequently.
- Withdraw over 1 to 2 wk after long-term therapy, as ordered.

piperacillin sodium
Pipracil, Pipril‡
Extended-spectrum penicillin/acylaminopenicillin
Antibiotic
Pregnancy Risk Category: B

Systemic infections due to susceptible strains of gram-positive and gram-negative organisms — **Adults and children > 12 yr:** 100 to 300 mg/kg I.V. or I.M. q.d. in divided doses q 4 to 6 hr. Maximum 24 g q.d. *Prophylaxis of surgical infections* — **Adults:** 2 g I.V. 30 to 60 min before surgery.

- Obtain specimen for culture and sensitivity tests before first dose.
- Monitor for superinfection.
- Give ≥ 1 hr before bacteriostatic antibiotics.
- Monitor serum potassium.
- Alter dosage as ordered in impaired renal function.

piperacillin sodium and tazobactam sodium
Zosyn
Extended-spectrum penicillin/beta-lactamase inhibitor

Appendicitis; skin; skin-structure infections; postpartum endometritis; pelvic inflammatory disease; moderately severe community-acquired pneumonia — **Adults:** 3 g piperacillin and 0.375 g tazobactam I.V. q 6 hr. *Renal impairment:* **Adults:** if creatinine clearance 20 to 40 ml/min, 2 g piperacillin

- Obtain specimen for culture and sensitivity tests before 1st dose.
- Superinfection may occur, especially in elderly, debilitated, or immunosuppressed patients. Observe closely.

(continued)

†Canadian ‡Australian

DRUG/CLASS/ CATEGORY	INDICATIONS/ DOSAGES	KEY NURSING CONSIDERATIONS
piperacillin sodium and tazobactam sodium *(continued)* Antibiotic Pregnancy Risk Category: B	and 0.25 g tazobactam I.V. q 6 hr; if < 20 ml/min, 2 g piperacillin and 0.25 g tazobactam I.V. q 8 hr. *Moderate to severe nosocomial pneumonia* — **Adults:** initially, 3.375 g I.V. over 30 min q 4 hr. Give with aminoglycoside. *Adjust-a-dose:* If creatinine clearance 20 to 40 ml/min, give 2 g piperacillin and 0.25 g tazobactam I.V. q 6 hr; if < 20 ml/min, 2 g piperacillin and 0.25 g tazobactam I.V. q 8 hr.	• Infuse over ≥ 30 min. Don't mix with other drugs. Discard unused drug after 24 hr if stored at room temperature; after 48 hr if refrigerated. Once diluted, drug stable in I.V. bags for 24 hr at room temperature or 1 wk if refrigerated.
pirbuterol acetate Maxair, Maxair Autohaler *Beta-adrenergic agonist Bronchodilator* Pregnancy Risk Category: C	*Prevention and reversal of bronchospasm, asthma* — **Adults and children ≥ 12 yr:** 1 or 2 inhalations (0.2 to 0.4 mg) repeated q 4 to 6 hr. Maximum 12 inhalations q.d.	• If > 1 inhalation ordered, tell patient to wait at least 2 min before repeating procedure. • If patient also using steroid inhaler, instruct to use bronchodilator first, then wait 5 min before using steroid.
piroxicam Apo-Piroxicam†, Feldene, Novo-Pirocam† *NSAID Nonnarcotic analgesic/antipyretic/anti-inflammatory* Pregnancy Risk Category: NR	*Osteoarthritis; rheumatoid arthritis* — **Adults:** 20 mg P.O. q.d. If desired, may divide dosage b.i.d.	• May lead to reversible renal impairment. • Check renal, hepatic, and auditory function and CBC during prolonged therapy. • May mask infection.
plicamycin (mithramycin)	Dosage and indications vary. *Hypercalcemia and hypercalciuria associat-*	• To reduce nausea, give antiemetic before administering. Infuse over 4 to 6 hr.

Mithracin *Antibiotic antineoplastic (cell cycle-phase nonspecific)* *Antineoplastic/hypocalcemic agent* Pregnancy Risk Category: X	ed with advanced malignant disease — **Adults:** 25 mcg/kg/day I.V. for 3 to 4 days. Repeat dosage at weekly intervals until response. *Testicular cancer* — **Adults:** 25 to 30 mcg/kg/day I.V. for 8 to 10 days or until toxicity occurs.	▪ If solution extravasates, stop immediately, notify doctor, and use ice packs. ▪ Monitor CBC, platelets, and PT. ▪ Monitor for tetany, carpopedal spasm, Chvostek's sign, and muscle cramps.
pneumococcal vaccine, polyvalent Pneumovax 23, Pnu-Imune 23 *Vaccine* *Bacterial vaccine* Pregnancy Risk Category: C	*Pneumococcal immunization* — **Adults and children ≥ 2 yr:** 0.5 ml I.M. or S.C. Not recommended for children < 2 yr.	▪ Check immunization history to avoid re-vaccination within 3 yr. ▪ Obtain history of allergies and reaction to immunization. Egg protein not used during manufacture; contains phenol. ▪ Keep epinephrine 1:1,000 available. ▪ Inject in deltoid or midlateral thigh.
poliovirus vaccine, live, oral, trivalent (TOPV) Orimune *Vaccine* *Viral vaccine* Pregnancy Risk Category: C	*Poliovirus immunization (TOPV)* — **Children and nonimmunized adults:** 0.5 ml P.O., then 0.5 ml in 6 to 8 wk, then 0.5 ml 6 to 12 mo later. Give 0.5 ml before school entry. **Infants:** 0.5 ml P.O. at 2, 4, and 18 mo. *Poliovirus immunization (IPV)* — **Adults:** 0.5 ml S.C.; then 2nd dose in 4 to 8 wk. 3rd dose in 6 to 12 mo. **Children:** 0.5 ml S.C. at 2 mo and 4 mo. 3rd dose at 15 to 18 mo. Give dose of 0.5 ml S.C. before school entry.	▪ Obtain history of allergies and reaction to immunization. ▪ Don't administer oral form parenterally. ▪ Keep TOPV frozen until used. Once thawed, if unopened, may refrigerate up to 30 days; if opened, up to 7 days. Thaw before administration. ▪ Give parenteral form to patients with altered immune status. ▪ Don't administer to neonates < 6 wk.
poliovirus vaccine, inactivated (IPV) IPOL *Vaccine* *Viral vaccine* Pregnancy Risk Category: C		
polymyxin B sulfate *Polymyxin antibiotic*	*Alone or with other agents to treat superficial eye infections from Pseudomonas or other gram-negative organisms* — **Adults**	▪ Don't touch dropper tip to eye or surrounding tissue. *(continued)*

†Canadian ‡Australian

DRUG/CLASS/ CATEGORY	INDICATIONS/ DOSAGES	KEY NURSING CONSIDERATIONS
polymyxin B sulfate *(continued)* *Ophthalmic antibiotic* Pregnancy Risk Category: C	**and children:** 1 to 3 drops of 0.1% to 0.25% (10,000 to 25,000 U/ml) q hr. Increase interval according to response; or up to 10,000 U injected subconjunctivally q.d.	▪ Apply light pressure on tear duct for 1 min after drops instilled. ▪ Tell patient not to share drug, washcloths, or towels and to notify doctor if anyone in household develops same symptoms.
potassium bicarbonate K + Care ET, K-Ide, Klor-Con/EF, K-Lyte *Potassium supplement Therapeutic agent for electrolyte balance* Pregnancy Risk Category: NR	*Hypokalemia* — **Adults:** 25 to 50 mEq dissolved in half-glass to full glass of water (120 to 240 ml) q.d. to q.i.d.	▪ Dissolve tablets in 6 to 8 oz (180 to 240 ml) cold water. ▪ Monitor BUN, serum potassium and creatinine, and I&O. ▪ Tell patient to take with meals and sip slowly. ▪ Warn patient not to use salt substitutes, except with doctor's permission.
potassium chloride K-10, Kaochlor 10%, K-Dur, K-Lyte/Cl, K-Tab, Slow-K K-Lyte/Cl *Potassium supplement Therapeutic agent for electrolyte balance* Pregnancy Risk Category: C	*Hypokalemia* — **Adults:** 40 to 100 mEq P.O. q.d. in 3 or 4 divided doses or 10 to 20 mEq for prevention. **Children:** 3 mEq/kg q.d. Maximum daily dose 40 mEq/m². If potassium < 2 mEq/ml, maximum infusion rate 40 mEq/hr; maximum infusion concentration 80 mEq/L; maximum 24-hr dose 400 mEq. If potassium > 2 mEq/ml, maximum infusion rate 10 mEq/hr; maximum infusion concentration 40 mEq/L; maximum 24-hr dose 200 mEq.	▪ Never switch potassium products without doctor's order. ▪ *I.V. use:* Give by infusion only. Give slowly as dilute solution. ▪ Make sure powder is completely dissolved before administering. ▪ Monitor ECG and serum electrolytes.

potassium gluconate
Glu-K, Kaon Liquid
Potassium supplement
Therapeutic agent for electrolyte balance
Pregnancy Risk Category: C

Hypokalemia — **Adults:** 40 to 100 mEq P.O. q.d. in 3 or 4 divided doses for treatment; 10 to 20 mEq q.d. for prevention. Further dosage adjustments based on serum potassium levels.

- Don't administer potassium supplements postoperatively until urine flow established.
- Instruct patient to take with or after meals with full glass of water or fruit juice.
- Caution patient not to use salt substitutes, except with doctor's permission.

potassium iodide
Pima, Thyro-Block
potassium iodide, saturated solution (SSKI), strong iodine solution
Electrolyte
Antihyperthyroid agent
Pregnancy Risk Category: D

Preparation for thyroidectomy — **Adults and children:** strong iodine solution (USP), 0.1 to 0.3 ml P.O. t.i.d., or SSKI, 1 to 5 drops in water P.O. t.i.d. after meals for 10 to 14 days before surgery.
Thyrotoxic crisis — **Adults and children:** 500 mg P.O. q 4 hr (SSKI) or 1 ml strong iodine solution t.i.d.
Radiation protectant for thyroid gland — **Adults and children ≥ 1 yr:** 130 mg P.O. q.d. for 7 to 14 days after radiation exposure.
Children < 1 yr: 65 mg P.O. q.d. for 7 to 14 days after exposure.

- Doctor may avoid prescribing enteric-coated tablets, which can lead to perforation, hemorrhage, or obstruction.
- Dilute oral solutions in water, milk, or fruit juice; give after meals to prevent gastric irritation, hydrate patient, and mask salty taste.
- Give iodides through straw to avoid tooth discoloration.
- Irritation and swollen eyelids are earliest signs of delayed hypersensitivity reactions to iodides.

pramipexole dihydrochloride
Mirapex
Nonergot dopamine agonist
Antiparkinsonian
Pregnancy Risk Category: C

Treatment of signs and symptoms of idiopathic Parkinson's disease — **Adults:** 0.375 mg P.O. q.d. in divided doses t.i.d.; increase q 5 to 7 days. Maintenance range 1.5 to 4.5 mg/day in 3 divided doses.
Adjust-a-dose: In patients with creatinine clearance > 60 ml/min, give 0.125 mg P.O.

- Withdraw drug over 1-wk period if drug needs to be discontinued.
- Know that drug may cause orthostatic hypotension, especially during dose escalation. Monitor patient carefully.

(continued)

†Canadian ‡Australian

DRUG/CLASS/ CATEGORY	INDICATIONS/ DOSAGES	KEY NURSING CONSIDERATIONS
pramipexole dihydrochloride *(continued)*	t.i.d., up to 1.5 mg t.i.d.; in those with clearance 35 to 59 ml/min, give 1.25 mg P.O. b.i.d., up to 1.5 mg b.i.d.; in those with clearance 15 to 34 ml/min, give 0.125 mg P.O. q.d., up to 1.5 mg q.d.	▪ Adjust dose gradually to achieve maximum therapeutic effect balanced against adverse effects of dyskinesia, hallucinations, somnolence, and dry mouth.
pravastatin sodium (eptastatin) Pravachol HMG-CoA reductase inhibitor Antilipemic Pregnancy Risk Category: X	*Reduction of LDL and total cholesterol levels in primary hypercholesterolemia (types IIa and IIb)* — **Adults:** 10 or 20 mg P.O. q.d. h.s. Adjust q 4 wk per response; maximum 40 mg q.d. Most elderly patients respond to ≤ 20 mg q.d.	▪ Initiate only after other nonpharmacologic therapies prove ineffective. ▪ Test liver function at start of therapy and periodically thereafter. ▪ Instruct patient to take in evening.
prazosin hydrochloride Minipress Alpha-adrenergic blocker Antihypertensive Pregnancy Risk Category: C	*Mild to moderate hypertension* — **Adults:** P.O. test dose 1 mg h.s. Initial dose 1 mg P.O. b.i.d. or t.i.d. Increase slowly. Maximum 20 mg q.d. Maintenance 6 to 15 mg q.d. in 3 divided doses.	▪ Monitor BP and HR frequently. Elderly patients may be more sensitive to hypotensive effects. ▪ Give 1st dose of each increment h.s. to reduce episodes of syncope.
prednisolone Delta-Cortef **prednisolone sodium phosphate** Hydeltrasol, Key-Pred-SP **prednisolone tebutate**	*Severe inflammation or immunosuppression* — **Adults:** 2.5 to 15 mg P.O. b.i.d., t.i.d., or q.i.d.; 2 to 30 mg I.M. (phosphate) or I.V. (phosphate) q 12 hr; or 2 to 30 mg (phosphate) into joints (depending on joint size), lesions, or soft tissue; or 4 to 40 mg	▪ Give oral dose with food to reduce GI irritation. ▪ Give I.M. injection deeply into gluteal muscle. Rotate injection sites to prevent muscle atrophy. Avoid S.C. injection. ▪ Monitor weight, BP, and serum electrolytes.

Hydeltra-T.B.A., Nor-Pred T.B.A.
Glucocorticoid
Anti-inflammatory/immunosuppressant
Pregnancy Risk Category: C

prednisolone acetate (suspension)
Econopred Plus, Pred-Forte
prednisolone sodium phosphate
AK-Pred, Inflamase Forte
Corticosteroid
Ophthalmic anti-inflammatory
Pregnancy Risk Category: C

prednisone
Liquid Pred, Meticorten, Panasol, Prednicen-M, Prednisone Intensol
Adrenocortical
Anti-inflammatory/immunosuppressant
Pregnancy Risk Category: C

primaquine phosphate
8-Aminoquinoline

(tebutate) into joints (depending on joint size) and lesions, p.r.n.

Inflammation — **Adults and children:** 1 to 2 drops instilled into eye. In severe conditions, may use hourly, tapering to discontinuation as inflammation subsides. In mild conditions, may use b.i.d. to q.i.d.

Severe inflammation or immunosuppression — **Adults:** 5 to 60 mg P.O. q.d. in 2 to 4 divided doses. Give maintenance dose q.d. or q.o.d. Dosage individualized. **Children:** 0.14 to 2 mg/kg or 4 to 60 mg/m² P.O. q.d. in 4 divided doses.

Radical cure for relapsing P. vivax malaria; prevention of relapse — **Adults:** 15 mg (base) P.O. q.d. for 14 days. (26.3-mg tablet

- Wash hands before and after applying. Don't touch dropper tip to eye or surrounding area.
- Apply light pressure on lacrimal sac for 1 min after instillation.
- Instruct patient to notify doctor if anyone in household develops same symptoms.
- Shake suspension. Store in tightly covered container.

- Monitor BP, sleep patterns, and serum potassium. Weigh patient daily; report sudden weight gain.
- Watch for depression or psychotic episodes, especially with high-dose therapy.
- Diabetic patients may need more insulin.
- May mask or exacerbate infections, including latent amebiasis.

- Give with fast-acting antimalarial to reduce risk of drug-resistant strains.

(continued)

259

†Canadian ‡Australian

DRUG/CLASS/ CATEGORY	INDICATIONS/ DOSAGES	KEY NURSING CONSIDERATIONS
primaquine phosphate *(continued)* *Antimalarial* Pregnancy Risk Category: C	provides 15 mg of base.) **Children:** 0.5 mg/kg/day (0.3 mg base/kg/day; maximum 15 mg base/dose) P.O. for 14 days.	• Monitor for sudden fall in Hgb, erythrocyte, or leukocyte count and for marked urine darkening. Discontinue immediately and notify doctor.
primidone Apo-Primidone†, Mysoline, PMS Primidone†, Sertan† *Barbiturate analogue* *Anticonvulsant* Pregnancy Risk Category: NR	*Tonic-clonic, complex partial, and simple partial seizures —* **Adults and children ≥ 8 yr:** initially, 100 to 125 mg P.O. h.s. on days 1 to 3; 100 to 125 mg P.O. b.i.d. on days 4 to 6; 100 to 125 mg P.O. t.i.d. on days 7 to 9; followed by dose of 250 mg P.O. t.i.d. Dose increased to 250 mg q.i.d., p.r.n. Maximum 2 g q.d. in divided doses. **Children < 8 yr:** 50 mg P.O. h.s. for 3 days, then 50 mg P.O. b.i.d. for days 4 to 6, 100 mg P.O. b.i.d. for days 7 to 9, followed by dose of 125 to 250 mg P.O. t.i.d.	• Don't withdraw suddenly; seizures may worsen. Call doctor if adverse reactions develop. • Therapeutic primidone blood level 5 to 12 mcg/ml; therapeutic phenobarbital level 15 to 40 mcg/ml. • Monitor CBC and routine blood chemistry q 6 mo.
probenecid Benemid, Benuryl† *Sulfonamide derivative* *Uricosuric* Pregnancy Risk Category: NR	*Gonorrhea —* **Adults:** 3.5 g ampicillin P.O. with 1 g probenecid P.O. given together; or 1 g probenecid P.O. 30 min before dose of 4.8 million U of aqueous penicillin G procaine I.M., injected at two different sites. *Hyperuricemia of gout, gouty arthritis —* **Adults:** 250 mg P.O. b.i.d. for 1st wk, then 500 mg b.i.d., to maximum 2 g q.d. *Prevention of renal failure caused by cidofo-*	• Give with milk, food, or antacids. • Monitor periodic BUN and renal function tests with long-term therapy. • Force fluids to maintain minimum output of 2 to 3 L/day. • May increase frequency, severity, and length of gout attacks during first 6 to 12 mo.

vir — **Adults:** 2 g P.O. 3 hr before cidofovir infusion, then 1 g P.O. 2 and 8 hr after infusion.

**procarbazine
hydrochloride**
Matulane, Natulant

*Antibiotic antineoplastic
(cell cycle–phase specific,
S phase)*

Antineoplastic

Pregnancy Risk Category: D

Adjunct treatment of Hodgkin's disease — **Adults:** 2 to 4 mg/kg/day P.O. q.d. for 1st wk. Then, 4 to 6 mg/kg/day until WBC count < 4,000/mm³ or platelet count < 100,000/mm³. After bone marrow recovers, resume maintenance of 1 to 2 mg/kg/day. For MOPP regimen, 100 mg/m²/day P.O. for 14 days. **Children:** 50 mg/m² P.O. q.d. for 1st wk; then 100 mg/m² until response or toxicity occurs. Maintenance dosage 50 mg/m² P.O. q.d. after bone marrow recovery.

- Monitor CBC and platelet counts.
- Be prepared to discontinue if confusion or paresthesia or other neuropathies develop. Notify doctor.
- Give h.s. and in divided doses.
- Watch for signs of infection and bleeding. Take temperature daily.
- Warn patient to avoid alcohol. Urge him to stop drug and call doctor immediately if disulfiram-like reaction occurs.

**procainamide
hydrochloride**
Procanbid, Promine,
Pronestyl

Procaine derivative

*Ventricular antiarrhythmic/
supraventricular anti-
arrhythmic*

Pregnancy Risk Category: C

Life-threatening ventricular arrhythmias — **Adults:** 100 mg slow I.V. push q 5 min, until arrhythmias disappear, adverse reactions develop, or 1 g given. Then give continuous infusion of 1 to 6 mg/min. If arrhythmias recur, repeat bolus and increase infusion rate. Or, 0.5 to 1 g I.M. q 4 to 8 hr until oral therapy begins. Oral: 50 mg/kg q.d. in divided doses q 3 hr. May divide sustained-release oral forms q 6 or 12 hr, depending on product.

- **I.V. use:** Monitor BP and ECG continuously. If prolonged QT intervals and QRS complexes, heart block, or increased arrhythmias occur, withhold drug and notify doctor.
- To suppress ventricular arrhythmias, drug levels 4 to 8 mcg/ml; NAPA levels 10 to 30 mcg/ml.

---

prochlorperazine
Compazine, PMS Prochlor-
perazine†, Prorazin†,
Stemetil†

**prochlorperazine
edisylate**

Preoperative nausea control — **Adults:** 5 to 10 mg I.M. 1 to 2 hr before anesthesia; repeat once in 30 min, p.r.n. Or, 5 to 10 mg I.V. 15 to 30 min before anesthesia; repeat once, p.r.n.

- Dilute oral solution with tomato or fruit juice, milk, coffee, carbonated beverage, tea, water, or soup or mix with pudding.

(continued)

261

---

†Canadian ‡Australian

DRUG / CLASS / CATEGORY	INDICATIONS / DOSAGES	KEY NURSING CONSIDERATIONS
prochlorperazine *(continued)* Compa-Z, Compazine, Co-tranzine, Ultrazine-10 **prochlorperazine maleate** Compazine, PMS Prochlor-perazine†, Prorazin†, Stemetil† *Phenothiazine (piperazine derivative)* Antipsychotic/antiemetic/antianxiety agent Pregnancy Risk Category: NR	*Severe nausea and vomiting —* **Adults:** 5 to 10 mg P.O. t.i.d. or q.i.d.; 25 mg P.R., b.i.d., p.r.n. 5 to 10 mg I.M. repeated q 3 to 4 hr, p.r.n. Or, 2.5 to 10 mg I.V. at maximum rate 5 mg/min. **Children 9 to 13 kg (20 to 29 lb):** 2.5 mg P.O. or P.R. q.d. or b.i.d. Or 0.132 mg/kg by I.M. injection. **Children 14 to 17 kg (31 to 38 lb):** 2.5 mg P.O. or P.R., b.i.d. or t.i.d. Or 0.132 mg/kg by deep I.M. injection. **Children 18 to 39 kg (40 to 86 lb):** 2.5 mg P.O. or P.R., t.i.d.; or 5 mg P.O. or P.R., b.i.d. or 0.132 mg/kg by deep I.M. injection. *To manage symptoms of psychotic disorders —* **Adults:** 5 to 10 mg P.O., t.i.d. or q.i.d. **Children 2 to 12 yr:** 2.5 mg P.O. or P.R., b.i.d. or t.i.d. Maximum 10 mg on day 1. Increase dose gradually, p.r.n. In children 2 to 10 yr, maximum 25 mg q.d. *Nonpsychotic anxiety —* **Adults:** 5 to 10 mg by deep I.M. injection q 3 to 4 hr, not to exceed 20 mg q.d. or for > 12 wk; or 5 to 10 mg P.O. t.i.d. or q.i.d. Or, 15 mg extended-release capsules q.d. or 10 mg extended-release capsules q 12 hr.	• *I.V. use:* 15 to 30 min before induction, add 20 mg prochlorperazine/L D_5W and 0.9% NaCl solution. Maximum infusion rate 5 mg/min. Maximum parenteral dose 40 mg q.d. Infuse slowly, never as bolus. • Avoid getting concentrate or injection solution on hands or clothing. • Watch for orthostatic hypotension, especially when giving I.V. • For I.M. use, inject deeply into upper outer quadrant of gluteal region. • Don't give S.C. or mix in syringe with another drug. • Used only when vomiting can't be controlled by other measures. Notify doctor if > 4 doses needed in 24 hr. • Advise patient to wear protective clothing when exposed to sunlight. • Store in light-resistant container. Slight yellowing does not affect potency; discard extremely discolored solutions.
progesterone Gesterol 50	*Amenorrhea —* **Adults:** 5 to 10 mg I.M. q.d. for 6 to 8 days, beginning 8 to 10 days be-	• Give oil solutions (peanut oil or sesame oil) via deep I.M. injection. Check sites fre-

Progestin
Progestin/contraceptive
Pregnancy Risk Category: X

fore anticipated start of menstruation.
Dysfunctional uterine bleeding — **Adults:** 5 to 10 mg I.M. q.d. for 6 doses.

- quently for irritation.
- Rotate injection sites.

promethazine hydrochloride
Anergan 25, Histantil†, Pentazine, Phenazine 25, Phencen-50, Phenergan, Phenergan Fortis, Phenoject-50, PMS-Promethazine†, Prothazine†, V-Gan-25

promethazine theoclate
Avomine‡
Phenothiazine derivative
Antiemetic/antivertigo agent/antihistamine (H₁-receptor antagonist)/preoperative, postoperative, or obstetric sedative and adjunct to analgesics
Pregnancy Risk Category: C

Motion sickness — **Adults:** 25 mg P.O. b.i.d. **Children:** 12.5 to 25 mg P.O., I.M., or P.R. b.i.d.
Nausea — **Adults:** 12.5 to 25 mg P.O., I.M., or P.R. q 4 to 6 hr, p.r.n. **Children:** 12.5 to 25 mg I.M. or P.R. q 4 to 6 hr, p.r.n.
Rhinitis; allergy symptoms — **Adults:** 12.5 mg P.O. q.i.d.; or 25 mg I.M. h.s. **Children:** 6.25 to 12.5 mg P.O. t.i.d. or 25 mg P.O. or P.R. h.s.
Sedation — **Adults:** 25 to 50 mg P.O. or I.M. h.s. or p.r.n. **Children:** 12.5 to 25 mg P.O., I.M., or P.R. h.s.
Routine preoperative or postoperative sedation; adjunct to analgesics — **Adults:** 25 to 50 mg I.M., I.V., or P.O. **Children:** 12.5 to 25 mg I.M., I.V., or P.O.

- Used as adjunct to analgesics; has no analgesic activity.
- Don't administer S.C.
- In patients scheduled for myelogram, discontinue drug 48 hr before procedure and don't resume until 24 hr after procedure.
- *I.V. use:* Don't give concentration > 25 mg/ml or give faster than 25 mg/min.
- May cause pronounced sedation. Warn patient to avoid alcohol and activities requiring alertness until CNS effects known.

propafenone hydrochloride
Rythmol
Sodium channel antagonist
Antiarrhythmic (class IC)
Pregnancy Risk Category: C

Suppression of life-threatening ventricular arrhythmias, such as supraventricular tachycardia — **Adults:** initially, 150 mg P.O. q 8 hr. May increase dose at 3- to 4-day intervals to 225 mg q 8 hr; if necessary, increase to 300 mg q 8 hr. Maximum 900 mg q.d.

- Continuous cardiac monitoring recommended during initiation and dosage adjustments. If PR interval or QRS complex increases by > 25%, expect to reduce dose.
- During use with digoxin, frequently monitor ECG and serum digoxin.

263

†Canadian ‡Australian

DRUG / CLASS / CATEGORY	INDICATIONS / DOSAGES	KEY NURSING CONSIDERATIONS
propantheline bromide Pro-Banthine *Anticholinergic* *Antimuscarinic/GI antispasmodic* Pregnancy Risk Category: C	*Adjunctive treatment of peptic ulceration —* **Adults:** 15 mg P.O. t.i.d. before meals and 30 mg h.s. **Elderly:** 7.5 mg P.O. t.i.d. before meals.	• Give 30 min to 1 hr before meals and h.s. Bedtime doses can be larger; give at least 2 hr after last meal of day. • Advise patient to avoid hazardous activities if drowsiness, dizziness, or blurred vision occurs; to drink plenty of fluids; and to report skin eruptions.
propofol Diprivan *Phenol derivative* *Anesthetic* Pregnancy Risk Category: B	*Initiation and maintenance of intensive care unit sedation in intubated, mechanically ventilated patients —* **Adults:** usually, 5 mcg/kg/min for 5 min. Increase rate at 5- to 10-min intervals in increments of 5 to 10 mcg/kg/min until desired response. Rates of 5 to 50 mcg/kg/min or higher may be required.	• Use cautiously in patients with seizures. • Allow adequate interval between dosage adjustments to assess effects. • Titrate drug daily to achieve only minimum effective drug concentration. • Don't administer in same I.V. line with blood or plasma. • Consult references for anesthesia dosages.
propoxyphene hydrochloride Darvon, 692† **propoxyphene napsylate** Darvon-N, Doloxene‡ *Narcotic analgesic* *Opioid analgesic* Pregnancy Risk Category: C	*Mild to moderate pain —* **Adults:** 65 mg (hydrochloride) P.O. q 4 hr, p.r.n. Maximum 390 mg/day. *Mild to moderate pain —* **Adults:** 100 mg (napsylate) P.O. q 4 hr, p.r.n. Maximum 600 mg/day.	• Mild narcotic analgesic. • Warn patient not to exceed recommended dosage. Respiratory depression, hypotension, profound sedation, and coma may result if used in excessive doses or with other CNS depressants. • Advise patient to avoid alcohol or other CNS-type drugs.

propranolol hydrochloride

Deralin‡, Detensol†, Inderal, Inderal LA, Novopranol†

Beta blocker

Antihypertensive/antianginal/antiarrhythmic/ adjunctive therapy for MI

Pregnancy Risk Category: C

Angina pectoris — **Adults:** total daily dose, 80 to 320 mg P.O. b.i.d., t.i.d., or q.i.d.; or one 80-mg extended-release capsule q.d. Increase dose at 7- to 10-day intervals.

Mortality reduction after MI — **Adults:** 180 to 240 mg P.O. t.i.d. or q.i.d. 5 to 21 days after MI.

Supraventricular and ventricular arrhythmias; tachyarrhythmias due to excessive catecholamine action during anesthesia or in hyperthyroidism or pheochromocytoma — **Adults:** 0.5 to 3 mg by slow I.V. push (≤ 1 mg/min). After 3 mg, give next dose in 2 min; other doses > q 4 hr. Maintenance 10 to 30 mg P.O. t.i.d. or q.i.d.

Hypertension — **Adults:** 80 mg P.O. q.d. in 2 to 4 divided doses or extended-release q.d. Increase at 3- to 7-day intervals. Maximum 640 mg q.d. Maintenance 160 to 480 mg q.d.

Essential tremor — **Adults:** 40 mg P.O. b.i.d. Maintenance 120 to 320 mg q.d. in 3 divided doses.

Hypertrophic subaortic stenosis — **Adults:** 20 to 40 mg P.O. t.i.d. or q.i.d., or 80 to 160 mg extended-release capsules once daily.

Adjunct therapy in pheochromocytoma — **Adults:** 60 mg P.O. q.d. in divided doses with an alpha blocker 3 days before surgery.

- Check apical pulse before giving drug. If extremes detected, stop drug and call doctor at once.
- Double-check dose and route.
- *I.V. use:* Give by direct injection into a large vessel or into the tubing of a free-flowing, compatible I.V. solution; continuous I.V. infusion generally is not recommended. Or, dilute drug with 0.9% NaCl solution and give by intermittent infusion over 10 to 15 min in 0.1- to 0.2-mg increments. Drug is compatible with D_5W and 0.45% and 0.9% NaCl and lactated Ringer's solutions.
- Give drug with meals.
- If severe hypotension occurs, notify doctor.
- Drug masks common signs of shock and hypoglycemia.
- For I.V. use, may be diluted and infused slowly.

DRUG/CLASS/ CATEGORY	INDICATIONS/ DOSAGES	KEY NURSING CONSIDERATIONS
propylthiouracil (PTU) Propyl-Thyracil† *Thyroid hormone antagonist* *Antihyperthyroid agent* Pregnancy Risk Category: D	*Hyperthyroidism* — **Adults:** 100 to 150 mg P.O. t.i.d.; up to 1,200 mg q.d. Maintenance 100 to 150 mg q.d. in divided doses t.i.d. **Children > 10 yr:** 150 to 300 mg P.O. q.d. in divided doses t.i.d. **Children 6 to 10 yr:** 50 to 150 mg P.O. q.d. in divided doses t.i.d. *Thyrotoxic crisis* — **Adults and children:** 200 mg P.O. q 4 to 6 hr on first day. Reduce dose gradually to maintenance level.	• Monitor thyroid function studies in pregnant patients. Thyroid may be added to regimen. Drug may be stopped during last few weeks of pregnancy. • Watch for hypothyroidism (depression; cold intolerance; hard, nonpitting edema); adjust dosage as ordered.
protamine sulfate *Antidote* *Heparin antagonist* Pregnancy Risk Category: C	*Heparin overdose* — **Adults:** dosage based on blood coagulation studies, usually 1 mg for each 90 to 115 U heparin. Maximum 50 mg.	• *I.V. use:* Give slowly over 10 min. Have emergency equipment available. • May act as anticoagulant in high doses.
pseudoephedrine hydrochloride Children's Sudafed, Drixoral, Efidac/24, Pedia Care Infant's Decongestant, Sudafed **pseudoephedrine sulfate** Afrin, Drixoral *Adrenergic* *Decongestant* Pregnancy Risk Category: C	*Nasal and eustachian tube decongestion* — **Adults:** 60 mg P.O. q 4 hr. Maximum 240 mg q.d. Or, 120 mg extended-release tablets P.O. q 12 hr or 240 mg extended-release q.d. **Children > 12 yr:** 120 mg P.O. q 12 hr, or 240 mg P.O. q.d. **Children 6 to 12 yr:** 30 mg P.O. regular-release form q 4 to 6 hr. Maximum 120 mg q.d. **Children 2 to 6 yr:** 15 mg P.O. regular-release form q 4 to 6 hr. Maximum 60 mg/day. **Children 1 to 2 yr:** 7 drops (0.2 ml)/kg q 4 to 6 hr, up to 4 doses/day. **Children 3 to 12 mo:** 3 drops/kg q 4 to 6 hr,	• Elderly patients more sensitive to drug effects. • Warn patient against using OTC products containing other sympathomimetics. • Tell patient not to take within 2 hr of bedtime. • Don't use with MAO inhibitors. • Tell patient not to crush or break forms. • Instruct patient to stop drug and notify doctor if unusual restlessness occurs.

up to 4 doses/day.

psyllium

Fiberall, Maalox Daily Fiber
Therapy, Metamucil, Mylanta
Natural Fiber Supplement,
Pro-Lax
Absorbent
Bulk laxative
Pregnancy Risk Category: NR

Constipation; bowel management — **Adults:**
1 to 2 tsp (rounded) P.O. in full glass of liquid q.d., b.i.d., or t.i.d.; or 1 packet dissolved in water q.d., b.i.d., or t.i.d. **Children > 6 yr:**
1 tsp (level) P.O. in half glass of liquid h.s.

- Mix with at least 8 oz (240 ml) of cold, pleasant-tasting liquid, such as orange juice, to mask grittiness; stir only few sec. Have patient drink immediately. Follow with additional glass of liquid.

pyrazinamide

Pyrazinamide†, Tebrazid†
Synthetic pyrazine analogue
Antituberculotic
Pregnancy Risk Category: C

Adjunctive treatment of TB — **Adults:** 15 to 30 mg/kg P.O. q.d. Maximum 2 g q.d. If patient noncompliant, 50 to 70 mg/kg P.O. twice weekly.

- Given for initial 2 mo if ≥ 6-mo regimen. Patients with HIV may require longer course.
- Watch for signs of gout and liver impairment.

pyridostigmine bromide

Mestinon, Mestinon-SR,
Mestinon Timespans,
Regonol
Cholinesterase inhibitor
Muscle stimulant
Pregnancy Risk Category: NR

Antidote for nondepolarizing neuromuscular blockers — **Adults:** 10 to 20 mg I.V. preceded by atropine sulfate 0.6 to 1.2 mg I.V.
Myasthenia gravis — **Adults:** 60 to 120 mg P.O. q 3 or 4 hr. Usual dose, 600 mg q.d.; higher dose may be needed. For I.M. or I.V. use, give 1/30 of oral dose. Or, 180 to 540 mg extended-release tablets (1 to 3 tablets) P.O. b.i.d., with at least 6 hr between doses. **Children:** 7 mg/kg P.O. or 200 mg/m2 P.O. q.d. in 5 or 6 divided doses.
Supportive treatment of neonates born to myasthenic mothers — **Neonates:** 0.05 to

- Stop other cholinergics before giving drug.
- ***I.V. use:*** Give I.V. injection no faster than 1 mg/min. Monitor vital signs. Position patient to ease breathing. Be ready to give atropine injection; provide respiratory support, p.r.n.
- Don't crush extended-release (Timespans) tablets.
- Test dose of edrophonium I.V. aggravates drug-induced weakness but temporarily relieves weakness caused by disease.

(continued)

267

†Canadian ‡Australian

DRUG / CLASS / CATEGORY	INDICATIONS / DOSAGES	KEY NURSING CONSIDERATIONS
pyridostigmine bromide *(continued)*	0.15 mg/kg I.M. q 4 to 6 hr. Decrease dose q.d. until drug can be stopped.	• Regonol (U.S. only) contains benzyl ethanol that may cause toxicity in neonates if given in high doses.
pyridoxine hydrochloride (vitamin B₆) Beesix, Nestrex, Rodex *Water-soluble vitamin* *Nutritional supplement* Pregnancy Risk Category: A	*Dietary vitamin B₆ deficiency* — **Adults:** 10 to 20 mg P.O., I.M. or I.V. q.d. for 3 wk; then 2 to 5 mg q.d. as supplement to proper diet. *Seizures related to vitamin B₆ deficiency or dependency* — **Adults and children:** 100 mg I.M. or I.V. in single dose. *Isoniazid poisoning (> 10 g)* — **Adults:** give equal amount of pyridoxine: 4 g I.V. followed by 1 g I.M. q 30 min.	• Protect from light. Don't use solution if it contains precipitate, although slight darkening acceptable. • High doses (2 to 6 g/day) may cause difficulty walking. • Monitor diet. Excessive protein intake increases daily pyridoxine requirements.
pyrimethamine Daraprim **pyrimethamine with sulfadoxine** Fansidar *Aminopyrimidine derivative (folic acid antagonist)* *Antimalarial* Pregnancy Risk Category: C	*Malaria prophylaxis and transmission control (pyrimethamine)* — **Adults and children ≥ 10 yr:** 25 mg P.O. weekly. **Children 4 to 10 yr:** 12.5 mg P.O. weekly. **Children < 4 yr:** 6.25 mg P.O. weekly. Continue 6 to 10 wk after leaving endemic areas. *Acute attacks of malaria (Fansidar)* — **Adults and children ≥ 14 yr:** 2 to 3 tablets as single dose. **Children 9 to 14 yr:** 2 tablets/wk. **Children 4 to 8 yr:** 1 tablet/wk. **Children < 4 yr:** ¾ tablet/wk. *Malaria prophylaxis (Fansidar)* — **Adults and children ≥ 14 yr:** 1 tablet/wk. **Children 9 to 14	• Obtain twice-weekly blood counts, including platelets, for toxoplasmosis patient. • Fansidar should be used in areas where chloroquine-resistant malaria prevalent and if traveler plans to stay > 3 wk. • Tell patient to take with meals. • Instruct patient to stop drug and notify doctor at first sign of rash. • Not recommended alone in nonimmune patients; use with faster-acting antimalarials for 2 days to initiate transmission control and suppressive cure.

yr: ¾ tablet/wk. **Children 4 to 8 yr:** ½ tablet/wk. **Children < 4 yr:** ¼ tablet/wk.

Acute attacks of malaria (pyrimethamine) — **Adults and children ≥ 15 yr:** 25 mg P.O. q.d. for 2 days. **Children < 15 yr:** 12.5 mg P.O. q.d. for 2 days.

Toxoplasmosis (pyrimethamine) — **Adults:** 50 to 75 mg P.O. q.d. for 1 to 3 wk, then reduce dose by 50% and continue for additional 4 to 5 wk. **Children:** 1 mg/kg P.O. (< 100 mg) in 2 equally divided doses for 2 to 4 days, then 0.5 mg/kg q.d. for 4 wk.

- Sulfadiazine given with pyrimethamine to treat toxoplasmosis.

---

quetiapine fumarate
Seroquel
Dibenzothiazipine derivative
Antipsychotic
Pregnancy Risk Category: C

Management of manifestations of psychotic disorders — **Adults:** 25 mg b.i.d. Increase by 25 to 50 mg b.i.d. or t.i.d. on days 2 and 3, as tolerated. Target dose range of 300 to 400 mg q.d., divided b.i.d. or t.i.d., by day 4. Further dose adjustments should occur at intervals of ≥ 2 days, p.r.n. **Elderly:** give lower doses, slow titration, and carefully monitor in the initial dosing period.

Adjust-a-dose: In patients with hepatic impairment or hypotension or in debilitated patients, use lower doses and slower titration.

- Use with caution in patients with CV or cerebrovascular disease, conditions that predispose patients to hypotension, or a history of seizures or conditions that lower the seizure threshold.
- Use with caution in patients who will experience conditions in which the core body temperature may be elevated.
- Watch for symptoms of neuroleptic malignant syndrome (extrapyramidal effects, hyperthermia, autonomic disturbance).
- Monitor patient for tardive dyskinesia.

---

quinapril hydrochloride
Accupril, Asig‡
ACE inhibitor

Hypertension — **Adults:** initially, 10 mg P.O. q.d. or 5 mg q.d. if patient takes diuretic. Adjust based on response at 2-wk intervals.

- Advise patient to report angioedema (including laryngeal edema).
- Monitor BP for effectiveness.

(continued)

269

†Canadian ‡Australian

DRUG/CLASS/ CATEGORY	INDICATIONS/ DOSAGES	KEY NURSING CONSIDERATIONS
quinapril hydrochloride *(continued)* *Antihypertensive* Pregnancy Risk Category: C (first trimester); D (second and third trimesters)	*Heart failure* — **Adults:** 5 to 10 mg P.O. b.i.d. Increase at weekly intervals.	▪ Observe for light-headedness and syncope. ▪ Monitor serum potassium.
quinidine gluconate Quinaglute Dura-Tabs, Quinalan, Quinate† **quinidine sulfate** Apo-Quinidine†, Cin-Quin, Quinidex Extentabs *Cinchona alkaloid* *Antitachyarrhythmic* Pregnancy Risk Category: C	*Atrial flutter or fibrillation* — **Adults:** 200 mg P.O. q 2 to 3 hr for 5 to 8 doses, then increase q.d. Maximum 3 to 4 g q.d. *Paroxysmal supraventricular tachycardia* — **Adults:** 400 to 600 mg I.M. or P.O. q 2 to 3 hr. *Premature atrial contractions; premature ventricular contractions; paroxysmal atrial tachycardia; paroxysmal ventricular tachycardia; maintenance after cardioversion of atrial fibrillation* — **Adults:** test dose 200 mg P.O. or I.M. Then 200 to 400 mg (sulfate or equivalent base) P.O. q 4 to 6 hr; or 600 mg (gluconate) I.M. then 400 mg q 2 hr, p.r.n.; or 800 mg (gluconate) in 40 ml D_5W I.V. infusion at 16 mg/min. **Children:** test dose 2 mg/kg P.O.; then 30 mg/kg/24 hr P.O. or 900 mg/m²/24 hr P.O. in 5 divided doses.	▪ Use cautiously in impaired renal or hepatic function, asthma, muscle weakness, or infection with fever. ▪ Check apical pulse and BP before therapy. ▪ Adverse GI reactions signal toxicity. Check blood drug levels; > 8 mcg/ml toxic. ▪ Give with meals to prevent GI symptoms. ▪ Give sulfate or equivalent base for atrial flutter or fibrillation only if AV node has been blocked by another agent to prevent increased AV conduction.

raloxifene hydrochloride

Evista

Selective estrogen receptor modulator

Antiosteoporotic

Pregnancy Risk Category: X

Prevention of osteoporosis in postmenopausal women — **Adults:** 60 mg P.O. q.d.

- Use cautiously in those with liver disease.
- Greatest risk for thromboembolic events occurs during first 4 mo of treatment.
- Discontinue at least 72 hr before prolonged immobilization and resume after patient is fully mobilized.
- Report unexplained uterine bleeding.

---

ramipril

Altace, Ramace‡, Tritace‡

ACE inhibitor

Antihypertensive

Pregnancy Risk Category: C (first trimester); D (second and third trimesters)

Hypertension — **Adults:** initially, 2.5 mg P.O. q.d. for patient not taking diuretic; 1.25 mg P.O. q.d. for patient taking diuretic. Increase, p.r.n., based on response. Maintenance 2.5 to 20 mg q.d. as single or divided doses.

Heart failure — **Adults:** 2.5 mg P.O. b.i.d. If hypotension, decrease to 1.25 mg P.O. b.i.d. May increase slowly to maximum 5 mg P.O. b.i.d., p.r.n.

Adjust-a-dose: In patients with creatinine clearance < 40 ml/min, give 1.25 mg P.O. q.d. Adjust gradually according to response.

- Advise patient to report angioedema (including laryngeal edema).
- Monitor BP regularly.
- Watch for light-headedness and syncope.
- Monitor serum potassium.

---

ranitidine hydrochloride

Apo-Ranitidine†, Zantac, Zantac-C†, Zantac 75

H₂-receptor antagonist

Antiulcerative

Pregnancy Risk Category: B

Duodenal and gastric ulcer (short-term treatment); pathologic hypersecretory conditions, such as Zollinger-Ellison syndrome — **Adults:** 150 mg P.O. b.i.d. or 300 mg q.d. h.s. Or: 50 mg I.V. or I.M. q 6 to 8 hr. Patients with Zollinger-Ellison syndrome may need up to 6 g P.O. q.d.

Maintenance therapy for duodenal or gastric ulcer — **Adults:** 150 mg P.O. h.s.

- **I.V. use:** When giving I.V. push, dilute to total volume of 20 ml and inject over 5 min.
- For intermittent I.V. infusion, dilute 50 mg in 100 ml compatible solution, and infuse over 15 to 20 min.
- For continuous I.V. infusion: 150 mg in 250 ml compatible solution. Administer at 6.25 mg/hr using infusion pump.

(continued)

DRUG/CLASS/ CATEGORY	INDICATIONS/ DOSAGES	KEY NURSING CONSIDERATIONS
ranitidine hydrochloride *(continued)*	*Gastroesophageal reflux disease* — **Adults:** 150 mg P.O. b.i.d. **Adjust-a-dose:** In patients with creatinine clearance < 50 ml/min, give 150 mg P.O. q 24 hr or 50 mg I.V. q 18 to 24 hr.	• Incompatible with aluminum.
ranitidine bismuth citrate Tritec *H₂-receptor agonist Antiulcerative* Pregnancy Risk Category: C	*In combination with clarithromycin for treatment of active duodenal ulcer associated with H. pylori infection* — **Adults:** 400 mg P.O. b.i.d with clarithromycin.	• Don't use with clarithromycin in patients with history of acute porphyria. • Shouldn't be used alone for treatment of active duodenal ulcers. • May cause temporary and harmless darkening of the tongue or stool.
repaglinide Prandin *Meglitinide Antidiabetic* Pregnancy Risk Category: C	*Adjunct to diet and exercise in lowering blood glucose in patients with type 2 diabetes mellitus whose hyperglycemia cannot be controlled by diet and exercise alone; in combination with metformin to lower blood glucose in patients whose hyperglycemia cannot be controlled by exercise, diet, and either repaglinide or metformin alone* — **Adults:** for patients not previously treated or whose glycosylated hemoglobin (HbA1c) is < 8%, 0.5 mg P.O. taken immediately to 30 min before each meal; for those previously treated with glucose-lowering drugs and whose HbA1c is ≥ 8%, 1 to 2 mg P.O., taken	• Use cautiously in elderly, debilitated, or malnourished patients and in those with adrenal or pituitary insufficiency because they're more susceptible to the hypoglycemic effect of glucose-lowering drugs. • Increase dosage carefully in patients with impaired renal function or renal failure requiring dialysis. • Adjust dosage by blood glucose response. May double dose up to 4 mg with each meal until patient achieves satisfactory response. At least 1 wk should elapse between dosage adjustments.

Drug	Indications & Dosages	Nursing Considerations
	immediately to 30 min before each meal. Recommended dose range is 0.5 to 4 mg with meals, divided b.i.d., t.i.d., or q.i.d. Maximum daily dose is 16 mg.	■ Be aware that loss of glycemic control can occur during stress. ■ Hypoglycemia may be difficult to recognize in the elderly and in patients taking beta blockers.
respiratory syncytial virus immune globulin intravenous, human (RSV-IGIV) RespiGam *Immunoglobulin G* *Immune serum* Pregnancy Risk Category: C	*Prevention of serious lower respiratory tract infections caused by RSV in children with bronchopulmonary dysplasia (BPD) or premature infants and children < 2 yr:* single infusion monthly. Give 1.5 ml/kg/hr I.V. for 15 min; then may increase to 3 ml/kg/hr for 15 min until infusion ends. Maximum 6 ml/kg/hr until infusion ends. Maximum total per monthly infusion 750 mg/kg.	■ Assess cardiopulmonary status and vital signs before infusion, each rate increase, and q 30 min until 30 min after infusion. ■ May use slower rate in critically ill children with BPD. ■ Monitor for fluid overload. ■ *I.V. use:* Enter single-use vial only once; don't shake, avoid foaming. Begin infusion within 6 hr and complete by 12 hr.
reteplase, recombinant Retavase *Tissue plasminogen activator* *Thrombolytic* Pregnancy Risk Category: C	*Management of acute MI —* **Adults:** double-bolus of 10 + 10 U. Give each bolus I.V. over 2 min. If no complications after first bolus, give second bolus 30 min after start of first.	■ Carefully monitor ECG during treatment. ■ Monitor for bleeding and mental status changes. Avoid I.M. injections, invasive procedures, and nonessential patient handling. If bleeding or anaphylactoid reactions occur after first bolus, notify doctor. ■ Don't give with other I.V. medications.
ribavirin Virazole *Synthetic nucleoside* *Antiviral* Pregnancy Risk Category: X	*Hospitalized infants and young children infected by RSV —* **Infants and young children:** solution in concentration of 20 mg/ml delivered via Viratek Small Particle Aerosol Generator (SPAG-2) and mechanical	■ Administer aerosol form by SPAG-2 only. ■ Use sterile USP water for injection only. ■ Discard solutions placed in SPAG-2 unit ≥ 24 hr before adding newly reconstituted solution.

(continued)

†Canadian ‡Australian

DRUG/CLASS/CATEGORY	INDICATIONS/DOSAGES	KEY NURSING CONSIDERATIONS
ribavirin *(continued)*	ventilation, or via oxygen mask, hood, or tent at flow rate of 12.5 L/min mist. Treat for 12 to 18 hr/day for 3 to 7 days, with flow rate of 12.5 L/min of mist.	• Eye irritation and headache reported in health care personnel exposed to aerosolized drug. • Monitor ventilator function frequently.
riboflavin (vitamin B₂) *Water-soluble vitamin* *Vitamin B complex vitamin* Pregnancy Risk Category: NR	Riboflavin deficiency or adjunct to thiamine treatment for polyneuritis or cheilosis secondary to pellagra — **Adults and children ≥ 12 yr:** 5 to 30 mg P.O. q.d., depending on severity. **Children < 12 yr:** 3 to 10 mg P.O. q.d., depending on severity.	• Deficiency often accompanies other vitamin B complex deficiencies; may require multivitamin therapy. • Tell patient to take with meals; food increases absorption. • Urine may appear bright yellow.
rifabutin *Mycobutin* *Semisynthetic ansamycin* *Antibiotic* Pregnancy Risk Category: B	Prevention of disseminated MAC in advanced HIV infection — **Adults:** 300 mg P.O. q.d. as single dose or divided b.i.d., with food.	• Use cautiously in preexisting neutropenia and thrombocytopenia. • Perform baseline hematologic studies; repeat periodically. • May stain soft contact lenses.
rifampin (rifampicin) *Rifadin, Rifadin IV, Rimactane, Rimycin‡, Rofact†* *Semisynthetic rifamycin B derivative (macrocyclic antibiotic)* *Antituberculotic* Pregnancy Risk Category: C	Pulmonary TB — **Adults:** 600 mg/day P.O. or I.V. in single dose 1 hr before or 2 hr after meals. **Children > 5 yr:** 10 to 20 mg/kg P.O. or I.V. in single dose 1 hr before or 2 hr after meals. Maximum 600 mg/day. Give with other antituberculotics. Meningococcal carriers — **Adults:** 600 mg P.O. or I.V. b.i.d. for 2 days, or 600 mg/day P.O. or I.V. for 4 days. **Children 1 mo to 12 yr:** 10	• Give 1 hr before or 2 hr after meals. • *I.V. use:* Reconstitute with 10 ml sterile water for injection to make solution containing 60 mg/ml. Add to 100 ml D₅W and infuse over 30 min, or add to 500 ml D₅W and infuse over 3 hr. • Give with ≥ one other antituberculotic. • May discolor urine, feces, saliva, sweat, sputum, and tears red-orange.

		■ May stain soft contact lenses.

mg/kg P.O. or I.V. b.i.d. for 2 days, ≤ 600 mg/day, or 10 to 20 mg/kg/day for 4 days. **Neonates:** 5 mg/kg P.O. or I.V. b.i.d. for 2 days. *Prophylaxis of* H. influenzae type b — **Adults and children:** 20 mg/kg/day P.O. for 4 days; maximum 600 mg/day.

---

rifapentine
Priftin
RNA polymerase inhibitor
Antituberculotic
Pregnancy Risk Category: C

Pulmonary tuberculosis, in conjunction with at least one other antituberculotic — **Adults:** during intensive phase of short-course therapy, 600 mg P.O. twice weekly for 2 mo, with an interval between doses of ≥ 3 days (≥ 72 hr). During continuation phase of short-course therapy, 600 mg P.O. once weekly for 4 mo with another antituberculotic.

- Monitor liver function tests before therapy.
- Must give with appropriate daily companion drugs. Compliance crucial for early sputum conversion and protection from relapse of tuberculosis.
- Giving during last 2 wk of pregnancy may lead to postnatal hemorrhage in mother or infant.
- Notify doctor of persistent or severe diarrhea.

---

riluzole
Rilutek
Benzothiazole
Neuroprotector
Pregnancy Risk Category: C

Amyotrophic lateral sclerosis — **Adults:** 50 mg P.O. q 12 hr, on empty stomach.

- Tell patient to take at same time daily.
- Instruct patient to report fever.
- Caution patient to avoid hazardous activities.
- Perform liver function tests periodically.

---

rimantadine hydrochloride
Flumadine
Adamantine
Antiviral
Pregnancy Risk Category: C

Influenza A (preventive) — **Adults and children ≥ 10 yr:** 100 mg P.O. b.i.d. **Children < 10 yr:** 5 mg/kg (maximum 150 mg) P.O. q.d. **Elderly:** 100 mg P.O. q.d.
Influenza A — **Adults:** 100 mg P.O. b.i.d., within 24 to 48 hr of symptom onset and for 48 hr after symptoms disappear.

- Use cautiously in renal or hepatic impairment and in history of seizures. Pregnant patients should compare risks versus benefits before starting.
- Tell patient to take several hr before bedtime.

(continued)

†Canadian ‡Australian

DRUG / CLASS / CATEGORY	INDICATIONS / DOSAGES	KEY NURSING CONSIDERATIONS
rimantadine hydrochloride *(continued)*	*Adjust-a-dose:* In patients with severe hepatic or renal dysfunction or those who experience adverse effects at normal dosage, give 100 mg P.O. q.d.	▪ Tell patient to take infection-control precautions. ▪ Resistant strains may emerge during therapy.
risperidone Risperdal Benzisoxazole derivative Antipsychotic Pregnancy Risk Category: C	*Psychosis —* **Adults:** initially, 1 mg P.O. b.i.d., increased in 1-mg increments b.i.d. on days 2 and 3 to 3 mg b.i.d. Wait ≥ 1 wk before adjusting dose. Safety of > 16 mg/day not known. *Adjust-a-dose:* In debilitated patients or those with hypotension or severe renal or hepatic impairment, give 0.5 mg P.O. b.i.d. Increase by 0.5-mg increments b.i.d. on days 2 and 3 to 1.5 mg P.O. b.i.d. Wait ≥ 1 wk before increasing.	▪ Obtain baseline BP; monitor often. ▪ Look for orthostatic hypotension and tardive dyskinesia. ▪ Assess for neuroleptic malignant syndrome. ▪ Use lower dose in elderly patients.
ritonavir Norvir Human immunodeficiency virus protease inhibitor Antiviral Pregnancy Risk Category: B	*Treatment of HIV infection with nucleoside analogues; as monotherapy when antiretroviral therapy needed —* **Adults:** 600 mg b.i.d. before meals. If nausea occurs, adjust dosage: 300 mg b.i.d. for 1 day, 400 mg b.i.d. for 2 days, 500 mg b.i.d. for 1 day, and 600 mg b.i.d. thereafter.	▪ Give before meals to decrease nausea. ▪ May be given alone or with nucleoside analogues. ▪ With combination regimen, patient may benefit by taking ritonavir alone and then adding nucleosides before completing 2 wk of ritonavir.
rituximab Rituxan	*B-cell malignant lymphoma with relapsed or refractory low-grade or follicular, CD20 posi-*	▪ Monitor patient closely for signs and symptoms of hypersensitivity reaction.

Monoclonal antibody
Antineoplastic
Pregnancy Risk Factor: C

tive disease — **Adults:** 375 mg/m² as I.V. infusion once weekly for 4 doses (days 1, 8, 15, and 22). Start initial infusion at 50 mg/hr. If hypersensitivity or infusion-related events don't occur, increase to 50 mg/hr q 30 min, to maximum of 400 mg/hr. Can give subsequent infusions, initially, at 100 mg/hr and increase by 100 mg/hr at 30-min intervals, to maximum of 400 mg/hr, as tolerated.

- Premedicate with acetaminophen and diphenhydramine before each infusion.
- Obtain CBC at regular intervals.
- Don't give as I.V. push or bolus.
- Monitor BP closely during infusion. If hypotension, bronchospasm, or angioedema occurs, stop and restart at 50% rate reduction when symptoms resolve. Stop infusion if serious arrhythmias occur.

---

rizatriptan benzoate
Maxalt, Maxalt-MLT
Serotonin receptor agonist
Antimigraine agent
Pregnancy Risk Category: C

Treatment of acute migraine headaches with or without aura — **Adults:** 5 or 10 mg P.O. If 1st dose ineffective, can give another dose 2 hr after first. Maximum dose is 30 mg/24 hr. For patients receiving propranolol, give 5 mg P.O. up to maximum of 3 doses (15 mg) in 24 hr.

- Use cautiously in patients with hepatic or renal impairment or risk of CAD.
- Don't use for prophylactic therapy or in patients with hemiplegic or basilar migraine or cluster headaches.

---

ropinirole hydrochloride
Requip
Nonergoline dopamine agonist
Antiparkinsonian
Pregnancy Risk Category: C

Idiopathic Parkinson's disease — **Adults:** 0.25 mg P.O. t.i.d. Adjust q wk. After wk 4, may increase by 1.5 mg/day q wk up to 9 mg/day, then increase q wk up to 3 mg/day. Maximum 24 mg/day.

- Monitor patient carefully for orthostatic hypotension, especially during dose escalation. May cause syncope.
- Can potentiate adverse effects of levodopa and may cause or exacerbate dyskinesia.
- May cause hallucinations.
- Withdraw gradually over 7 days.

---

rotavirus vaccine, live, oral, tetravalent
RotaShield

Prevention of gastroenteritis caused by rotavirus serotypes contained in vaccine — **Infants < 6 mo born ≥ 37 wk gestation:** 2.5 ml P.O. at 2, 4, and 6 mo. Or, may give 1st

- May give with standard childhood vaccines, including OPV, HIB, and whole-cell DTP.

(continued)

†Canadian ‡Australian

DRUG / CLASS / CATEGORY	INDICATIONS / DOSAGES	KEY NURSING CONSIDERATIONS
rotavirus vaccine (continued) Live vaccine Oral vaccine Pregnancy Risk Category: C	dose as early as 6 wk of age, with subsequent doses at least 3 wk apart.	▪ Repeat dosing isn't indicated if infant regurgitates vaccine. ▪ Keep vaccinated children from contact with immunocompromised persons at high risk for up to 4 wk.
rubella and mumps virus vaccine, live Biavax II Vaccine Viral vaccine Pregnancy Risk Category: C	*Rubella and mumps immunization* — **Adults and children ≥ 1 yr:** 0.5 ml S.C.	▪ Obtain history of allergies and reaction to antibiotics or immunization. ▪ Keep epinephrine 1:1,000 available. ▪ Use only diluent supplied. Discard 8 hr after reconstituting. ▪ Inject S.C. into outer upper arm.
rubella virus vaccine, live attenuated (RA 27/3) Meruvax II Vaccine Viral vaccine Pregnancy Risk Category: C	*Rubella immunization* — **Adults and children ≥ 1 yr:** 0.5 ml (1,000 U) S.C.	▪ Obtain history of allergies and reaction to immunization. ▪ Keep epinephrine 1:1,000 available. ▪ Use only diluent supplied. Discard 8 hr after reconstituting. ▪ Inject S.C. into outer upper arm.
salmeterol xinafoate Serevent, Serevent Diskus Selective beta₂-adrenergic stimulating agonist Bronchodilator	*Long-term maintenance of asthma; prevention of bronchospasm for nocturnal asthma or reversible obstructive airway disease* — **Adults and children > 12 yr:** 2 inhalations b.i.d. *Prevention of exercise-induced broncho-*	▪ Use cautiously in CV disorders, thyrotoxicosis, or seizure disorders and in patients unusually responsive to sympathomimetics. ▪ Tell patient to take at 12-hr intervals. ▪ Instruct patient to use 30 to 60 min before

Pregnancy Risk Category: C	spasm — **Adults and children ≥ 12 yr:** 2 inhalations 30 to 60 min before exercise.	• Monitor hydration if adverse GI reactions occur. • Adverse reactions include headache, nausea, and diarrhea.
saquinavir Fortovase **saquinavir mesylate** Invirase *Protease inhibitor* *Antiviral* Pregnancy Risk Category: B	*Adjunct treatment of advanced HIV infection in selected patients* — **Adults:** 600 mg (Invirase) or 1,200 mg (Fortovase) P.O. t.i.d. within 2 hr after full meal and with nucleoside analogue.	
sargramostim (granulocyte-macrophage colony-stimulating factor, GM-CSF) Leukine *Biologic response modifier* *Colony-stimulating factor* Pregnancy Risk Category: C	*Acceleration of hematopoietic reconstitution after autologous bone marrow transplantation (BMT)* — **Adults:** 250 mcg/m²/day for 21 days given as 2-hr I.V. infusion starting 2 to 4 hr after BMT. *BMT failure or engraftment delay* — **Adults:** 250 mcg/m²/day for 14 days as 2-hr I.V. infusion. May repeat dose after 7 days of no therapy.	• Don't add other medications to infusion solution. • Don't give within 24 hr of last chemotherapy dose or within 12 hr of last radiotherapy dose. • Monitor CBC with differential. • Transient rash and local reactions at injection site may occur. • Duration of therapy based on indications and response.
scopolamine (hyoscine) Isopto Hyoscine, Transderm-Scōp, Transderm-V† **scopolamine butylbromide (hyoscine butylbromide)**	*Spastic states* — **Adults:** 10 to 20 mg P.O. t.i.d. or q.i.d. Adjust dosage, p.r.n. Or 10 to 20 mg (butylbromide) S.C., I.M., or I.V. t.i.d. or q.i.d. *Delirium; preanesthetic sedation and obstetric amnesia with analgesics* — **Adults:** 0.3 to 0.65 mg I.M., S.C., or I.V. **Children:** 0.006 mg/kg I.M., S.C., I.V.; maximum 0.3 mg.	• Use cautiously in autonomic neuropathy, hyperthyroidism, CAD, arrhythmias, heart failure, hypertension, hiatal hernia associated with reflux esophagitis, hepatic or renal disease, or ulcerative colitis; in children < 6 yr; or in hot or humid environments. *(continued)*

†Canadian ‡Australian

DRUG/CLASS / CATEGORY	INDICATIONS / DOSAGES	KEY NURSING CONSIDERATIONS
scopolamine (continued) Buscopan‡ **scopolamine hydrobromide (hyoscine hydrobromide; systemic])** *Anticholinergic* *Antimuscarinic/cycloplegic mydriatic* Pregnancy Risk Category: C	*Prevention of motion sickness* — **Adults:** 1 Transderm-Scop or Transderm-V patch applied to skin behind ear several hr before antiemetic required. Or 300 to 600 mcg (hydrobromide) S.C., I.M., or I.V. **Children:** 6 mcg/kg or 200 mcg/m² (hydrobromide) S.C., I.M., or I.V.	• *I.V. use:* Avoid intermittent and continuous infusions. For direct I.V. use, dilute with sterile water. • Protect I.V. solutions from freezing and light; store at room temperature. • Tolerance may develop with long-term use.
scopolamine hydrobromide Isopto Hyoscine *Anticholinergic* *Antimuscarinic/cycloplegic mydriatic* Pregnancy Risk Category: NR	*Cycloplegic refraction* — **Adults:** 1 to 2 drops 0.25% solution 1 hr before refraction. **Children:** 1 drop 0.25% solution b.i.d. for 2 days before refraction. *Iritis; uveitis* — **Adults:** 1 to 2 drops 0.25% solution q.d. to q.i.d. **Children:** 1 drop q.d. to q.i.d.	• Warn patient to avoid hazardous activities until temporary blurring subsides. • Observe for adverse CNS effects. • Advise patient to wear dark glasses. • May use in patients sensitive to atropine. • Compress lacrimal sac by distal pressure for several min after installation.
secobarbital sodium Novosecobarb†, Seconal Sodium *Barbiturate* *Sedative-hypnotic/anticonvulsant*	*Preoperative sedation* — **Adults:** 200 to 300 mg P.O. 1 to 2 hr before surgery or 1 mg/kg I.M. 15 min before procedure. **Children:** 2 to 6 mg/kg P.O. Maximum single dose 100 mg. *Insomnia* — **Adults:** 100 to 200 mg P.O. or I.M. *Status epilepticus* — **Adults:** 250 to 350 mg	• *I.V. use:* I.V. injection for emergency use; give by direct injection. Administer at rate not > 50 mg/15 sec. • I.V. use may cause respiratory depression, laryngospasm, or hypotension; keep emergency resuscitation equipment available.

Pregnancy Risk Category: D Controlled Substance Schedule: II	I.M. or I.V. **Children:** 15 to 20 mg/kg I.V. over 15 min.	▪ Assess mental status before initiating.
selegiline hydrochloride Eldepryl *MAO-B inhibitor* *Antiparkinsonian* Pregnancy Risk Category: C	*Adjunctive treatment with carbidopa-levodopa in managing Parkinson's disease* — **Adults:** 10 mg/day P.O. (5 mg at breakfast and 5 mg at lunch). After 2 or 3 days, slowly decrease carbidopa-levodopa dose.	▪ Some patients may experience more adverse reactions with levodopa and need 10% to 30% reduction of carbidopa-levodopa dose. ▪ May cause dizziness at start of therapy.
senna Fletcher's Castoria, Senexon, Senokot *Anthraquinone derivative* *Stimulant laxative* Pregnancy Risk Category: C	*Acute constipation; preparation for bowel or rectal exam* — **Adults:** 1 to 8 tablets (Senokot) P.O.; ½ to 4 tsp granules added to liquid P.O.; 1 to 2 suppositories P.R. h.s.; or 1 to 4 tsp syrup P.O. h.s.	▪ Don't expose drug to excessive heat or light.
sertraline hydrochloride Zoloft *Serotonin uptake inhibitor* *Antidepressant* Pregnancy Risk Category: B	*Depression* — **Adults:** 50 mg/day P.O.; adjust dosage as tolerated and needed at ≥ 1-wk intervals. *Obsessive-compulsive disorder* — **Adults:** 50 mg/day P.O. Maximum 200 mg/day. Adjust dosage at ≥ 1-wk intervals.	▪ Use cautiously in patients at risk for suicide and in seizure disorders, major affective disorder, or conditions that affect metabolism or hemodynamic responses. ▪ Monitor for suicidal tendencies and allow minimum drug supply.
sibutramine hydrochloride monohydrate Meridia	*Management of obesity* — **Adults:** 10 mg P.O. q.d. May increase to 15 mg P.O. q.d. after 4 wk, p.r.n. Patients who do not tolerate 10 mg dose may receive 5 mg P.O. q.d. Maximum 15 mg q.d.	▪ Use cautiously in patients with history of seizures or narrow angle-glaucoma. ▪ Rule out organic causes of obesity before starting therapy. *(continued)*

†Canadian ‡Australian

DRUG / CLASS / CATEGORY	INDICATIONS / DOSAGES	KEY NURSING CONSIDERATIONS
sibutramine hydrochloride monohydrate *(continued)* *Norepinephrine, serotonin, and dopamine reuptake inhibitor* Antiobesity agent Pregnancy Risk Category: C Controlled Substance Schedule: IV		• Measure BP and pulse before starting therapy, with dose changes, and at regular intervals during therapy. • Allow at least 2 wk to elapse between stopping an MAO inhibitor and starting drug therapy, and vice versa.
sildenafil citrate Viagra *Selective cyclic guanosine monophosphate-specific phosphodiesterase type 5 inhibitor* Erectile dysfunction therapy Pregnancy Risk Category: B	*Treatment of erectile dysfunction* — **Adults** **< 65 yr:** 50 mg P.O., p.r.n., about 1 hr before sexual activity. Dose range is 25 mg to 100 mg. Maximum 1 dose q.d. **Elderly:** 25 mg P.O., p.r.n., about 1 hr before sexual activity. Adjust p.r.n., based on patient response. Maximum 1 dose q.d. ***Adjust-a-dose:*** In adults with hepatic or severe renal impairment, 25 mg P.O., about 1 hr before sexual activity. Adjust p.r.n., based on patient response. Maximum 1 dose q.d.	• Systemic vasodilatory effects cause transient decreases in supine blood pressure and cardiac output (about 2 hr after ingestion). • May cause serious CV events. • Don't give with nitrates.
silver sulfadiazine Flamazine†, Flint SSD, Silvadene, Thermazene	*Prevention and treatment of wound infection in second- and third-degree burns —*	• Use sterile application technique. • Use only on affected areas; keep medicated at all times.

	- Inspect skin daily, and note changes. Notify doctor of burning or excessive pain. - Discard darkened cream.
Synthetic anti-infective *Topical antibacterial* Pregnancy Risk Category: B	**Adults:** apply ¹⁄₁₆" thickness to clean, debrided burn q.d. or b.i.d.	

simethicone Gas-X, Mylanta Gas, Mylicon *Dispersant* *Antiflatulent* Pregnancy Risk Category: NR	*Flatulence; functional gastric bloating —* **Adults and children > 12 yr:** 40 to 160 mg before meals and h.s.; **Children 2 to 12 yr:** 40 mg (drops) P.O. q.i.d.; **Children < 2 yr:** 20 mg (drops) P.O. q.i.d. up to 240 mg/day.	- Don't use for infant colic. - Doesn't prevent gas formation.

simvastatin (syvinolin) Lipex‡, Zocor *HMG-CoA reductase inhibitor* *Antilipemic* Pregnancy Risk Category: X	*Reduction of LDL and total cholesterol levels in primary hypercholesterolemia (types IIa and IIb) —* **Adults:** initially, 5 to 10 mg/day P.O. in evening. Adjust dose q 4 wk based on tolerance and response; maximum 80 mg/day.	- Use cautiously in patients who use excessive alcohol or in history of liver disease. - Assess liver function before therapy and periodically thereafter; if liver enzyme elevations persist, liver biopsy may be done.

sodium bicarbonate Bell/ans, Citrocarbonate†, Soda Mint *Alkalinizing agent* *Systemic and urinary alkalinizer* Pregnancy Risk Category: C	*Cardiac arrest —* **Adults and children:** 1 mEq/kg I.V. of 7.5% or 8.4% solution, followed by 0.5 mEq/kg I.V. q 10 min, based on ABGs. If ABG unavailable, use 0.5 mEq/kg I.V. q 10 min until spontaneous circulation returns. **Infants < 2 yr:** ≤ 8 mEq/kg/day I.V. of 4.2% solution. *Metabolic acidosis —* **Adults and children:** 2 to 5 mEq/kg I.V. over 4 to 8 hr. *Systemic or urinary alkalinization —* **Adults:** 4 g P.O., then 1 to 2 g q 4 hr. **Children:** 84 to 840 mg/kg/day P.O.	- **I.V. use:** Don't mix with I.V. norepinephrine, dopamine, or calcium. - Obtain blood pH, Pao_2, $Paco_2$, and serum electrolytes; report results to doctor. - Not routinely used in cardiac arrest or during early resuscitation stages unless pre-existing acidosis exists. - When used as urinary alkalinizer, monitor urine pH. - Dosage based on blood carbon dioxide content, pH, and clinical condition.

283

†Canadian ‡Australian

DRUG / CLASS / CATEGORY	INDICATIONS / DOSAGES	KEY NURSING CONSIDERATIONS
sodium chloride *Electrolyte* *Sodium and chloride replacement* Pregnancy Risk Category: C	*Hyponatremia caused by electrolyte loss or in severe salt depletion* — **Adults:** Use 3% or 5% solution only with frequent electrolyte determination. With 0.45% solution: 3% to 8% of body weight, according to deficiencies, over 18 to 24 hr; with 0.9% solution: 2% to 6% of body weight, according to deficiencies, over 18 to 24 hr. *Heat cramp caused by excessive perspiration* — **Adults:** 1 g P.O. with water.	▪ Never give concentrated solutions (> 5%) without diluting. Read labels carefully. ▪ *I.V. use:* Infuse 3% and 5% solutions slowly and cautiously. Use only for critical situations. Observe patient continually. ▪ Monitor serum electrolytes, acid-base balance, and changes in fluid balance. ▪ Never use bacteriostatic NaCl injection with newborns.
sodium phosphates Fleet Enema *Acid salt* *Saline laxative* Pregnancy Risk Category: C	*Constipation* — **Adults:** 20 ml solution mixed with 120 ml cold water P.O., or as enema, 120 ml P.R. **Children:** 5 to 10 ml solution mixed with 120 ml cold water P.O.; or as enema, 60 ml P.R.	▪ Use cautiously in patients with large hemorrhoids or anal excoriations. ▪ Before giving for constipation, assess for adequate fluid intake, exercise, and diet. ▪ Up to 10% of sodium content may be absorbed.
sodium polystyrene sulfonate Kayexalate, Resonium A, SPS *Cation-exchange resin* *Potassium-removing resin* Pregnancy Risk Category: C	*Hyperkalemia* — **Adults:** 15 g P.O. q.d. to q.i.d. in water or sorbitol (3 to 4 ml/g of resin). Or, mix powder with appropriate medium and instill through NG tube. Or, 30 to 50 g/100 ml of sorbitol q 6 hr as warm emulsion deep into sigmoid colon (20 cm). **Children:** 1 g/kg or body weight/dose P.O. or P.R., p.r.n. P.O. route preferred (drug should be in intestine ≥ 30 min).	▪ Monitor serum potassium at least daily. Stop drug when level falls to 4 or 5 mEq/L. Monitor serum calcium in patients receiving drug for > 3 days. ▪ Watch for signs of hypokalemia and digitalis toxicity in digitalized patients. ▪ Monitor for other electrolyte deficiencies. ▪ Prevent fecal impaction in elderly patients by giving resin P.R.

sotalol
Betapace, Sotacort‡
Beta blocker
Antiarrhythmic
Pregnancy Risk Category: B

Documented, life-threatening ventricular arrhythmias — **Adults:** initially, 80 mg P.O. b.i.d. Increase q 2 to 3 days as needed and tolerated; most respond to 160 to 320 mg/day.

Adjust-a-dose: In patients with creatinine clearance 30 to 60 ml/min, increase dosage interval to q 24 hr; if between 10 and 30 ml/min, increase to q 36 to 48 hr; if < 10 ml/min, individualize dosage.

- Proarrhythmic events may occur at start of therapy and at dosage adjustments. Use cardiac rhythm monitoring.
- Withdraw other antiarrhythmics first.
- Monitor serum electrolytes regularly.

sparfloxacin
Zagam
Fluoroquinolone
Anti-infective
Pregnancy Risk Category: C

Community-acquired pneumonia and acute bacterial exacerbation of chronic bronchitis caused by susceptible organisms — **Adults > 18 yr:** 400 mg P.O. on day 1 as loading dose, then 200 mg/day for 10 days.

Adjust-a-dose: In patients with creatinine clearance < 50 ml/min, 400 mg loading dose P.O.; then 200 mg P.O. q 48 hr for 9 days.

- Use cautiously in patients with renal impairment.
- If patient experiences excessive CNS stimulation, discontinue and notify doctor. Institute seizure precautions.

spironolactone
Aldactone, Novo-Spiroton†
Potassium-sparing diuretic
Management of edema/antihypertensive/treatment of diuretic-induced hypokalemia
Pregnancy Risk Category: NR

Edema — **Adults:** 25 to 200 mg P.O. q.d. or in divided doses. **Children:** 3.3 mg/kg P.O. q.d. or in divided doses.
Hypertension — **Adults:** 50 to 100 mg P.O. q.d. or in divided doses.
Diuretic-induced hypokalemia — **Adults:** 25 to 100 mg P.O. q.d.

- Instruct patient to take in morning; if 2nd dose needed, tell him to take in early evening. Tell patient to take with food.
- Warn patient to avoid excessive ingestion of potassium-rich foods, salt substitutes, and potassium supplements.
- Notify doctor if breast enlargement occurs in men.

285

DRUG/CLASS/ CATEGORY	INDICATIONS/ DOSAGES	KEY NURSING CONSIDERATIONS
stavudine (d4T) Zerit Synthetic thymidine nucleoside analogue Antiviral Pregnancy Risk Category: C	*Treatment of HIV-infected patients who have received prolonged zidovudine therapy* — **Adults ≥ 60 kg (132 lb):** 40 mg P.O. q 12 hr. **Adults < 60 kg:** 30 mg P.O. q 12 hr.	• Monitor CBC, serum creatinine, AST, ALT, and alkaline phosphatase levels. • Instruct patient not to take with other drugs for HIV or AIDS unless doctor approves. • Instruct patient to tell doctor if peripheral neuropathy occurs.
streptokinase Kabikinase, Streptase Plasminogen activator Thrombolytic enzyme Pregnancy Risk Category: C	*Arteriovenous cannula occlusion* — **Adults:** 250,000 IU in 2 ml I.V. solution by I.V. pump infusion into each occluded limb of cannula over 25 to 35 min. Clamp off cannula for 2 hr. Then aspirate, flush, and reconnect. *Venous thrombosis; pulmonary embolism (PE); arterial thrombosis and embolism* — **Adults:** loading dose 250,000 IU I.V. over 30 min. Sustaining dose 100,000 IU/hr I.V. for 72 hr for deep vein thrombosis and 100,000 IU/hr I.V. over 24 to 72 hr for PE and arterial thrombosis or embolism. *Lysis of coronary artery thrombi* — **Adults:** loading dose 20,000 IU bolus via coronary catheter; then 2,000 IU/min infusion over 60 min. Or, give as I.V. infusion. Usual adult dose 1.5 million IU I.V. over 60 min.	• Before initiating, draw blood for coagulation studies, Hct, platelet count, and type and crossmatching. Keep aminocaproic acid and corticosteroids available. • Avoid I.M. injections and other invasive procedures during therapy. • Check for hypersensitivity reactions. Monitor vital signs, particularly BP and pulse, and neurologic status often. • Monitor closely for excessive bleeding. If bleeding occurs, stop therapy and notify doctor. • Monitor pulses, color, and sensation of extremities q hr. • Avoid unnecessary patient handling; pad side rails.
streptozocin Zanosar	*Metastatic islet cell carcinoma of pancreas* — **Adults and children:** 500 mg/m² I.V. for 5	• Monitor CBC and liver function ≥ weekly. • Check urine protein and glucose q shift.

Antibiotic antineoplastic nitrosurea (cell cycle-phase nonspecific) *Antineoplastic* Pregnancy Risk Category: C	consecutive days q 6 wk until maximum benefit or toxicity observed. Or, 1,000 mg/m² at weekly intervals for first 2 wk. Maximum single dose 1,500 mg/m². Infuse diluted solution over ≥ 15 min. Give with antiemetic.	• If extravasation, stop infusion; notify doctor. • Obtain urinalysis, BUN, creatinine, and electrolyte levels ≥ weekly and for 4 wk after each course.
sucralfate Carafate, SCF†, Sulcrate† *Pepsin* *Antiulcer agent* Pregnancy Risk Category: B	*Short-term (≤ 8 wk) treatment of duodenal ulcer* — **Adults:** 1 g P.O. q.i.d. 1 hr after meals and h.s. *Maintenance therapy for duodenal ulcer* — **Adults:** 1 g P.O. b.i.d.	• Monitor for severe, persistent constipation. • May be as effective as cimetidine in healing duodenal ulcers. • Avoid giving within 2 hr of quinolone antibiotics.
sulfamethoxazole Apo-Sulfamethoxazole†, Gantanol *Sulfonamide* *Antibiotic* Pregnancy Risk Category: C (contraindicated at term)	*UTIs and systemic infections* — **Adults:** initially, 2 g P.O., then 1 g P.O. b.i.d. or t.i.d. for severe infections. *C. trachomatis* — **Adults:** 1 g P.O. b.i.d. for 21 days. **Children and infants > 2 mo:** initially, 50 to 60 mg/kg P.O., then 25 to 30 mg/kg b.i.d. Maximum dose 75 mg/kg/day.	• Monitor urine cultures, CBC, and urinalysis before and during therapy. • Monitor fluid I&O. Intake should be sufficient to produce output of 1,500 ml/day. If fluid intake not adequate, may give sodium bicarbonate. Monitor urine pH daily.
sulfasalazine (salazosulfapyridine, sulphasalazine) Azulfidine, EN-tab† *Sulfonamide* *Antibiotic* Pregnancy Risk Category: B	*Mild to moderate ulcerative colitis; adjunctive therapy in severe ulcerative colitis; Crohn's disease* — **Adults:** 3 to 4 g/day P.O. in evenly divided doses; usual maintenance: 2 g/day P.O. in divided doses q 6 hr. **Children > 2 yr:** 40 to 60 mg/kg/day P.O., divided into 3 to 6 doses; then 30 mg/kg/day in 4 doses. *Rheumatoid arthritis* — **Adults:** 2 to 3 g q.d. in 2 divided doses.	• Administer after food; space doses evenly. • May start at lower dose if GI intolerance occurs. • Advise patient to maintain adequate fluid intake. • Discontinue immediately and notify doctor if hypersensitivity occurs. • Warn patient to avoid ultraviolet light.

†Canadian ‡Australian

DRUG/CLASS/ CATEGORY	INDICATIONS/ DOSAGES	KEY NURSING CONSIDERATIONS
sulfinpyrazone Anturan?, Anturane *Uricosuric agent Renal tubular-blocking agent/platelet aggregation inhibitor* Pregnancy Risk Category: NR	*Intermittent or chronic gouty arthritis —* **Adults:** 200 to 400 mg P.O. b.i.d. 1st wk, then 400 mg b.i.d. Maximum 800 mg/day.	▪ Give with milk, food, or antacids. ▪ Monitor I&O closely. Force fluids to maintain minimum output of 2 to 3 L/day. ▪ May increase severity of acute gout attacks during first 6 to 12 mo. ▪ Instruct patient to take drug regularly.
sulfisoxazole Gantrisin, Novo-Soxazole† **sulfisoxazole acetyl** Gantrisin Pediatric *Sulfonamide Antibiotic* Pregnancy Risk Category: C (contraindicated at term)	*UTIs; systemic infections —* **Adults:** initially, 2 to 4 g P.O., then 4 to 8 g/day divided in 4 to 6 doses. **Children >2 mo:** initially, 75 mg/kg/day P.O. or 2 g/m² P.O., then 150 mg/kg or 4 g/m² P.O. q.d. in divided doses q 6 hr. Maximum total dose 6 g/day. *C. trachomatis —* **Adults:** 500 mg P.O. for 10 to 21 days. **Adjust-a-dose:** Increase dosage interval if creatinine clearance < 50 ml/min.	▪ Obtain specimen for culture and sensitivity tests before 1st dose. ▪ Monitor urine cultures, CBC, PT, and urinalyses before and during therapy. ▪ Watch for superinfection. ▪ Monitor fluid I&O. Intake should be sufficient to produce output of 1,500 ml/day. If fluid intake not adequate, may give sodium bicarbonate. Monitor urine pH daily.
sulindac Aclin‡, Apo-Sulin†, Clinoril, Novo-Sundac† *NSAID Nonnarcotic analgesic/anti-inflammatory* Pregnancy Risk Category: NR	*Osteoarthritis; rheumatoid arthritis; ankylosing spondylitis —* **Adults:** initially, 150 mg P.O. b.i.d.; increase to 200 mg b.i.d., p.r.n. *Acute subacromial bursitis or supraspinatus tendinitis; acute gouty arthritis —* **Adults:** 200 mg P.O. b.i.d. for 7 to 14 days. Reduce dose as symptoms subside.	▪ Give with food, milk, or antacids. ▪ May mask signs and symptoms of infection. ▪ May cause peptic ulceration and bleeding. ▪ Periodically monitor hepatic and renal function and CBC with long-term therapy.

sumatriptan succinate
Imitrex
Selective 5-hydroxytryptamine receptor agonist
Antimigraine agent
Pregnancy Risk Category: C

Acute migraine attacks (with or without aura) — **Adults:** 6 mg S.C. Maximum dose two 6-mg injections q.d., at least 1 hr apart. Or, initial dose of 25 to 100 mg P.O. and 2nd dose of up to 100 mg P.O. in 2 hr, p.r.n. Further doses may be given q 2 hr, p.r.n., to maximum oral dose 300 mg/day.

- Instruct patient to immediately report persistent or severe chest pain.
- Tell patient to stop taking drug and report if pain, tightness in throat, wheezing, heart throbbing, rash, lumps, hives, or swelling of eyelids, face, or lips develops.

tacrine hydrochloride
Cognex
Cholinesterase inhibitor
Psychotherapeutic agent
Pregnancy Risk Category: C

Mild to moderate dementia of Alzheimer's type — **Adults:** initially, 10 mg P.O. q.i.d. After 6 wk and if tolerated with no rise in transaminase, increase to 20 mg q.i.d. After 6 wk, adjust to 30 mg q.i.d. If still tolerated, increase to 40 mg q.i.d. after another 6 wk.

- Abrupt discontinuation or large reduction in daily dose (≥ 80 mg/day) may cause behavioral disturbances and loss of cognitive function.
- Monitor liver function, as ordered.

tacrolimus
Prograf
Bacteria-derived macrolide
Immunosuppressant
Pregnancy Risk Category: C

Prophylaxis of organ rejection in allogenic liver transplantation — **Adults:** 0.05 to 0.1 mg/kg/day I.V. as controlled infusion ≥ 6 hr after transplantation. Initial P.O. dosage 0.15 to 0.3 mg/kg/day in 2 divided doses q 12 hr. Start 8 to 12 hr after stopping I.V. Adjust per response. **Children:** 0.1 mg/kg/day I.V., then 0.3 mg/kg/day P.O. on schedule similar to adults, adjusted p.r.n.

- Monitor for anaphylaxis continuously during first 30 min and frequently thereafter. Keep epinephrine 1:1,000 available.
- Observe for hyperkalemia.
- Monitor for neurotoxicity and nephrotoxicity.
- Check blood glucose regularly.
- Increases risk for infections, lymphomas, and other malignant diseases.

tamoxifen citrate
Nolvadex, Nolvadex-D†‡,
Nonsteroidal antiestrogen
Antineoplastic
Pregnancy Risk Category: D

Advanced premenopausal and postmenopausal breast cancers — **Adults:** 10 to 20 mg P.O. b.i.d.

- Monitor serum calcium. May compound hypercalcemia at start of therapy.
- Monitor CBC.
- Exacerbation of bone pain during therapy often indicates good response.

289

†Canadian ‡Australian

DRUG/CLASS/ CATEGORY	INDICATIONS/ DOSAGES	KEY NURSING CONSIDERATIONS
tamsulosin hydrochloride Flomax *Alpha 1a-antagonist* *BPH agent* Pregnancy Risk Category: B	*BPH* — **Adults:** 0.4 mg P.O. q.d. If no response after 2 to 4 wk, may increase to 0.8 mg P.O. q.d. If treatment interrupted for several days, restart therapy at 1 capsule daily.	▪ Tell patient to swallow capsules whole and to take 30 min after same meal daily. ▪ Monitor BP. ▪ Instruct patient not to perform hazardous tasks for 12 hr after dose changes.
telmisartan Micardis *Selective angiotensin II blocker* *Antihypertensive* Pregnancy Risk Category: C (D in second and third trimesters)	*Hypertension* — **Adults:** 40 mg P.O. q.d. BP response is dose-related over range of 20 to 80 mg q.d.	▪ Use cautiously in patients with biliary obstruction disorders or renal and hepatic insufficiency and in those who are volume- or salt-depleted. ▪ Monitor for hypotension. ▪ Most of antihypertensive effect occurs within 2 wk. Maximal BP reduction may take 4 wk.
temazepam Restoril *Benzodiazepine* *Sedative-hypnotic* Pregnancy Risk Category: X Controlled Substance Schedule: IV	*Insomnia* — **Adults:** 7.5 to 30 mg P.O. h.s. **Elderly:** 7.5 mg P.O. h.s.	▪ Assess mental status before initiating therapy. Elderly patients more sensitive to adverse CNS effects. ▪ Prevent hoarding or self-overdosing by depressed, suicidal, or drug-dependent patients or those with drug abuse history.
terazosin hydrochloride Hytrin	*Hypertension* — **Adults:** initially, 1 mg P.O. h.s. Adjust dose gradually based on re-	▪ Monitor BP frequently. ▪ If discontinued for several days, readjust using initial dosing regimen.

Drug / Classification	Indications & Dosage	Nursing Considerations
Selective alpha₁ blocker *Antihypertensive* Pregnancy Risk Category: C	sponse. Usual range 1 to 5 mg/day; maximum, 20 mg/day. *Symptomatic BPH* — **Adults:** initially, 1 mg P.O. h.s. Increase in stepwise fashion to 2, 5, or 10 mg/day; most need 10 mg/day.	• Advise patient not to discontinue suddenly and to call doctor if adverse reactions occur. • Caution patient to avoid hazardous activities for 12 hr after 1st dose.
terbinafine hydrochloride (oral) Lamisil *Synthetic allylamine derivative* *Antifungal* Pregnancy Risk Category: B	*Treatment of fingernail onychomycosis due to dermatophytes (tinea unguium)* — **Adults:** 250 mg P.O. q.d. for 6 wk. *Treatment of toenail onychomycosis due to dermatophytes (tinea unguium)* — **Adults:** 250 mg P.O. q.d. for 12 wk.	• Not recommended during pregnancy or in breast-feeding patients. • Successful treatment may not be noticed for 10 wk for toenails and 4 wk for fingernails.
terbinafine hydrochloride (topical) Lamisil *Synthetic allylamine derivative* *Antifungal* Pregnancy Risk Category: B	*Interdigital tinea pedis; tinea cruris; tinea corporis* — **Adults:** cover affected and immediate surrounding area with cream b.i.d. for at least 1 wk.	• Use as directed for full course, even if symptoms disappear. • Don't apply near eyes, mouth, or mucous membranes or use occlusive dressings. • Tell patient to discontinue and contact doctor if irritation or sensitivity develops. • Therapy shouldn't exceed 4 wk.
terbutaline sulfate Brethaire, Brethine, Bricanyl‡ *Adrenergic (beta₂ agonist)* *Bronchodilator/premature labor inhibitor (tocolytic)* Pregnancy Risk Category: B	*Bronchospasm in patients with reversible obstructive airway disease* — **Adults and children ≥ 12 yr:** *Aerosol inhaler* — 2 inhalations separated by 60-sec interval; repeat q 4 to 6 hr. *Injection* — 0.25 mg S.C.; repeat in 15 to 30 min. p.r.n. Maximum 0.5 mg in 4 hr. *Tablets in adults* — 2.5 to 5 mg P.O. q 6 hr t.i.d. Maximum 15 mg/day. *Tablets in children 12*	• Use cautiously in CV disorders, hyperthyroidism, diabetes, or seizure disorders. • Give S.C. injections in lateral deltoid area. • Protect injection from light; discard if discolored. • May use tablets and aerosol together.

(continued)

†Canadian ‡Australian

DRUG/CLASS/CATEGORY	INDICATIONS/DOSAGES	KEY NURSING CONSIDERATIONS
terbutaline sulfate *(continued)*	*to 15 yr* — 2.5 mg P.O. q 6 hr t.i.d. while awake. Maximum 7.5 mg/day.	▪ Teach patient to perform oral inhalation correctly. ▪ Advise patient to discontinue drug and call doctor if paradoxal bronchospasm occurs.
terconazole Terazol 3 Vaginal Ovules, Terazol 7 Vaginal Ovules Cream *Triazole derivative* *Antifungal* Pregnancy Risk Category: C	*Vulvovaginal candidiasis* — **Adults:** 1 applicatorful of cream or 1 suppository inserted into vagina h.s. 0.4% Cream used for 7 days; 0.8% cream or 80-mg suppository for 3 days. Course repeated, p.r.n., after reconfirmation by smear or culture.	▪ Discontinue and notify doctor if fever, chills, flulike symptoms, or signs of sensitivity develop. ▪ Persistent infection may be caused by reinfection. Evaluate for possible sources. ▪ Continue treatment during menses. Avoid tampons.
testosterone Andro 100, Testamone 100 **testosterone cypionate** Depo-Testosterone **testosterone propionate** Testex **testosterone transdermal system** Androderm, Testoderm *Androgen* *Androgen replacement/antineoplastic*	*Male hypogonadism* — **Adults:** 10 to 25 mg (testosterone or propionate) I.M. two to three times/wk or 50 to 400 mg (cypionate) I.M. q 2 to 4 wk. *Metastatic breast cancer in women 1 to 5 yr postmenopausal* — **Adults:** 100 mg I.M. two times weekly; 50 to 100 mg (propionate) I.M. 3 times weekly; or 200 to 400 mg (cypionate) I.M. q 2 to 4 wk. *Primary or hypogonadotropic hypogonadism in men* — **Adults:** (Testoderm) one 4- to 6-mg/day patch on scrotal area q.d. Patch worn for 22 to 24 hr/day. **Adults:** (Androderm) 2 systems applied	▪ Use cautiously in elderly patients and in patients with renal, hepatic, or cardiac disease. ▪ Don't use in women of childbearing age until pregnancy ruled out. ▪ Give daily dosage requirement in divided doses for best results. ▪ Assess liver function tests, serum lipid profiles, Hgb and Hct, and prostate antigen levels.

Pregnancy Risk Category: X
Controlled Substance
Schedule: III

tetracycline hydrochloride (oral)
Achromycin V, Panmycin P‡, Robitet, Sumycin, Tetracyn
Tetracycline
Antibiotic
Pregnancy Risk Category: D

Infections — **Adults:** 250 to 500 mg P.O. q 6 hr. **Children > 8 yr:** 25 to 50 mg/kg/day P.O., in divided doses q 6 hr.
C. trachomatis infections — **Adults:** 500 mg P.O. q.i.d. for 7 to 21 days.
Brucellosis — **Adults:** 500 mg P.O. q 6 hr for 3 wk, given with streptomycin I.M.

- Use with extreme caution in patients with impaired renal or hepatic function. Use with extreme caution (if at all) during last half of pregnancy and in children < 9 yr.
- Check tongue for candidal infection. Emphasize good oral hygiene.

tetracycline hydrochloride (topical)
Topicycline
Tetracycline
Antibiotic
Pregnancy Risk Category: B

Acne vulgaris — **Adults and children > 11 yr:** use b.i.d. on affected areas.
Superficial skin infections caused by susceptible bacteria — **Adults:** apply to affected area b.i.d. in morning and evening or t.i.d.

- Wash area before applying.
- Tell patient not to share drug, towels, or washcloths.
- Explain how to adjust applicator pressure against skin to control flow rate.

theophylline
Immediate-release tablets and capsules: Bronkodyl, Slo-Phyllin; *timed-release tablets:* Theo-Dur; *timed-release capsules:* Aerolate

Acute bronchospasm if not on drug — For I.V., loading dose 4.7 mg/kg slowly; then maintenance. **Adults (nonsmokers):** 6 mg/kg P.O., then 2 to 3 mg/kg q 6 hr for 2 doses. Maintenance: 3 mg/kg q 8 hr. Or, 0.55 mg/kg/hr I.V. for 12 hr, then 0.39 mg/kg/hr. **Adults (healthy smokers):** 6 mg/kg P.O., then 3 mg/

- For acute bronchospasm in patient already receiving drug, dose adjusted per current level. Note that each 0.5 mg/kg I.V. or P.O. (load) increases levels by 1 mcg/ml.
- Extended-release preparations not for use in treatment of acute bronchospasm.

(continued)

293

†Canadian ‡Australian

DRUG/CLASS/CATEGORY

theophylline
(continued)
**theophylline
sodium glycinate**
Xanthine derivative
Bronchodilator
Pregnancy Risk Category: C

INDICATIONS/DOSAGES

kg q 4 hr for 3 doses. Maintenance: 3 mg/kg q 6 hr. Or, 0.79 mg/kg/hr I.V. for 12 hr; then 0.63 mg/kg/hr. **Adults with heart failure or liver disease:** 6 mg/kg P.O., then 2 mg/kg q 8 hr for 2 doses. Maintenance: 1 to 2 mg/kg q 12 hr. Or, 0.39 mg/kg/hr I.V. for 12 hr; then 0.08 to 0.16 mg/kg/hr. **Children 9 to 16 yr:** 6 mg/kg P.O., then 3 mg/kg q 4 hr for 3 doses. Maintenance: 3 mg/kg q 6 hr. Or, 0.79 mg/kg/hr I.V. for 12 hr; then 0.63 mg/kg/hr. **Children 6 mo to 9 yr:** 6 mg/kg P.O., then 4 mg/kg q 4 hr for 3 doses. Maintenance: 4 mg/kg q 6 hr. Or, 0.95 mg/kg/hr I.V. for 12 hr; then 0.79 mg/kg/hr.
Chronic bronchospasm — **Adults and children:** 16 mg/kg or 400 mg P.O. q.d. in 3 to 4 divided doses q 6 to 8 hr; or, 12 mg/kg or 400 mg P.O. q.d. in extended-release preparation in 2 to 3 divided doses q 8 or 12 hr. Increase as tolerated q 2 to 3 days to maximum. **Adolescents > 16 yr:** 13 mg/kg or 900 mg P.O. q.d. in divided doses. **Children 12 to 16 yr:** 18 mg/kg P.O. q.d. in divided doses. **Children 9 to 12 yr:** 20 mg/kg P.O. q.d. in divided doses. **Children < 9 yr:** 24 mg/kg/day P.O. in divided doses.

KEY NURSING CONSIDERATIONS

- Monitor vital signs; measure and record fluid I&O. Clinical effects include improved pulse quality and respirations.
- Don't confuse extended-release and regular form.
- *I.V. use:* Use commercially available infusion solution, or mix in D₅W. Use infusion pump for continuous infusion.
- Give around-the-clock, using extended-release product h.s.
- Xanthine metabolism varies; dose based on response, tolerance, pulmonary function, and theophylline levels (10 to 20 mcg/ml); toxicity reported with levels > 20 mcg/ml.
- Teach patient to swallow extended-release preparations whole. For children who can't swallow, sprinkle contents over soft food.
- Dose in chronic bronchospasm adjusted for minimum necessary for response. Also adjust dose for older adult with cor pulmonale.

thiamine hydrochloride (vitamin B₁)
Betamin, Biamine
Water-soluble vitamin
Nutritional supplement
Pregnancy Risk Category: A

Beriberi — **Adults:** 10 to 20 mg I.M. t.i.d. for 2 wk, then diet correction and multivitamin supplement containing 5 to 10 mg/day thiamine for 1 mo. **Children:** depending on severity, 10 to 50 mg/day I.M. for several wk with adequate diet.
Wernicke's encephalopathy — **Adults:** initially, 100 mg I.V., followed by 50 to 100 mg/day I.V. or I.M. until patient eats balanced diet.

- **I.V. use:** Dilute before giving. Administer large doses cautiously; give skin test before therapy in history of hypersensitivity reactions. Have epinephrine available.
- Accurate dietary history important.
- Significant deficiency can occur in 3 wk of thiamine-free diet. Thiamine deficiency usually requires concurrent treatment for multiple deficiencies.

---

thioridazine hydrochloride
Aldazine‡, Apo-Thioridazine†, Mellaril, Mellaril Concentrate, Novo-Ridazine†, PMS Thioridazine†
Phenothiazine (piperidine derivative)
Antipsychotic
Pregnancy Risk Category: NR

Psychosis — **Adults:** 50 to 100 mg P.O. t.i.d., with gradual increases to 800 mg/day in divided doses, p.r.n. Dosage varies.
Short-term treatment of moderate to marked depression with variable degrees of anxiety; treatment of multiple symptoms in geriatric patients — **Adults:** 25 mg P.O. t.i.d. Maintenance 20 to 200 mg/day. Maximum 200 mg/day. **Children 2 to 12 yr:** 0.5 to 3 mg/kg P.O. q.d. in divided doses.

- Different liquid formulations have different concentrations. Check dosage carefully.
- Keep drug away from skin and clothes; wear gloves when preparing liquid forms.
- Monitor for tardive dyskinesia.
- Shake suspension well before use.
- Dilute liquid concentrate with water or fruit juice before use.
- Advise patient to rise slowly to avoid dizziness from orthostatic hypotension.

---

thiotepa (TESPA, triethylenethio-phosphoramide, TSPA)
Thioplex
Alkylating agent (cell cycle–phase nonspecific)
Antineoplastic
Pregnancy Risk Category: D

Breast and ovarian cancers; lymphoma; Hodgkin's disease — **Adults and children > 12 yr:** 0.3 to 0.4 mg/kg I.V. q 1 to 4 wk or 0.2 mg/kg for 4 to 5 days at 2- to 4-wk intervals.

- If pain occurs at insertion site, dilute further or use local anesthetic.
- Monitor CBC weekly for 3 wk after last dose. Notify doctor if WBC count < 3,000/mm³ or if platelet count < 150,000/mm³.
- Monitor serum uric acid.
- Tell patient to watch for signs of infection and bleeding and take temperature daily.

†Canadian ‡Australian

295

DRUG/CLASS/ CATEGORY	INDICATIONS/ DOSAGES	KEY NURSING CONSIDERATIONS
thiothixene Navane **thiothixene hydrochloride** Navane *Thioxanthene* *Antipsychotic* Pregnancy Risk Category: NR	*Mild to moderate psychosis* — **Adults:** 2 mg P.O. t.i.d. Increase gradually to 15 mg/day. *Severe psychosis* — **Adults:** initially, 5 mg P.O. b.i.d. Increase slowly to 20 to 30 mg/ day. Maximum recommended 60 mg/day. Or, 4 mg I.M. b.i.d. or q.i.d. Maximum 30 mg/day I.M. P.O. should replace I.M. promptly.	• Watch for orthostatic hypotension. Keep patient supine for 1 hr afterward. • Keep drug off skin and clothes. Wear gloves when preparing liquid forms. • Dilute liquid concentrate with fruit juice, milk, or semisolid food before use. • Monitor for tardive dyskinesia.
tiagabine hydrochloride Gabitril *Gamma aminobutyric acid enhancer* *Anticonvulsant* Pregnancy Risk Category: C	*Adjunctive therapy in treatment of partial seizures* — **Adults:** initially, 4 mg P.O. q.d. May increase total daily dose by 4 to 8 mg q wk until clinical response or up to 56 mg/day, given in divided doses b.i.d. to q.i.d. **Children 12 to 18 yr:** 4 mg P.O. q.d. May increase total daily dose by 4 mg at start of wk 2, then by 4 to 8 mg/wk until clinical response or up to 32 mg/day, given in divided doses b.i.d. to q.i.d. ***Adjust-a-dose:*** In patients with impaired liver function, reduce initial and maintenance doses or lengthen dosing intervals, p.r.n.	• Withdraw drug gradually unless safety concerns require a more rapid withdrawal. • May cause status epilepticus and sudden unexpected death in epilepsy. • Patients who aren't receiving at least one concomitant enzyme-inducing antiepilepsy drug at the time of tiagabine initiation may require lower doses or a slower adjustment. • May cause moderately severe to incapacitating generalized weakness. Usually, weakness resolves after dosage reduction or discontinuation of drug.
ticarcillin disodium Ticar, Ticillin‡ *Extended-spectrum penicillin/alpha-carboxypenicillin*	*Severe systemic infections caused by susceptible organisms* — **Adults:** 18 g/day I.V. or I.M., in divided doses q 4 to 6 hr. **Children:** 50 to 300 mg/kg/day I.V. or I.M. in di-	• Before giving, ask about previous allergic reactions to penicillin. • Avoid continuous infusion. Change site q 48 hr.

Antibiotic
Pregnancy Risk Category: B

vided doses q 4 to 6 hr.
Adjust-a-dose: In patients with renal failure, if creatinine clearance 30 to 60 ml/min, give 2 g I.V. q 4 hr; 10 to 29 ml/min, give 2 g I.V. q 8 hr; < 10 ml/min, give 2 g I.V. q 12 hr, or 1 g I.M. q 6 hr.

- For I.M. use 2 ml diluent per g of drug. Inject deep I.M. into large muscle. Don't exceed 2/injection.

**ticarcillin disodi-
um/clavulanate
potassium**
Timentin
Beta-lactamase inhibitor
Antibiotic
Pregnancy Risk Category: B

Lower respiratory tract, urinary tract, bone and joint, and skin and skin-structure infections and septicemia when caused by beta-lactamase-producing strains of bacteria or by ticarcillin-susceptible organisms — **Adults:** 3.1 g (3 g ticarcillin and 100 mg clavulanic acid) by I.V. infusion q 4 to 6 hr.
Adjust-a-dose: In patients with renal failure, if creatinine clearance 30 to 60 ml/min, give 2 g I.V. q 4 hr; 10 to 29 ml/min, give 2 g I.V. q 8 hr; < 10 ml/min, give 2 g I.V. q 12 hr.

- Before giving, ask about previous allergic reactions to penicillin.
- Check CBC and platelet counts frequently. May cause thrombocytopenia.
- With large doses and prolonged therapy, bacterial or fungal superinfection may occur.

**ticlopidine
hydrochloride**
Ticlid
Platelet aggregation inhibitor
Antithrombotic agent
Pregnancy Risk Category: B

To reduce risk of thrombotic stroke in patients with history of stroke or with stroke precursors — **Adults:** 250 mg P.O. b.i.d. with meals.

- Instruct patient to avoid aspirin and aspirin-containing products unless ordered by doctor and to check with doctor or pharmacist before taking OTC products.
- Report unusual or prolonged bleeding.
- Report signs of infection immediately.

**tiludronate
disodium**
Skelid
Biphosphonate analogue

Paget's disease of bone in patients who have serum alkaline phosphatase level at least twice the upper limit of normal, who are symptomatic, or who are at risk for fu-

- Use cautiously in upper GI disease.
- Correct hypocalcemia and mineral metab-

(continued)

297

†Canadian ‡Australian

DRUG / CLASS / CATEGORY	INDICATIONS / DOSAGES	KEY NURSING CONSIDERATIONS
tiludronate disodium *(continued)* *Antihypercalcemic* Pregnancy Risk Category: C	*ture complications of their disease* — **Adults:** 400 mg P.O. once daily for 3 mo.	olism disturbances (such as vitamin D deficiency) before initiating therapy. • Tell patient to take with full glass of plain water (6 to 8 oz) 2 hr before or after meals.
timolol maleate (systemic) Apo-Timol†, Blocadren *Beta blocker* *Antihypertensive/adjunct in MI* Pregnancy Risk Category: C	*Hypertension* — **Adults:** 10 mg P.O. b.i.d. Maximum 60 mg/day. Increase q wk, p.r.n. *MI (long-term prophylaxis in patients who have survived acute phase)* — **Adults:** 10 mg P.O. b.i.d. *Migraine headache prophylaxis* — **Adults:** 20 mg P.O. q.d. in 1 or divided doses b.i.d. Increase, p.r.n., to maximum 30 mg/day.	• Use cautiously in compensated heart failure, diabetes, hyperthyroidism, and hepatic, renal, or respiratory disease. • Check apical pulse before giving and monitor BP closely. • May mask signs and symptoms of hypoglycemia. Monitor blood glucose in diabetic patients.
timolol maleate (ophthalmic) Betimol, Timoptic Solution, Timoptic-XE *Beta blocker* *Antiglaucoma agent* Pregnancy Risk Category: C	*Chronic open-angle, secondary, and aphakic glaucomas; ocular hypertension* — **Adults:** initially, 1 drop 0.25% solution in each affected eye b.i.d.; maintenance, 1 drop/day. If no response, 1 drop 0.5% solution b.i.d. If IOP controlled, reduce to 1 drop/day. Or, 1 drop gel q.d.	• Administer other ophthalmic agents ≥ 10 min before gel drop. • Can mask hypoglycemia signs. • Some patients may need a few wk of treatment to stabilize pressure-lowering response. Determine IOP after 4 wk.
tirofiban hydrochloride Aggrastat *Human platelet glycoprotein*	*Treatment of acute coronary syndrome, with heparin, to be managed medically and those undergoing PTCA or atherectomy* — **Adults:** I.V. loading dose of	• Use cautiously in patients with increased risk of bleeding, including those with hemorrhagic retinopathy or platelet count below 150,000/mm³.

receptor binder
Platelet aggregation inhibitor
Pregnancy Risk Category: B

0.4 mcg/kg/min for 30 min, followed by continuous infusion of 0.1 mcg/kg/min. Continue infusion through angiography and for 12 to 24 hr after angioplasty or artherectomy.
Adjust-a-dose: In patients with creatinine clearance < 30 ml/min, give loading dose of 0.2 mcg/kg/min for 30 min, followed by continuous infusion of 0.05 mcg/kg/min. Continue infusion as described above.

- Monitor Hct, Hgb, and platelet counts before starting therapy, 6 hr after loading dose, and at least daily during therapy.
- Minimize injection and avoid noncompatible I.V. sites.
- Administer drug with aspirin and heparin.

---

tioconazole
Vagistat-1
Imidazole derivative
Antifungal
Pregnancy Risk Category: C

Vulvovaginal candidiasis — **Adults:** 1 applicatorful (about 4.6 g) inserted intravaginally h.s. once.

- Review proper use of drug. Written instructions available with product. Tell patient to insert drug high into vagina.
- Report irritation or sensitivity.
- Tell patient to open applicator just before use.

---

tobramycin
AKTob, Tobrex
Aminoglycoside
Antibiotic
Pregnancy Risk Category: B

External ocular infections caused by susceptible bacteria — **Adults and children:** in mild to moderate infections, 1 or 2 drops into affected eye q 4 hr, or thin strip (1 cm long) of ointment q 8 to 12 hr. In severe infections, instill 2 drops into infected eye q 30 to 60 min until improvement; then reduce frequency. Or, thin strip of ointment q 3 to 4 hr until improvement; then reduce frequency.

- Clean eye area before application.
- Advise patient to watch for itching lids, swelling, or constant burning. Tell him to discontinue and notify doctor if these occur.
- Instruct patient not to share drug, washcloths, or towels and to notify doctor if family member develops same symptoms.
- Discontinue if keratitis; erythema, lacrimation, edema, or lid itching occurs.

DRUG/CLASS/ CATEGORY	INDICATIONS/ DOSAGES	KEY NURSING CONSIDERATIONS
tobramycin sulfate Nebcin *Aminoglycoside* *Antibiotic* Pregnancy Risk Category: D	*Serious infections* — **Adults:** 3 mg/kg/day I.M. or I.V. divided q 8 hr. Up to 5 mg/kg/day divided q 6 to 8 hr for life-threatening infec- tions; reduce to 3 mg/kg/day as soon as indi- cated. **Children:** 6 to 7.5 mg/kg/day I.M. or I.V. in 3 or 4 equally divided doses. **Neonates** **< 1 wk or premature infants:** up to 4 mg/kg/ day I.V. or I.M. in 2 equal doses q 12 hr.	▪ *I.V. use:* Infuse over 20 to 60 min. ▪ Notify doctor if tinnitus, vertigo, or hear- ing loss occurs. ▪ Obtain blood for peak level 1 hr after I.M. injection and ½ hr after infusion ends; trough level just before next dose. ▪ Monitor renal function.
tocainide hydrochloride Tonocard *Anesthetic* *Ventricular antiarrhythmic* Pregnancy Risk Category: C	*Suppression of symptomatic life-threaten- ing ventricular arrhythmias* — **Adults:** ini- tially, 400 mg P.O. q 8 hr. Usual dosage 1,200 to 1,800 mg P.O. q.d. in 3 divided doses. May treat patients with renal or hepatic im- pairment with 1,200 mg/day.	▪ May ease transition from I.V. lidocaine to oral antiarrhythmic. Monitor carefully. ▪ Correct potassium deficit. ▪ Observe for tremor. ▪ Monitor blood levels. Therapeutic range 4 to 10 mcg/ml.
tolcapone Tasmar *Catechol-O-methyltrans- ferase inhibitor* *Antiparkinsonian* Pregnancy Risk Category: C	*Adjunct to carbidopa-levodopa for treatment of signs and symptoms of idiopathic Parkin- son's disease* — **Adults:** 100 mg P.O. t.i.d. (with carbidopa-levodopa). Recommended daily dose 100 mg P.O. t.i.d.; 200 mg P.O. t.i.d. can be given if anticipated clinical ben- efit is justified. If giving 200 mg t.i.d. and dyskinesia occurs, levodopa dose reduction may be necessary. Maximum 600 mg q.d. *Adjust-a-dose:* Don't use doses > 100 mg t.i.d. in patients with severe renal dysfunction.	▪ Obtain written informed consent from pa- tient before drug is used. ▪ Monitor liver function tests before starting drug; then q 2 wk for 1st yr of therapy; then q 4 wk for next 6 mo, and q 8 wk thereafter. ▪ Administer 1st dose of day with first daily dose of levodopa-carbidopa. ▪ Diarrhea is common and usually resolves with drug discontinuation. ▪ Stop drug if no benefit within 3 wk.

tolterodine tartrate
Detrol
Muscarinic receptor antagonist
Anticholinergic
Pregnancy Risk Category: C

Treatment of patients with overactive bladder with symptoms of urinary frequency, urgency, or urge incontinence — **Adults:** 2 mg P.O. b.i.d. Decrease to 1 mg P.O. b.i.d. based on response and tolerance.

Adjust-a-dose: In adults with significantly reduced hepatic function or in those who are currently taking drug that inhibits cytochrome P-450 3A4 isoenzyme system, give 1 mg P.O. b.i.d.

- Use with caution in patients with significant bladder outflow obstruction, GI obstructive disorders (such as pyloric stenosis), or controlled narrow-angle glaucoma, and hepatic or renal impairment.
- Assess baseline bladder function and monitor therapeutic effects.
- Tell patient to avoid driving and other potentially hazardous activities until visual effects of drug are known.

topiramate
Topamax
Sulfamate-substituted monosaccharide
Antiepileptic
Pregnancy Risk Category: C

Adjunctive therapy for adults with partial onset seizures — **Adults:** adjust up to maximum daily dose of 400 mg P.O. in divided doses b.i.d. Schedule is as follows: wk 1, 50 mg P.O. q evening; wk 2, 50 mg P.O. b.i.d.; wk 3, 50 mg P.O. q morning and 100 mg P.O. q evening; wk 4, 100 mg P.O. b.i.d.; wk 5, 100 mg P.O. q morning and 150 mg P.O. q evening; wk 6, 150 mg P.O. b.i.d.; wk 7, 150 mg P.O. q morning and 200 mg P.O. q evening; wk 8, 200 mg P.O. b.i.d.

Adjust-a-dose: In patients with creatinine clearance < 70 ml/min, reduce dose by 50%.

- Use with caution in breast-feeding or pregnant patients and in those with hepatic impairment.
- Withdraw gradually to minimize risk of increased seizure activity.
- Monitor liver enzymes.
- Be aware that drug rapidly cleared by dialysis. Prolonged period of dialysis may result in low drug levels and seizures.

topotecan hydrochloride
Hycamtin
Semisynthetic camptothecin derivative

Metastatic carcinoma of ovary after failure of initial or subsequent chemotherapy — **Adults:** 1.5 mg/m² I.V. infusion over 30 min q.d. for 5 days, starting on day 1 of 21-day cycle. Give minimum 4 cycles. Reduce dose

- Before first course, baseline neutrophil count > 1,500 cells/mm³ and platelet count > 100,000 cells/mm³ required. Monitor CBC.

(continued)

†Canadian ‡Australian

DRUG/CLASS/ CATEGORY	INDICATIONS / DOSAGES	KEY NURSING CONSIDERATIONS
topotecan hydrochloride *(continued)* *Antineoplastic* Pregnancy Risk Category: D	for subsequent course if severe neutropenia occurs.	• Use reconstituted product immediately.
toremifene citrate Fareston *Nonsteroidal antiestrogen* *Antineoplastic* Pregnancy Risk Category: D	*Metastatic breast cancer in postmenopausal women with estrogen-receptor positive or unknown tumors —* **Adults:** 60 mg P.O. q day.	• Obtain periodic CBC, calcium levels, and liver function tests. • Monitor for hot flashes and vaginal bleeding. • Monitor PT and INR closely.
torsemide Demadex *Loop diuretic* *Diuretic/antihypertensive* Pregnancy Risk Category: B	*Diuresis in patients with heart failure —* **Adults:** 10 to 20 mg/day P.O. or I.V. If response inadequate, double dose until response obtained. Maximum 200 mg/day. *Diuresis in patients with chronic renal failure —* **Adults:** 20 mg/day P.O. or I.V. If response inadequate, double dose until response obtained. Maximum 200 mg/day. *Hypertension —* **Adults:** 5 mg/day P.O. Increase to 10 mg, p.r.n.	• **I.V. use:** May give by direct injection over at least 2 min. Rapid injection may cause ototoxicity. Don't give > 200 mg at a time. Immediately report ringing in ears. • Monitor I&O, serum electrolytes, BP, weight, and HR. • Watch for hypokalemia. • Tell patient to take in morning to prevent nocturia.
tramadol hydrochloride Ultram *Synthetic derivative*	*Moderate to moderately severe pain —* **Adults:** 50 to 100 mg P.O. q 4 to 6 hr, p.r.n. Maximum 400 mg/day. **Elderly:** in patients > 75 yr, maximum 300 mg/day in divided	• Monitor CV and respiratory status. Withhold dose and notify doctor if respirations fall or respiratory rate < 12. • Monitor bowel and bladder function.

Analgesic
Pregnancy Risk Category: C

doses.

Adjust-a-dose: In patients with creatinine clearance < 30 ml/min, increase dose interval to q 12 hr. In patients with cirrhosis, give 50 mg q 12 hr.

- Give before onset of intense pain.
- Monitor patients at risk for seizures.

---

trandolapril
Mavik
ACE inhibitor
Antihypertensive
Pregnancy Risk Category: C (D in second and third trimesters)

Hypertension — **Adults:** for patients not receiving diuretics, initially 1 mg for nonblack patient and 2 mg for black patient P.O. q.d. If control not adequate, can increase dosage at ≥ 1-wk intervals. Maintenance doses generally 2 to 4 mg/day. Some patients receiving 4 mg/day may need b.i.d. doses. For patient receiving diuretic, give initial dose of 0.5 mg/day P.O. Dosage per BP response.
Heart failure post-MI or left-sided heart failure post-MI — **Adults:** initially, 1 mg/day P.O., adjusted to 4 mg/day, as tolerated.

- Angioedema associated with involvement of tongue, glottis, or larynx may be fatal.
- Monitor serum potassium closely.
- Monitor for hypotension. If possible, discontinue diuretics 2 to 3 days before starting trandolapril. If drug doesn't control BP, diuretics may be reinstituted cautiously.
- Assess renal function before and during therapy.

---

trastuzumab
Herceptin
Monoclonal antibody
Antineoplastic
Pregnancy Risk Category: B

Single-agent treatment of metastatic breast cancer in patients whose tumors overexpress human epidermal growth factor receptor 2 protein (HER2) and who have received one or more chemotherapy regimens for their metastatic disease; in combination with paclitaxel for metastatic breast cancer in patients whose tumors overexpress HER2 protein and who have not received chemotherapy for their metastatic disease — **Adults:** initial loading dose 4 mg/kg I.V. over

- Assess for cardiac dysfunction, especially if patient is receiving drug with anthracyclines and cyclophosphamide.
- Monitor for dyspnea, increased cough, paroxysmal nocturnal dyspnea, peripheral edema, or S₃ gallop. May stop treatment in patients who develop clinically significant decrease in left ventricular function.
- Monitor for first-infusion symptom complex (chills or fever, nausea, vomiting, *(continued)*

303

†Canadian ‡Australian

DRUG / CLASS / CATEGORY	INDICATIONS / DOSAGES	KEY NURSING CONSIDERATIONS
trastuzumab *(continued)*	90 min. Maintenance dose 2 mg/kg I.V. weekly as a 30-min I.V. infusion if initial loading dose is well tolerated.	pain, rigors, headache, dizziness, dyspnea, hypotension, rash, and asthenia.
trazodone hydrochloride Desyrel, Trazon, Trialodine *Triazolopyridine derivative* *Antidepressant* Pregnancy Risk Category: C	*Depression* — **Adults:** initially, 150 mg P.O. q.d. in divided doses; increased by 50 mg/ day q 3 to 4 days, p.r.n. Average dose 150 to 400 mg/day. Maximum daily dose for inpatients 600 mg; for outpatients, 400 mg.	▪ Administer before meals or with light snack. ▪ Monitor for suicidal tendencies and allow only minimum drug supply. ▪ Report presence of priapism immediately. ▪ Warn patient to avoid hazardous activities until CNS effects known.
tretinoin (retinoic acid, vitamin A acid; topical) Avita, Renova, Retin-A, StieVA-A† *Vitamin A derivative* *Antiacne agent* Pregnancy Risk Category: C	*Acne vulgaris* — **Adults and children:** clean affected area and lightly apply q.d. h.s. *Adjunct therapy to skin care and sun avoidance program* — **Adults:** apply to affected area q.d. h.s.	▪ Clean area thoroughly before application. Avoid getting in eyes, mouth, or mucous membranes. Instruct to wash face with mild soap no more than b.i.d. or t.i.d. ▪ Instruct patient to minimize exposure to sunlight, ultraviolet rays, wind, cold temperatures.
tretinoin (oral) Vesanoid *Retinoid* *Antineoplastic* Pregnancy Risk Category: D	*Induction of remission in patients with acute promyelocytic leukemia, French-American-British classification M3 (including M3 variant), when anthracycline chemotherapy contraindicated or unsuccessful* — **Adults and children ≥ 1 yr:** 45 mg/m²/day P.O. in 2 even doses. Discontin-	▪ Notify doctor if fever, dyspnea, or weight gain occurs. ▪ Monitor CBC and platelet counts regularly. ▪ Maintain infection control and bleeding precautions. ▪ Watch for infection or bleeding.

ue 30 days after complete remission or after 90 days of treatment, whichever is first.

triamcinolone acetonide (systemic)
Azmacort, Kenalog-10, Triamonide 40, Trilog
Glucocorticoid
Anti-inflammatory/anti-asthmatic
Pregnancy Risk Category: C

Severe inflammation or immunosuppression — **Adults:** 4 to 48 mg/day P.O. in divided doses; 40 mg I.M. weekly; 1 mg into lesions; 2.5 to 40 mg into joints or soft tissue. *Persistent asthma* — **Adults:** Azmacort 2 inhalations t.i.d. or q.i.d. Maximum 16 inhalations q.d. Total daily dose may be given b.i.d. for maintenance. **Children 6 to 12 yr:** Azmacort 1 to 2 inhalations t.i.d. or q.i.d. Maximum 12 inhalations q.d.

- For better results and less toxicity, give daily dose in morning with food.
- Don't use diluents with preservatives.
- Monitor weight, BP, and serum electrolytes.

triamcinolone acetonide (topical)
Aristocort, Flutex, Kenalog, Kenalonet, Triacet
Topical adrenocorticoid
Anti-inflammatory
Pregnancy Risk Category: C

Inflammation associated with corticosteroid-responsive dermatoses — **Adults and children:** apply sparingly b.i.d. to q.i.d. *Inflammation associated with oral lesions* — **Adults and children:** apply paste h.s. and, if needed, b.i.d. or t.i.d., preferably after meals.

- Wash skin before applying. Rub in gently, leaving thin coat. Apply directly to lesions.
- Stop drug if infection, striae, or atrophy occurs.
- Don't leave occlusive dressing in place > 16 hr each day or use on infected or exudative lesions.

triamcinolone acetonide (nasal)
Nasacort
Glucocorticoid
Anti-inflammatory
Pregnancy Risk Category: C

Relief from symptoms of seasonal or perennial allergic rhinitis — **Adults and children ≥ 12 yr:** 2 sprays (110 mcg) in each nostril q.d. Increase, p.r.n. to 440 mcg/day as daily dose or in divided doses ≤ q.i.d. Then decrease, if possible, to as little as 1 spray in each nostril q.d.

- Instruct patient to instill properly.
- Stress importance of using regularly. Warn patient not to exceed dosage prescribed.
- Instruct patient to report nasal infection.
- Tell patient to notify doctor if symptoms worsen or don't diminish within 2 to 3 wk.
- Discard canister after 100 actuations.

DRUG/CLASS/ CATEGORY	INDICATIONS/ DOSAGES	KEY NURSING CONSIDERATIONS
triamterene Dyrenium *Potassium-sparing diuretic* *Diuretic* Pregnancy Risk Category: B	*Edema* — **Adults:** initially, 100 mg P.O. b.i.d. after meals. Maximum total dose 300 mg/day.	▪ Monitor BP, blood uric acid, CBC, blood glucose, BUN, and serum electrolytes. ▪ Warn patient to avoid excessive ingestion of potassium-rich foods and supplements. ▪ Inform patient that urine may turn blue.
triazolam Apo-Triazo†, Halcion *Benzodiazepine* *Sedative-hypnotic* Pregnancy Risk Category: X Controlled Substance Schedule: IV	*Insomnia* — **Adults:** 0.125 to 0.5 mg P.O. h.s. **Adults > 65 yr:** 0.125 mg P.O. h.s.; increased, p.r.n., to 0.25 mg P.O. h.s.	▪ Assess mental status before initiating therapy. Elderly patients more sensitive to CNS effects. ▪ Prevent hoarding or self-overdosing if patient is depressed, suicidal, or drug-dependent or has drug abuse history.
trifluoperazine hydrochloride Apo-Trifluoperazine†, Solazine†, Stelazine†, Terfluzine† *Phenothiazine (piperazine derivative)* *Antipsychotic/antiemetic* Pregnancy Risk Category: NR	*Anxiety states* — **Adults:** 1 to 2 mg P.O. b.i.d. Maximum 6 mg/day. Don't give > 12 wk. *Schizophrenia; other psychotic disorders* — **Adults:** 2 to 5 mg P.O. b.i.d., gradually increased until response. Or 1 to 2 mg deep I.M. q 4 to 6 hr, p.r.n. More than 6 mg I.M. in 24 hr rarely required. **Children 6 to 12 yr (hospitalized or under close supervision):** 1 mg P.O. q.d. or b.i.d.; may increase gradually to 15 mg q.d.	▪ Wear gloves when preparing liquid forms. ▪ Watch for orthostatic hypotension. Keep patient supine for 1 hr after administration. ▪ Dilute liquid concentration with 60 ml tomato or fruit juice, carbonated beverages, coffee, tea, milk, water, or semisolid food. ▪ Protect from light. Slight yellowing of injection or concentration common. Discard markedly discolored solutions.
trihexyphenidyl hydrochloride	*All forms of parkinsonism, drug-induced parkinsonism, and adjunctive treatment to*	▪ Dose may need to be increased if tolerance develops.

Aparkane†, Apo-Trihex†, Artane, Novohexidyl†, Trihexane *Anticholinergic* *Antiparkinsonian* Pregnancy Risk Category: NR	*levodopa in parkinsonism management* — **Adults:** 1 mg P.O. 1st day, 2 mg 2nd day; then increased in 2-mg increments q 3 to 5 days until total of 6 to 10 mg/day. Usually given t.i.d. with meals or q.i.d. or switched to extended-release form b.i.d. Postencephalitic parkinsonism may require 12- to 15-mg total daily dose.	■ Adverse reactions dose-related and transient. Monitor patient. ■ May cause nausea if given after meals. ■ Gonioscopic evaluation and IOP monitoring required, especially in patients > 40 yr.
trimethoprim Proloprim, Trimpex, Triprim† *Synthetic folate antagonist* *Antibiotic* Pregnancy Risk Category: C	*Uncomplicated UTIs caused by susceptible organisms* — **Adults:** 200 mg P.O. as single dose or in divided doses q 12 hr for 10 days. Don't use in children < 12 yr. **Adjust-a-dose:** For patients with creatinine clearance 15 to 30 ml/min, give 50 mg P.O. q 12 hr; if < 15 ml/min, don't use.	■ Obtain urine specimen for culture and sensitivity tests before 1st dose. ■ Monitor CBC routinely. Sore throat, fever, pallor, and purpura may be early signs of serious blood disorders. ■ Prolonged use at high doses may cause bone marrow suppression.
trimipramine maleate Apo-Trimip†, Surmontil *TCA* *Antidepressant/antianxiety agent* Pregnancy Risk Category: C	*Depression* — **Adults:** 75 to 100 mg P.O. q.d. in divided doses, increased to 200 to 300 mg/day. Doses > 300 mg/day not recommended in hospitalized patients; ≤ 200 mg in outpatients. Total dose requirement may be given h.s. **Elderly and adolescent patients:** initially, 50 mg/day, gradually increased to 100 mg/day.	■ Gradually discontinue several days before surgery. ■ If signs of psychosis occur or increase, expect to reduce dose. Monitor for suicidal tendencies and allow only minimum drug supply. ■ Tell patient to relieve dry mouth with sugarless hard candy or gum.
troglitazone Rezulin *PPAR gamma activator*	*Adjunct to diet and insulin therapy in type 2 diabetes if hyperglycemia inadequately controlled with insulin > 30 U/day as multiple injections* — **Adults:** for patients on insulin,	■ Should be used by pregnant patient only if benefit justifies risk to fetus. *(continued)*

†Canadian ‡Australian

DRUG / CLASS / CATEGORY	INDICATIONS / DOSAGES	KEY NURSING CONSIDERATIONS
troglitazone *(continued)* *Antidiabetic* Pregnancy Risk Category: B	continue with current insulin dose and begin therapy with 200 mg/day P.O. with meal. May increase after 2 to 4 wk. Usual daily dose 400 mg; maximum 600 mg/day. Insulin dose may be decreased 10% to 25% when fasting glucose < 120 mg/dl in patients on troglitazone and insulin.	▪ Shouldn't be used to treat type 1 diabetes or ketoacidosis. ▪ Monitor for hypoglycemia. Insulin dose may need to be reduced. ▪ Monitor for liver abnormalities. ▪ Notify doctor if jaundice or dark urine occurs.
trovafloxacin mesylate Trovan Tablets **alatrofloxacin mesylate** Trovan I.V. *Fluoroquinolone derivative* *Antibiotic* Pregnancy Risk Category: C	*Nosocomial pneumonia; gynecologic, pelvic and complicated intra-abdominal infections—* **Adults:** 300 mg I.V. q.d.; then 200 mg P.O. q.d. for 7 to 14 days (10 to 14 days for pneumonia). *Community-acquired pneumonia; complicated skin infections—* **Adults:** 200 mg P.O. or I.V. q.d.; then 200 mg P.O. q.d. for 7 to 14 days (10 to 14 days for skin infections). *Prophylaxis of infection associated with colorectal surgery or hysterectomy—* **Adults:** 200 mg P.O. or I.V as single dose 30 min to 4 hr before surgery. *Acute sinusitis; chronic prostatitis, cervicitis, pelvic inflammatory disease (PID)—* **Adults:** 200 mg P.O. q.d. for 5 days (cervicitis), 10 days (sinusitis), 14 days (PID), or 28 days (prostatitis).	▪ Use cautiously in patients with CNS disorders and in those at increased risk for seizures. Drug may cause neurologic complications, such as seizures, psychosis, or increased intracranial pressure. Monitor patient with preexisting condition closely. ▪ Assess liver function periodically. ▪ May cause moderate to severe phototoxicity reactions if patient exposed to direct sunlight. ▪ No dosage adjustment necessary when switching from I.V. to oral form. ▪ May be used to treat diabetic foot infections but not osteomyelitis.

Uncomplicated UTIs, gonorrhea, and skin infections; acute bacterial exacerbation of chronic bronchitis — **Adults:** 100 mg P.O. q.d. for 3 days (UTIs), 7 to 10 days (skin infections, bronchitis) or single dose (gonorrhea).

Adjust-a-dose: For patients with mild to moderate cirrhosis, reduce 300-mg I.V. dose to 200-mg I.V. and 200-mg I.V. or P.O. dose to 100-mg I.V. or P.O.

urokinase
Abbokinase, Abbokinase Open-Cath, Ukidant‡
Thrombolytic enzyme
Thrombolytic enzyme
Pregnancy Risk Category: B

Lysis of acute massive pulmonary embolism (PE) or PE with unstable hemodynamics — **Adults:** for I.V. infusion *only* by infusion pump. Priming dose: 4,400 IU/kg with 0.9% NaCl or D_5W solution admixture over 10 min. Then 4,400 IU/kg/hr for 12 hr.

Coronary artery thrombosis — **Adults:** after bolus dose of heparin, infuse 6,000 IU/min of urokinase into occluded artery for up to 2 hr. Average total dose 500,000 IU. Initiate within 6 hr of symptoms.

Venous catheter occlusion — **Adults:** 5,000 IU/ml solution into occluded line; after 5 min, aspirate. Repeat aspiration attempts q 5 min for 30 min. If not patent, cap line and leave for 30 to 60 min before aspirating again. May require second instillation.

- Be prepared with RBCs, whole blood, plasma expanders other than dextran, and aminocaproic acid to treat bleeding, and corticosteroids, epinephrine, and antihistamines to treat allergic reactions.
- I.M. injections and other invasive procedures contraindicated during therapy.
- Monitor for excessive bleeding q 15 min for 1st hr; q 30 min for 2nd through 8th hr; then q 4 hr.
- Monitor pulses, color, and sensation of extremities q hr. Monitor vital signs and neurologic status as ordered.
- *I.V. use:* Reconstitute according to manufacturer's directions. Don't mix with other drugs. Administer through separate line.

†Canadian ‡Australian

DRUG/CLASS/ CATEGORY	INDICATIONS/ DOSAGES	KEY NURSING CONSIDERATIONS
valacyclovir hydrochloride Valtrex *Synthetic purine nucleoside* *Antiviral* Pregnancy Risk Category: B	*Herpes zoster infection (shingles) in patients with normal immune system* — **Adults:** 1 g P.O. t.i.d. for 7 days. Adjust for impaired renal function based on creatinine clearance. *For first episode of genital herpes in patients with normal immune system* — **Adults:** 1 g P.O. b.i.d. for 10 days. If creatinine clearance ≥ 30 ml/min, 1 g P.O. q 12 hr; for 10 to 29 ml/min, 1 g P.O. q 24 hr; for < 10 ml/min, 500 mg P.O. q 24 hr. *Recurrent genital herpes in patients with normal immune system* — **Adults:** 500 mg P.O. b.i.d. for 5 days, given at first sign.	▪ Use cautiously in renal impairment, elderly patients, and those receiving other nephrotoxic drugs, and in immunocompromised patients. ▪ Alert doctor if patient is breast-feeding. ▪ Inform patient that drug may be taken without regard to meals. ▪ Teach patient signs and symptoms of herpes infection and tell him to notify doctor if they occur. Treatment should begin within 48 hr.
valproate sodium Depakene Syrup, Epilim‡ **valproic acid** Depakene **divalproex sodium** Depakote, Depakote Sprinkle, Epival† *Carboxylic acid derivative* *Anticonvulsant* Pregnancy Risk Category: D	*Simple and complex absence seizures, mixed seizure types* — **Adults and children:** 15 mg/kg P.O. q.d., divided b.i.d. or t.i.d.; increase by 5 to 10 mg/kg q.d. q wk to maximum 60 mg/kg q.d. *Mania (delayed-release capsules)* — **Adults and children:** 750 mg q.d. in divided doses. Adjust per response; maximum 60 mg/kg/day. *Prophylaxis for migraine (Depakote only)* — **Adults:** initially, 250 mg P.O. b.i.d. Some patients may need up to 1,000 mg/day.	▪ Serious or fatal hepatotoxicity may follow nonspecific symptoms. Notify doctor; drug must be discontinued if hepatic dysfunction suspected. ▪ Administer with food or milk. ▪ Don't give syrup to patients on sodium restriction. ▪ Never withdraw suddenly. Call doctor if adverse reactions develop. ▪ Therapeutic serum levels 50 to 100 mcg/ml for most patients.

valsartan

Diovan

Angiotensin II antagonist

Antihypertensive

Pregnancy Risk Category: C (first trimester); D (second and third trimesters)

Hypertension — **Adults:** initially, 80 mg P.O. q.d. Expect BP reduction in 2 to 4 wk. For additional effect, increase to 160 or 320 mg q.d., or add diuretic. (Adding diuretic has greater effect than increases beyond 80 mg.) Usual dosage range: 80 to 320 mg q.d.

- Correct volume and salt depletions before starting. Monitor for hypotension.
- Advise patient to notify doctor if pregnancy occurs; drug must be discontinued.
- May be taken with or without food.

vancomycin hydrochloride

Lyphocin, Vancocin, Vancoled

Glycopeptide

Antibiotic

Pregnancy Risk Category: C

Serious infections — **Adults:** 1 to 1.5 g I.V. q 12 hr. **Children:** 10 mg/kg I.V. q 6 hr. **Neonates, young infants:** 15 mg/kg I.V. loading dose; then 10 mg/kg I.V. q 12 hr if < 1 wk, and 10 mg/kg I.V. q 8 hr if > 1 wk but < 1 mo. *Antibiotic-associated pseudomembranous and staphylococcal enterocolitis* — **Adults:** 125 to 500 mg P.O. q 6 hr for 7 to 10 days. **Children:** 40 mg/kg P.O. q.d. in divided doses q 6 hr for 7 to 10 days. Maximum 2 g/day. *Endocarditis prophylaxis for dental procedures* — **Adults:** 1 g I.V. slowly over 1 hr, starting 1 hr before procedure. **Children:** > 27 kg (60 lb), adult dose; < 27 kg, 20 mg/kg.

- Check daily for phlebitis and irritation. Report pain at infusion site. Avoid extravasation.
- Refrigerate I.V. solution after reconstitution; use within 96 hr.
- Monitor for red-neck syndrome. If present, stop infusion and report to doctor. Reaction usually stimulated by too rapid I.V. infusion rate.
- May need to reduce I.V. dose in renally impaired patients; monitor for changes in serum creatinine.

vasopressin (ADH)

Pitressin

Posterior pituitary hormone/

Antidiuretic hormone/

hemostatic agent

Pregnancy Risk Category: C

Nonnephrogenic, nonpsychogenic diabetes insipidus — **Adults:** 5 to 10 U I.M. or S.C. b.i.d. to q.i.d., p.r.n.; or intranasally in individualized doses, based on response. **Children:** 2.5 to 10 U I.M. or S.C. b.i.d. to q.i.d., p.r.n.; or intranasally in individualized doses.

- Never inject during first stage of labor.
- Monitor for signs of water intoxication.
- Monitor BP if patient taking b.i.d. Watch for elevated BP or lack of response.
- Monitor daily weight, urine specific gravity, and fluid I&O.

†Canadian ‡Australian

DRUG / CLASS / CATEGORY	INDICATIONS / DOSAGES	KEY NURSING CONSIDERATIONS
venlafaxine hydrochloride Effexor, Effexor XR *Serotonin, norepinephrine, dopamine reuptake inhibitor Antidepressant* Pregnancy Risk Category: C	*Depression* — **Adults:** initially, 75 mg P.O. q.d., in 2 or 3 divided doses with food. Increase, p.r.n., by 75 mg/day at intervals of ≥4 days. For certain patients, usual maximum 225 mg/day; certain severely depressed patients may receive 375 mg/day.	▪ Closely monitor BP. ▪ If patient has received drug for 6 wk or more, taper over 2 wk, as instructed by doctor. ▪ Warn patient to avoid hazardous activities until CNS effects known.
verapamil Apo-Verap†, Calan, Isoptin, Novo-Veramil†, Nu-Verap† **verapamil hydrochloride** Calan, Calan SR, Covera HS, Isoptin, Isoptin SR, Verelan *Calcium channel blocker Antianginal/antihypertensive/antiarrhythmic* Pregnancy Risk Category: C	*Vasospastic angina and classic chronic, stable angina pectoris; chronic atrial fibrillation* — **Adults:** 80 to 120 mg P.O. t.i.d. Increase, q wk, p.r.n. Maximum 480 mg q.d. *Supraventricular arrhythmias* — **Adults:** 0.075 to 0.15 mg/kg I.V. push over 2 min. 0.15 mg/kg in 30 min if no response. **Children 1 to 15 yr:** 0.1 to 0.3 mg/kg I.V. over 2 min. For children, may repeat in 30 min. **Children < 1 yr:** 0.1 to 0.2 mg/kg I.V. over 2 min. *Hypertension* — **Adults:** 80 mg P.O. t.i.d. Maximum 480 mg. Or, 120 to 240 mg extended-release tablets P.O. q.d. in morning. May add ½ tablet q.d.	▪ Monitor BP and ECG during and after I.V. administration. ▪ Assist with ambulation. ▪ *I.V. use:* Give by direct injection into vein or into tubing of free-flowing, compatible I.V. solution. Administer over ≥ 3 min to minimize adverse reactions. ▪ Monitor R-R interval for I.V. use. All patients should be on a cardiac monitor.
vidarabine Vira-A *Purine nucleoside Antiviral*	*Acute keratoconjunctivitis, superficial keratitis, and recurrent epithelial keratitis caused by herpes simplex* — **Adults and children:** 1 cm ointment into lower conjunctival sac 5	▪ Explain that ointment may produce temporary visual haze. ▪ Advise patient to watch for signs of sensitivity. Instruct him to discontinue and noti-

Pregnancy Risk Category: C	times q.d. at 3-hr intervals.	fy doctor if present.
vinblastine sulfate (VLB) Velban, Velbet‡ *Vinca alkaloid* *Antineoplastic* Pregnancy Risk Category: D	*Breast or testicular cancer; Hodgkin's disease; malignant lymphoma* — **Adults:** 3.7 mg/m² I.V. q 1 to 2 wk. Maximum 18.5 mg/m² I.V. q wk per response. Don't repeat if WBC < 4,000/mm³. **Children:** 2.5 mg/m² I.V. q wk. Increase by 1.25 mg/m² until WBC < 3,000/mm³ or tumor response seen. Maximum 12.5 mg/m² I.V. q wk. ***Adjust-a-dose:*** In patients with direct serum bilirubin > 3 mg/dl, can reduce dose by 50%.	- Give antiemetic first. - ***I.V. use:*** Inject directly into vein or tubing of running I.V. line over 1 min. If extravasation occurs, stop infusion and notify doctor. - Don't administer into limb with compromised circulation. - Monitor for acute bronchospasm. - Assess hands and feet for numbness and tingling. Assess gait for footdrop.
vincristine sulfate (VCR) Oncovin, Vincasar PFS *Vinca alkaloid* *Antineoplastic* Pregnancy Risk Category: D	*Acute lymphoblastic and other leukemias; Hodgkin's disease* — **Adults:** 1.4 mg/m² I.V. q wk. Maximum weekly 2 mg. **Children > 10 kg (22 lb):** 2 mg/m² I.V. q wk. **Children 10 kg and under or with body surface area < 1 m²:** initially, 0.05 mg/kg I.V. q wk.	- ***I.V. use:*** Inject into vein or tubing of running I.V. line slowly over 1 min. If extravasation occurs, stop and notify doctor. - Monitor for acute bronchospasm and hyperuricemia. Maintain adequate hydration. - Assess gait for footdrop.
vinorelbine tartrate Navelbine *Vinca alkaloid* *Antineoplastic* Pregnancy Risk Category: D	*Alone or with cisplatin for first-line treatment of ambulatory patients with nonresectable advanced non-small-cell lung cancer (NSCLC)* — *alone or with cisplatin in stage IV of NSCLC; with cisplatin in stage III of NSCLC* — **Adults:** 30 mg/m² I.V. q wk. ***Adjust-a-dose:*** Dosage modified if serum bilirubin > 2 mg/dl.	- Check granulocyte count. If < 1,000 cells/mm³, withhold and notify doctor. - Dilute before administering. - If extravasation occurs, stop and inject remaining dose into different vein. - Monitor deep tendon reflexes.

†Canadian ‡Australian

DRUG / CLASS / CATEGORY	INDICATIONS / DOSAGES	KEY NURSING CONSIDERATIONS
warfarin sodium Coumadin, Panwarfin, Sofarin, Warfilone Sodium† *Coumarin derivative* *Anticoagulant* Pregnancy Risk Category: X	*Pulmonary embolism with deep vein thrombosis; MI; rheumatic heart disease with heart valve damage; prosthetic heart valves; chronic atrial fibrillation —* **Adults:** 2 to 5 mg P.O. q.d. for 2 to 4 days, then dosage based on daily PT and INR. Usual maintenance dose 2 to 10 mg P.O. q.d.	▪ Monitor PT and INR. ▪ Assess patient for bleeding. ▪ Withhold and call doctor if fever or rash occurs. ▪ Anticoagulant can be neutralized by vitamin K injections.
xylometazoline hydrochloride 4-Way Long Acting, Neo-Synephrine II, Otrivin *Sympathomimetic* *Decongestant/Vasoconstrictor* Pregnancy Risk Category: NR	*Nasal congestion —* **Adults and children ≥ 12 yr:** 2 to 3 drops or sprays 0.1% solution in each nostril q 8 to 10 hr. **Children 2 to 12 yr:** 2 to 3 drops 0.05% solution in each nostril q 8 to 10 hr. **Children 6 mo to 2 yr:** 1 drop 0.05% solution in each nostril q 6 hr, p.r.n., under doctor supervision.	▪ Have patient hold head upright to minimize swallowing drug, then sniff spray briskly. ▪ Product should be used by only one person. ▪ Instruct patient to report insomnia, dizziness, weakness, tremor, or irregular heartbeat. ▪ Use only as needed ≤ 5 days.
zafirlukast Accolate *Antileukotriene* *Anti-inflammatory* Pregnancy Risk Category: B	*Prophylaxis and chronic treatment of asthma —* **Adults and children ≥ 12 yr:** 20 mg P.O. b.i.d. 1 hr before or 2 hr after meals.	▪ Not for reversing bronchospasm in acute asthma attacks. ▪ Advise patient to keep taking even if symptoms disappear. ▪ Give 1 hr before or 2 hr after meals.
zalcitabine (dideoxycytidine, ddC) Hivid *Nucleoside analogue*	*Monotherapy for advanced HIV disease in patients who can't tolerate zidovudine or with disease progression while on zidovudine —* **Adults and children ≥ 13 yr:** 0.75 mg P.O. q 8 hr.	▪ Don't give with food. ▪ Assess for peripheral neuropathy; can progress to sharp shooting pain or severe continuous burning pain. May not be reversible.

Antiviral
Pregnancy Risk Category: C

Combination therapy for advanced HIV disease — **Adults and children ≥ 13 yr:** 0.75 mg P.O. q 8 hr given with zidovudine 200 mg P.O. q 8 hr.

Adjust-a-dose: In patients with creatinine clearance 10 to 40 ml/min, give 0.75 mg P.O. q 12 hr; if < 10 ml/min, give 0.75 mg P.O. q 24 hr.

- Monitor for signs of pancreatitis such as increased serum amylase.

---

zidovudine (azidothymidine, AZT)
Apo-Zidovudine†, Novo-AZT†, Retrovir
Thymidine analogue
Antiviral
Pregnancy Risk Category: C

Symptomatic HIV infection, including AIDS — **Adults and children ≥ 12 yr:** 100 mg P.O. q 4 hr or 300 mg P.O. q 12 hr; I.V. infusion 1 mg/kg (over 1 hr) q 4 hr to 6 mg/kg/day. **3 mo to 12 yr:** 180 mg/m^2 P.O. q 6 hr (720 mg/m^2/day), ≤ 200 mg q 6 hr.
Asymptomatic HIV infection — **Adults and children ≥ 12 yr:** 100 mg P.O. q 4 hr while awake: I.V. infusion 1 mg/kg (over 1 hr) q 4 hr while awake to 5 mg/kg/day. **Children 3 mo to 12 yr:** 180 mg/m^2 P.O. q 6 hr (720 mg/m^2/day), maximum 200 mg q 6 hr.
To reduce risk of HIV transmission from mother with CD4$^+$ lymphocyte count > 200 cells/mm^3 to newborn — **Adults:** 100 mg P.O. 5 times q.d. between 14 and 34 wks' gestation and continued through pregnancy. During labor, loading dose of 2 mg/kg I.V. over 1 hr, followed by continuous I.V. infusion of 1 mg/kg/hr until umbilical cord clamped. **Neonates:** 2 mg/kg P.O. (syrup) q 6

- **I.V. use:** Dilute first. Infuse at constant rate over 1 hr. Avoid rapid infusion or bolus injection. Don't add to biological or colloidal fluids. After dilution, stable for 24 hr at room temperature and 48 hr if refrigerated at 35.6° to 46.4° F (2° to 8° C). Store undiluted vials at 59° to 77° F (15° to 25° C); protect from light.
- Monitor blood studies every 2 wk.
- Administer on empty stomach. Have patient sit up and drink adequate fluids.
- Monitor for superinfection. May cause overgrowth of nonsusceptible bacteria or fungi.
- Tell patient to continue to take drug as prescribed, even if he feels better.

(continued)

†Canadian ‡Australian

DRUG / CLASS / CATEGORY	INDICATIONS / DOSAGES	KEY NURSING CONSIDERATIONS
zidovudine *(continued)*	hr for 6 wk, starting within 12 hr of birth. Or, 1.5 mg/kg I.V. (infuse over 30 min) q 6 hr. ***Adjust-a-dose:*** In end-stage renal disease on hemodialysis or peritoneal dialysis, give 100 mg P.O. or 1 mg/kg I.V. q 6 to 8 hr.	▪ Caution that drug isn't bronchodilator and shouldn't be used to treat acute asthma attack.
zileuton Zyflo *S-lipoxygenase inhibitor Anti-inflammatory* Pregnancy Risk Category: C	*Prophylaxis and chronic treatment of asthma* — **Adults and children ≥ 12 yr:** 600 mg P.O. q.i.d.	
zolmitriptan Zomig *Selective 5-hydroxytryptamine receptor agonist Antimigraine agent* Pregnancy Risk Category: C	*Acute migraine headaches* — **Adults:** ≥ 2.5 mg P.O.; increase to 5 mg/dose, p.r.n. If headache returns after initial dose, 2nd dose may be given after 2 hr. Maximum dose is 10 mg in 24-hr period. ***Adjust-a-dose:*** In patients with moderate to severe hepatic impairment, use lower dose.	▪ Not intended for prophylactic therapy or for use in hemiplegic or basilar migraines. ▪ Safety not established for cluster headaches. ▪ Monitor for pain or tightness in the chest or throat, heart throbbing, rash, skin lumps, or swelling of the face, lips, or eyelids.
zolpidem tartrate Ambien *Imidazopyridine Hypnotic* Pregnancy Risk Category: B Controlled Substance Schedule: IV	*Short-term management of insomnia* — **Adults:** 10 mg P.O. immediately before bedtime. **Elderly:** 5 mg P.O. immediately before bedtime. Maximum 10 mg q.d. ***Adjust-a-dose:*** In patients with hepatic insufficiency, give 5 mg P.O. immediately before bedtime. Maximum 10 mg q.d.	▪ Give only for short-term management of insomnia, usually 7 to 10 days. ▪ Prevent hoarding or self-overdosing in depressed, suicidal, or drug-dependent patient or one with drug abuse history.

Selected narcotic analgesic combination products

Many common analgesics are combinations of two or more generic drugs. The following table details these drugs and their components.

Trade name	Generic drug combination
Aceta with Codeine (CSS III)	- acetaminophen 300 mg - codeine phosphate 30 mg
Anexia 7.5/650 (CSS III), Lorcet Plus (CSS III)	- acetaminophen 650 mg - hydrocodone bitartrate 7.5 mg
Azdone, Damason-P (CSS III)	- acetaminophen 500 mg - hydrocodone bitartrate 5 mg
Capital with Codeine (CSS V), Tylenol with Codeine Elixir (CSS V)	- acetaminophen 120 mg - codeine phosphate 12 mg/5 ml
Darvocet-N 50 (CSS IV)	- acetaminophen 325 mg - propoxyphene napsylate 50 mg
Darvocet-N 100, Propacet 100 (CSS IV)	- acetaminophen 650 mg - propoxyphene napsylate 100 mg
E-Lor, Wygesic (CSS IV)	- acetaminophen 650 mg - propoxyphene hydrochloride 65 mg
Empirin with Codeine No. 3 (CSS III)	- aspirin 325 mg - codeine phosphate 30 mg

*Available in Canada only.   CSS = Controlled Substance Schedule.

(continued)

Selected narcotic analgesic combination products

Trade name	Generic drug combination
Empirin with Codeine No. 4 (CSS III)	• aspirin 325 mg • codeine phosphate 60 mg
Fioricet with Codeine (CSS III)	• acetaminophen 325 mg • butalbital 50 mg • caffeine 40 mg • codeine phosphate 30 mg
Fiorinal with Codeine (CSS III)	• aspirin 325 mg • butalbital 50 mg • caffeine 40 mg • codeine phosphate 30 mg
Innovar Injection (CSS II)	• droperidol 2.5 mg • fentanyl citrate 0.05 mg/ml
Lorcet 10/650 (CSS III)	• acetaminophen 650 mg • hydrocodone bitartrate 10 mg
Lortab 2.5/500 (CSS III)	• acetaminophen 500 mg • hydrocodone bitartrate 2.5 mg
Lortab 5/500 (CSS III)	• acetaminophen 500 mg • hydrocodone bitartrate 5 mg
Lortab 7.5/500 (CSS III)	• acetaminophen 500 mg • hydrocodone bitartrate 7.5 mg
Percocet (CSS II)	• acetaminophen 325 mg

	- oxycodone hydrochloride 5 mg
Percodan-Demi (CSS II)	- aspirin 325 mg - oxycodone hydrochloride 2.25 mg - oxycodone terephthalate 0.19 mg
Percodan, Roxiprin (CSS II)	- aspirin 325 mg - oxycodone hydrochloride 4.5 mg - oxycodone terephthalate 0.38 mg
Phenaphen/Codeine No. 3 (CSS III)	- acetaminophen 325 mg - codeine phosphate 30 mg
Phenaphen/Codeine No. 4 (CSS III)	- acetaminophen 325 mg - codeine phosphate 60 mg
Propoxyphene Napsylate/Acetaminophen (CSS IV)	- propoxyphene napsylate 100 mg - acetaminophen 650 mg
Roxicet (CSS II)	- acetaminophen 325 mg - oxycodone hydrochloride 5 mg
Roxicet 5/500 (CSS II)	- acetaminophen 500 mg - oxycodone hydrochloride 5 mg
Roxicet Oral Solution (CSS II)	- acetaminophen 325 mg - oxycodone hydrochloride 5 mg/5 ml
Talacen (CSS IV)	- acetaminophen 650 mg - pentazocine hydrochloride 25 mg

(continued)

* Available in Canada only.   CSS = Controlled Substance Schedule.

Selected narcotic analgesic combination products

Trade name	Generic drug combination
Talwin Compound (CSS IV)	• aspirin 325 mg • pentazocine hydrochloride 12.5 mg
Tylenol with Codeine No. 2 (CSS III)	• acetaminophen 300 mg • codeine phosphate 15 mg
Tylenol with Codeine No. 3 (CSS III)	• acetaminophen 300 mg • codeine phosphate 30 mg
Tylenol with Codeine No. 4 (CSS III)	• acetaminophen 300 mg • codeine phosphate 60 mg
Tylox (CSS II)	• acetaminophen 500 mg • oxycodone hydrochloride 5 mg
Vicodin, Zydone (CSS III)	• acetaminophen 500 mg • hydrocodone bitartrate 5 mg
Vicodin ES (CSS III)	• acetaminophen 750 mg • hydrocodone bitartrate 7.5 mg

*Available in Canada only.   CSS = Controlled Substance Schedule.

Drugs that shouldn't be crushed

Many drug forms (such as slow release, enteric coated, encapsulated beads, wax matrix, sublingual, or buccal preparations) are formulated to release their active ingredient for a specified duration or at a predetermined time after administration. Disrupting these formulations by crushing can dramatically affect the drug absorption rate and increase the risk of
adverse effects. Certain drugs also should not be crushed for such reasons as taste, tissue irritation, and unusual formulation—for example, a capsule within a capsule, a liquid within a capsule, or a multiple, compressed tablet. Avoid crushing
the drugs listed below by brand name for the reasons noted beside them.

Accutane (mucous membrane
  irritant)
Actifed 12-Hour (slow release)
Acutrim (slow release)
Adalat CC (slow release)
Adipost capsules (slow release)
Aerolate Sr., Jr., III (slow release)
Aller-Chlor (slow release)
Allerest 12-Hour (slow release)
Ammonium Chloride Enseals (enteric
  coated)
Ansaid (taste)
Artane Sequels (slow release)
ASA Enseals (enteric coated)
Asacol (slow release)
Atrohist LA, Sprinkle (slow release)
Azulfidine EN-tabs (enteric coated)
Bellergal-S (slow release)
Betapen-VK (taste)
Bisacodyl (enteric coated)
Bisco-Lax (enteric coated)

Bontril Slow-Release (slow release)
Breonesin (liquid filled)
Brexin L.A. (slow release)
Bromfed (slow release)
Bromfed-PD (slow release)
Bromphen (slow release)
Bromophen T.D. (slow release)
Calan SR (slow release)
Carbiset-TR (slow release)
Cardizem (slow release)
Cardizem CD, SR (slow release)
Carter's Little Pills (enteric coated)
Ceftin (taste)
Cerespan (slow release)
Charcoal Plus (enteric coated)
Chloral Hydrate (liquid within a
  capsule, taste)
Chlor-Trimeton Allergy 12 Hour (slow
  release)
Chlor-Trimeton Repetabs (slow
  release)

Choledyl (enteric coated)
Choledyl SA (slow release)
Cipro (taste)
Codimal L.A. (slow release)
Colace (liquid within a capsule, taste)
Comhist LA (slow release)
Compazine Spansules (slow release)
Congess SR, JR (slow release)
Constant-T (slow release)
Contac 12-Hour, Maximum Strength
  (slow release)
Control (slow release)
Cotazym-S (enteric coated)
Creon (enteric coated)
Cystospaz-M (slow release)
Dallergy (slow release)
Dallergy-D, JR (slow release)
Deconamine SR (slow release)
Deconsal, Sprinkle, II (slow release)
Demazin Repetabs (slow release)

(continued)

Depakene (slow release, mucous membrane irritant)
Depakote (enteric coated)
Desoxyn Gradumets (slow release)
Desyrel (taste)
Dexatrim (slow release)
Dexedrine Spansule (slow release)
Diamox Sequels (slow release)
Dilatrate-SR (slow release)
Dimetapp Extentabs (slow release)
Disobrom (slow release)
Donnatal Extentabs (slow release)
Donnazyme (slow release)
Drisdol (liquid filled)
Drixoral (slow release)
Drize (slow release)
Dulcolax (enteric coated)
Duotrate (slow release)
Duraquin (slow release)
Dynabac (enteric coated)
DynaCirc CR (slow release)
Easprin (enteric coated)
Ecotrin (enteric coated)
Ecotrin Maximum Strength (enteric coated)
Efidac/24 (slow release)
Elixophyllin SR (slow release)
E-Mycin (enteric coated)
Endafed (slow release)
Entex LA (slow release)

Guaifed-PD (slow release)
Halfprin (enteric coated)
Humibid Sprinkle, DM, DM Sprinkle, L.A. (slow release)
Hydergine LC (liquid within a capsule)
Hydergine Sublingual (sublingual)
Hytakerol (liquid filled)
Iberet (slow release)
Iberet-500 (slow release)
Ilotycin (enteric coated)
IMDUR (slow release)
Inderal LA (slow release)
Inderide LA (slow release)
Indocin SR (slow release)
Ionamin (slow release)
Iso-Bid (slow release)
Isoptin SR (slow release)
Isordil Sublingual (sublingual)
Isordil Tembids (slow release)
Isosorbide Dinitrate SR (slow release)
Isosorbide Dinitrate Sublingual (sublingual)
Isuprel Glossets (sublingual)
Kaon-Cl (slow release)
K-Dur (slow release)
Klor-Con (slow release)
Klotrix (slow release)
K-Tab (slow release)

Optilets-500 (enteric coated)
Optilets-M-500 (enteric coated)
Oramorph SR (slow release)
Ornade Spansules (slow release)
Oruvail (slow release)
OxyContin (slow release)
Pabalate (enteric coated)
Pancrease (enteric coated)
Pancrease MT (enteric coated)
Papaverine Sustained Action (slow release)
Pavabid Plateau (slow release)
PBZ-SR (slow release)
PCE (slow release)
Pentasa (slow release)
Perdiem (wax coated)
Peritrate SA (slow release)
Phazyme (slow release)
Phazyme 95 (slow release)
Phenergan (taste)
Phyllocontin (slow release)
Plendil (slow release)
Polaramine Repetabs (slow release)
Poly-Histine-D (slow release)
Prelu-2 (slow release)
Prevacid (slow release)
Prilosec (slow release)
Pro-Banthine (taste)
Procanbid (slow release)
Procardia (delays absorption)

Entozyme (enteric coated)
Equanil (taste)
Ergostat (sublingual)
Eryc (enteric coated)
Ery-Tab (enteric coated)
Erythrocin Stearate (enteric coated)
Erythromycin Base (enteric coated)
Eskalith CR (slow release)
Extendryl SR, JR (slow release)
Fedahist Gyrocaps, Timecaps (slow release)
Feldene (mucous membrane irritant)
Feocyte (slow release)
Feosol (enteric coated)
Feosol Spansules (slow release)
Feratab (enteric coated)
Fergon (slow release)
Fero-Grad 500 (slow release)
Fero-Gradumet (slow release)
Ferralet Slow Release (slow release)
Ferralyn Lanacaps (slow release)
Ferro-Sequel (slow release)
Feverall Sprinkle Caps (taste)
Fumatinic (slow release)
Genabid (slow release)
Geocillin (taste)
Gris-PEG (crushing may cause precipitation as larger particles)
Guaifed (slow release)

K + 10 (slow release)
Levsinex Timecaps (slow release)
Levsinex Timecaps (slow release)
Lithobid (slow release)
Measurin (slow release)
Meprospan (slow release)
Mestinon Timespans (slow release)
Micro-K (slow release)
Micro-K Extencaps (slow release)
Motrin (taste)
MS Contin (slow release)
Naldecon (slow release)
Niac (slow release)
Nico-400 (slow release)
Nicobid (slow release)
Nicobid Tempules (slow release)
Nitro-Bid (slow release)
Nitroglyn (slow release)
Nitrong (sublingual)
Nitrospan (slow release)
Nitrostat (sublingual)
Nitrostat SR (slow release)
Noctec (liquid within a capsule)
Nolamine (slow release)
Nolex LA (slow release)
Norflex (slow release)
Norpace CR (slow release)
Novafed (slow release)
Novafed A (slow release)

Procardia XL (slow release)
Pronestyl-SR (slow release)
Proventil Repetabs (slow release)
Prozac (slow release)
Quibron-T/SR Dividose (slow release)
Quinaglute Dura-Tabs (slow release)
Quinalan (slow release)
Quinidex Extentabs (slow release)
Respaire SR (slow release)
Respbid (slow release)
Ritalin-SR (slow release)
Rondec-TR (slow release)
Ru-Tuss DE (slow release)
Sinemet CR (slow release)
Singlet (slow release)
Slo-bid Gyrocaps (slow release)
Slo-Niacin (slow release)
Slo-Phyllin GG, Gyrocaps (slow release)
Slow-Fe (slow release)
Slow-K (slow release)
Slow-Mag (slow release)
Sorbitrate SA (slow release)
Sorbitrate Sublingual (sublingual)
Span-FF (slow release)
Sparine (taste)
Sudafed 12 Hour (slow release)
Sustaire (slow release)
Tamine S.R. (slow release)

(continued)

Tavist-D (multiple compressed tablet)
Teldrin (slow release)
Teldrin Allergy (extended release)
Ten-K (slow release)
Tenuate Dospan (slow release)
Tepanil Ten-Tab (slow release)
Tessalon Perles (slow release)
Theobid (slow release)
Theobid Duracaps, Jr. Duracaps (slow release)
Theochron (slow release)
Theoclear L.A. (slow release)
Theo-Dur (slow release)
Theo-Dur Sprinkle (slow release)
Theolair-SR (slow release)
Theo-Sav (slow release)
Theospan-SR (slow release)
Theo-Time (slow release)
Theo-24 (slow release)
Theovent (slow release)
Theo-X (slow release)
Therapy Bayer Caplets (enteric coated)
Thorazine Spansule (slow release)
Toprol XL (slow release)
T-Phyl (slow release)
Tranxene-SD (slow release)
Trental (slow release)
Triaminic (slow release)

Triaminic TR (slow release)
Triaminic-12 (slow release)
Trinalin Repetabs (slow release)
Triptone Caplets (slow release)
Tuss-LA (slow release)
Tuss-Ornade Spansules (slow release)
ULR-LA (slow release)
Uniphyl (slow release)
Valrelease (slow release)
Verelan (slow release)
Voltaren (enteric coated)
Wellbutrin (mucous membrane anesthetic)
Wyamycin S (slow release)
Wygesic (taste)
ZORprin (slow release)
Zyban (slow release)
Zymase (enteric coated)

Dangerous drug interactions

The following table lists drug interactions for selected drugs. Especially dangerous interactions are shown in *italic* type.

Drug	Interacting drug	Possible effect
allopurinol	mercaptopurine	*Increased potential for bone marrow suppression*
atenolol	verapamil	Enhanced pharmacologic effects of beta blockers and verapamil
captopril	amiloride, spironolactone, triamterene	Possible hyperkalemia
	indomethacin	Decreased antihypertensive effect of ACE inhibitors
carbamazepine	erythromycin, isoniazid, propoxyphene	Increased risk of carbamazepine toxicity
carvedilol	MAO inhibitors, reserpine	Severe hypotension or bradycardia
cisapride	clarithromycin, erythromycin, fluconazole, itraconazole, ketoconazole, miconazole	Increased risk of arrhythmias
clonidine	sotalol	Enhanced rebound hypertension following clonidine withdrawal
cyclosporine	erythromycin	Possible elevated cyclosporine concentrations and nephrotoxicity
	phenytoin	Reduced plasma levels of cyclosporine
digoxin	amiodarone, verapamil	Elevated serum digoxin levels
	bendroflumethiazide, chlorothiazide, hydrochlorothiazide, methyclothiazide, metolazone, quinethazone, trichloromethiazide	Increased risk of cardiac arrhythmias due to hypokalemia
	quinidine	*Elevated serum digoxin levels*

(continued)

Drug	Interacting drug	Possible effect
enalapril	indomethacin	Decreased antihypertensive effect of ACE inhibitors
epinephrine	nadolol, pindolol, propranolol	*Increased systolic and diastolic pressures; marked decrease in heart rate*
esmolol	verapamil	Enhanced pharmacologic effects of beta blockers and verapamil
ethanol	acetohexamide, chlorpropamide, disulfiram, metronidazole, tolbutamide	*Acute alcohol intolerance reaction*
gentamicin	bumetanide, ethacrynic acid, furosemide	Possible enhanced ototoxicity
	ceftazidime, ceftizoxime, cephalothin	Possible enhanced nephrotoxicity
indinavir	benzodiazepines	Increased risk of sedation, respiratory impairment
lisinopril	indomethacin	Decreased antihypertensive effect of ACE inhibitors
lithium	bendroflumethiazide, chlorothiazide, hydrochlorothiazide, methyclothiazide, polythiazide, trichlormethiazide	*Decreased lithium excretion, which increases risk of lithium toxicity*
methotrexate	aspirin	*Increased risk of methotrexate toxicity*
	probenecid	*Decreased methotrexate elimination, increasing risk of methotrexate toxicity*
metoprolol	verapamil	Enhanced pharmacologic effects of beta blockers and verapamil
neomycin	bumetanide, ethacrynic acid, furosemide	Possible enhanced ototoxicity
	ceftazidime, ceftizoxime, cephalothin	Possible enhanced nephrotoxicity
penicillin	tetracycline	Reduced effectiveness of penicillins
potassium	amiloride, spironolactone, triamterene	*Increased risk of hyperkalemia*

propranolol	verapamil	Enhanced pharmacologic effects of beta blockers and verapamil
quinidine	amiodarone	Increased risk of quinidine toxicity
ritonavir	zolpidem	Increased sedation, respiratory impairment
	amiodarone, bepridil, cisapride, encainide, flecainide, propafenone, quinidine	Increased risks of arrhythmias
sildenafil	nitrates	Increased risk of hypotension
tetracyclines	aluminum carbonate, aluminum hydroxide, aluminum phosphate, calcium carbonate, dihydroxyaluminum sodium carbonate, magaldrate, magnesium oxide antacids	*Decreased plasma levels and effectiveness of tetracyclines*
tobramycin	ceftazidime, ceftizoxime, cephalothin	Possible enhanced nephrotoxicity
warfarin sodium	amiodarone, aspirin, cefamandole, cefoperazone, cefotetan, chloral hydrate, cimetidine, clofibrate, desipramine, erythromycin, glucagon, imipramine, nortriptyline, protriptyline, trimipramine	Increased risk of bleeding
	carbamazepine	Reduced effectiveness of warfarin
	cholestyramine	May bind with oral anticoagulants, resulting in impaired absorption
	co-trimoxazole, disulfiram, methimazole, metronidazole, propylthiouracil, sulfinpyrazone	*Increased risk of bleeding*
	griseofulvin	Decreased pharmacologic effect of oral anticoagulants
	rifampin	*Decreased pharmacologic effect of oral anticoagulants*

Table of equivalents

Metric system equivalents

Metric weight

1 kilogram (kg or Kg)	=	1,000 grams (g or gm)
1 gram	=	1,000 milligrams (mg)
1 milligram	=	1,000 micrograms (µg or mcg)
0.6 g	=	600 mg
0.3 g	=	300 mg
0.1 g	=	100 mg
0.06 g	=	60 mg
0.03 g	=	30 mg
0.015 g	=	15 mg
0.001 g	=	1 mg

Metric volume

1 liter (l or L)	=	1,000 milliliters (ml)*
1 milliliter	=	1,000 microliters (µl)

Household		Metric
1 teaspoon (tsp)	=	5 ml
1 tablespoon (T or tbs)	=	15 ml
2 tablespoons	=	30 ml
1 measuring cupful	=	240 ml
1 pint (pt)	=	473 ml
1 quart (qt)	=	946 ml
1 gallon (gal)	=	3,785 ml

*1 ml = 1 cubic centimeter (cc); however, ml is the preferred measurement term today.

Weight conversions

1 oz = 30 g	1 lb = 453.6 g	2.2 lb = 1 kg

Temperature conversions

FAHRENHEIT DEGREES	CELSIUS DEGREES	FAHRENHEIT DEGREES	CELSIUS DEGREES	FAHRENHEIT DEGREES	CELSIUS DEGREES
106.0	41.1	100.6	38.1	95.2	35.1
105.8	41.0	100.4	38.0	95.0	35.0
105.6	40.9	100.2	37.9	94.8	34.9
105.4	40.8	100.0	37.8	94.6	34.8
105.2	40.7	99.8	37.7	94.4	34.7
105.0	40.6	99.6	37.6	94.2	34.6
104.8	40.4	99.4	37.4	94.0	34.4
104.6	40.3	99.2	37.3	93.8	34.3
104.4	40.2	99.0	37.2	93.6	34.2
104.2	40.1	98.8	37.1	93.4	34.1
104.0	40.0	98.6	37.0	93.2	34.0
103.8	39.9	98.4	36.9	93.0	33.9
103.6	39.8	98.2	36.8	92.8	33.8
103.4	39.7	98.0	36.7	92.6	33.7
103.2	39.6	97.8	36.5	92.4	33.6
103.0	39.4	97.6	36.4	92.2	33.4
102.8	39.3	97.4	36.3	92.0	33.3
102.6	39.2	97.2	36.2	91.8	33.2
102.4	39.1	97.0	36.1	91.6	33.1
102.2	39.0	96.8	36.0	91.4	33.0
102.0	38.9	96.6	35.9	91.2	32.9
101.8	38.8	96.4	35.8	91.0	32.8
101.6	38.7	96.2	35.7	90.8	32.7
101.4	38.6	96.0	35.6	90.6	32.6
101.2	38.4	95.8	35.4	90.4	32.4
101.0	38.3	95.6	35.3	90.2	32.3
100.8	38.2	95.4	35.2	90.0	32.2

Managing anaphylaxis

Anaphylaxis, an immediate hypersensitivity reaction to an allergen, may occur from any I.V. drug, usually within seconds or minutes of administration. The severity of the reaction depends on the patient's sensitivity to the drug and the amount of drug injected. A severe reaction may precipitate vascular collapse.

Signs and symptoms

Signs and symptoms include angioedema, anxiety, arrhythmias, bronchospasm, chills, coughing, dizziness, dyspnea, flushing, GI disturbances, laryngeal edema (evident by voice change), nasal congestion, paresthesia, pounding headache, pruritus, hypotension, shock, stridor, sweating, thready pulse, urticaria, weakness, and wheezing.

Treatment

Anaphylaxis requires emergency treatment. Follow your facility's protocol. Your immediate priorities may include the following interventions:

- Prevent further exposure to the antigen. For anaphylaxis caused by I.V. drugs or contrast media, *stop the infusion immediately*. For venom-induced anaphylaxis, apply a tourniquet to the patient's arm or leg above the sting, if appropriate. If possible, remove the stinger by scraping the site with a dull object (grasping and pulling can compress the venom sac and release more toxin).
- Maintain airway patency and adequate ventilation, with intubation as necessary.

- As ordered, administer oxygen in high concentrations. (Watch for signs and symptoms of laryngeal edema.)
- Administer epinephrine to prevent further histamine release and counteract bronchoconstriction, hypotension, and vasodilation. In early anaphylaxis, the doctor may order an S.C. or I.M. injection of 0.3 to 0.5 ml of 1:1,000 solution (0.01 ml/kg for a child), repeated every 5 to 15 minutes if needed. For acute respiratory distress, expect to give up to 5 ml (0.5 mg) I.V. of a 1:10,000 solution. In children, expect to give 0.1 to 0.2 mg or 0.01 mg/kg/dose over 5 minutes; repeated every 30 minutes as needed. If vascular collapse prevents venous access, give epinephrine endotracheally if ordered.
- If bronchoconstriction persists, the doctor may order aminophylline, a longer-acting bronchodilator. Other drugs may include antihistamines (usually diphenhydramine), which help counteract peripheral signs and symptoms, and corticosteroids.
- Insert I.V. lines and administer I.V. crystalloid or I.V. colloid solutions to correct intravascular fluid loss from third-space shifts and vasodilation.
- If fluid therapy fails to maintain adequate BP, the doctor may order a vasopressor, such as norepinephrine or dopamine. However, vasopressors may not be effective in patients receiving beta blockers. In such patients, glucagon may be used to increase BP.
- Continue to observe the patient for several hours for indications of delayed reactions to anaphylaxis or its treatment.

Index

A

abacavir, 2
Abbokinase, 309
Abbokinase Open-Cath, 309
abciximab, 2
Abdominal distention, postoperative, neostigmine bromide/neostigmine methylsulfate for, 229
Abortion
  incomplete, oxytocin, synthetic injection, for, 241
  second-trimester, dinoprostone for, 110
Abrasions, bacitracin for, 32
acarbose, 2
Accolate, 314
Accupril, 269
Accutane, 182
acebutolol hydrochloride, 3
Acel-Imune, 112
Acephen, 3
Aceta, 3
acetaminophen, 3
Acetaminophen toxicity, acetylcysteine for, 5
Acetazolam, 4
acetazolamide, 4
acetazolamide sodium, 4
acetylcholine, 4
acetylcysteine, 5
acetylsalicylic acid, 27
Aches-N-Pain, 170
Achromycin V, 293
Aclin, 288
Acne
  clindamycin for, 83
  erythromycin for, 128
  metronidazole for, 215

Acne (continued)
  isotretinoin for, 182
  tetracycline for, 293
  tretinoin for, 304
Acquired immunodeficiency syndrome complications, dronabinol for, 121. See also HIV infection.
Acromegaly
  bromocriptine for, 42
  octreotide for, 235
ACTH, 88
Acthar, 88
Acthar Gel (H.P.), 88
ACTH Gel, 88
Acticort, 168
Actidose, 5
Actidose-Aqua, 5
Actilyse, 11
Actimmune, 178
actinomycin D, 96
Activase, 11
activated charcoal, 5
Actron, 183
ACT-3, 170
Acular, 184
Acute pyelonephritis, levofloxacin for, 189
acyclovir, 5
acyclovir sodium, 6
Adalat, 231
Adalat CC, 231
Adapine, 231
Adenocard, 6
adenosine, 6
ADH, 311
Adrenal cancer, aminoglutethimide for, 15
Adrenalin, 124
Adrenalin Chloride, 124, 125

adrenaline, 124-125
Adrenal insufficiency
  cortisone for, 89
  fludrocortisone for, 143-144
  hydrocortisone for, 167
Adrenocortical function, diagnosing, corticotropin for, 88
adrenocorticotropic hormone, 88
Adriamycin, 119
Adriamycin PFS, 119
Adriamycin RDF, 119
Adrucil, 146
Adsorbocarpine, 252
Advil, 170
AeroBid, 145
AeroBid-M, 145
Aerolate, 293
Aeroseb-Dex, 102
Afrin, 240, 266
Agenerase, 21
Aggrastat, 298
Agitation, lorazepam for, 195
Agrylin, 22
AHF, 22-23
A-hydroCort, 167
Airbron, 5
AK-Chlor, 72
AK-Dilate, 250
Akineton, 40
Akineton Lactate, 40
AK-Nefrin Ophthalmic, 250
Akne-Mycin, 128
AK-Pentolate, 92
AK-Pred, 259
AKTob, 299
AK-Tracin, 32
AK-Zol, 4
alatrofloxacin mesylate, 308-309
albumin 5%, 7
albumin 25%, 7

Albuminar 5, 7
Albuminar 25, 7
Albutein 5%, 7
Albutein 25%, 7
albuterol, 7-8
albuterol sulfate, 7-8
Alcoholism
  disulfiram for, 114
  mesoridazine for, 207
  naltrexone for, 225
Alcohol withdrawal
  chlordiazepoxide for, 73
  clorazepate for, 85
  oxazepam for, 239
Alconefrin, 251
Aldactone, 285
Aldazine, 295
aldesleukin, 8
Aldomet, 210
Aldomet Ester Injection, 210
alendronate sodium, 8
Alepam, 239
Aleve, 226
Alexan, 94
Alfenta, 9
alfentanil hydrochloride, 9
alitretinoin, 9
Alka-Mints, 49
Alkeran, 203
Allegra, 141
Allegron, 234
Aller-Chlor L, 74
Allerdryl, 110
Allerest, 225
Allerest 12 Hr Nasal Spray, 240
Allergic reactions
  dexamethasone for, 101
  epinephrine for, 124
Allergy symptoms
  brompheniramine for, 42-43
  budesonide for, 43
  cetirizine for, 71

Allergy symptoms *(continued)*
chlorpheniramine for, 74
clemastine for, 82
cortisone for, 89
cromolyn sodium for, 90
diphenhydramine for, 110
fexofenadine for, 141
flunisolide for, 145
fluticasone for, 150-151
loratadine for, 195
promethazine for, 263
triamcinolone for, 305
allopurinol, 9
Alopecia
finasteride for, 142
minoxidil for, 218
Alphapress, 166
Alphatrex, 38
alprazolam, 10
alprostadil, 10-11
Altace, 271
alteplase, 11-12
AlternaGEL, 12
Alu-Cap, 12
aluminum carbonate, 12
aluminum hydroxide, 12
aluminum-magnesium complex, 197
Alupent, 207
Alzapam, 195
Alzheimer's disease
donepezil for, 117
tacrine for, 289
amantadine hydrochloride, 13
Amaryl, 159
Ambien, 316
Amebiasis, metronidazole for, 214
Amen, 203
Amenorrhea
bromocriptine for, 42
~droxyprogesterone
for, 203

Amenorrhea *(continued)*
norethindrone for, 234
progesterone for, 262-263
Amerge, 227
A-methaPred, 212
amethopterin, 210
Amicar, 15
amifostine, 13
amikacin sulfate, 14
Amikin, 14
amiloride hydrochloride, 14
amino acid infusions, 14-15
aminocaproic acid, 15
aminoglutethimide, 15
aminophylline, 16
Aminosyn, 14
Aminosyn-HBC, 15
Aminosyn II in Dextrose, 14
Aminosyn II with Electrolytes in Dextrose, 14-15
Aminosyn-RF, 15
amiodarone hydrochloride, 17
amlodipine besylate, 17
amitriptyline hydrochloride, 17
amoxapine, 18
amoxicillin/clavulanate potassium, 18
amoxicillin trihydrate, 18-19
Amoxil, 18
amoxycillin/clavulanate potassium, 18
amoxycillin trihydrate, 18-19
Amphocin, 19
Amphojel, 12
Amphotec, 20
amphotericin B, 19

amphotericin B cholesteryl sulfate complex, 20
Amphotericin B for injection, 19
ampicillin sodium/sulbactam sodium, 20-21
Amprace, 123
amprenavir, 21
amrinone lactate, 21
Amyotrophic lateral sclerosis, riluzole for, 275
Anacin (aspirin free), 3
Anacobin, 91
Anafranil, 83
anagrelide hydrochloride, 22
Analgesic combination products, 317
Anandron, 231
Anaphylaxis
epinephrine for, 124
managing, 330
Anaprox, 226
Anaspaz, 169
anastrozole, 22
Ancalixir, 249
Ancef, 58
Ancobon, 143
Ancotil, 143
Andro 100, 292
Androderm, 292
Android, 212
Android-F, 147
Anemia
epoetin alfa for, 125-126
folic acid for, 152
leucovorin for, 188
Anergan 25, 263
Anesthesia
alfentanil for, 9
butorphanol for, 46
droperidol for, 121, 122
fentanyl for, 139-140
midazolam for, 216

Anesthesia *(continued)*
nalbuphine for, 224
Angina
amlodipine for, 17
atenolol for, 27
bepridil for, 37
diltiazem for, 109
eptifibatide for, 126-127
isosorbide for, 181-182
metoprolol for, 214
nadolol for, 223
nicardipine for, 229-230
nifedipine for, 231
nitroglycerin for, 232, 233
propranolol for, 265
verapamil for, 312
Anginine, 232
Angioedema, clemastine for, 82
Ankylosing spondylitis
diclofenac for, 105
indomethacin for, 173
naproxen for, 226
sulindac for, 288
Ansaid, 148
Antabuse, 114
Antiflux, 197
antihemophilic factor, 22-23
Antispas, 106
antithrombin III, human, 24
Anti-Tuss, 164
Antivert, 202
Anturane, 288
Anturane, 288
Anxiety
alprazolam for, 10
buspirone for, 45
chlordiazepoxide for, 73
diazepam for, 104
hydroxyzine for, 169
lorazepam for, 195
mesoridazine for, 207
oxazepam for, 239

Anxiety *(continued)*
  prochlorperazine for, 262
  trifluoperazine for, 306
Anzemet, 116
Apacet, 3
APAP, 3
Aparkane, 307
Apo-Alpraz, 10
Apo-Amitriptyline, 17
Apo-Atenolol, 27
Apo-Benztropine, 36
Apo-Capto, 52
Apo-Carbamazepine, 53
Apo-Cephalex, 69
Apo-Chlorthalidone, 75
Apo-Clorazepate, 85
Apo-Diazepam, 104
Apo-Diltiaz, 109
Apo-Ferrous Sulfate, 140
Apo-Flurazepam, 148
Apo-Flurbiprofen, 148
Apo-Furosemide, 154
Apo-Haloperidol, 164
Apo-Hydro, 167
Apo-Hydroxyzine, 169
Apo-Imipramine, 172
Apo-Indomethacin, 173
Apo-ISDN, 181
Apo-Lorazepam, 195
Apo-Methyldopa, 211
Apo-Metoclop, 213
Apo-Metoprolol, 214
Apo-Metronidazole, 214
Apo-Minocycline, 217
Apo-Napro-Na, 226
Apo-Nifed, 231
Apo-Perphenazine, 248
Apo-Pindol, 253
Apo-Piroxicam, 254
Apo-Primidone, 260
Apo-Quinidine, 270
Apo-Ranitidine, 271
Apo-Sulfamethoxazole, 287
Apo-Sulfatrim, 89
Apo-Sulin, 288

Apo-Thioridazine, 295
Apo-Timol, 298
Apo-Triazo, 306
Apo-Trifluoperazine, 306
Apo-Trihex, 307
Apo-Trimip, 307
Apo-Verap, 312
Apo-Zidovudine, 315
Appendicitis
  meropenem for, 206
  piperacillin and tazobactam for, 253-254
apraclonidine hydrochloride, 25
Apresoline, 166
aprotinin, 25
Aquachloral Supprettes, 71
Aquazide-H, 167
ara-C, 94
Aralen HCl, 73
Aralen Phosphate, 73
Aratac, 17
Arava, 187
ardeparin sodium, 26
Aredia, 241
Aricept, 117
Arimidex, 22
Aristocort, 305
Arrhythmias
  acebutolol for, 3
  adenosine form 6
  amiodarone for, 17
  atropine for, 28
  bretylium for, 41-42
  digoxin for, 107
  diltiazem for, 109
  disopyramide for, 113-114
  esmolol for, 129
  flecainide for, 142
  ibutilide for, 170-171
  isoproterenol for, 181
  lidocaine for, 190-191
  magnesium sulfate for, 200

Arrhythmias *(continued)*
  mexiletine for, 215
  moricizine for, 221
  procainamide for, 261
  propafenone for, 263
  propranolol for, 265
  quinidine for, 270
  sotalol for, 285
  tocainide for, 300
  verapamil for, 312
Artane, 307
Arterial thrombosis, streptokinase for, 286
Arteriovenous cannula occlusion
  streptokinase for, 286
  urokinase for, 309
Arthritis. *See also specific type.*
  ibuprofen for, 170
  magnesium salicylate for, 199
A.S.A., 27
Ascriptin, 27
Asendin, 18
Asig, 269
Asmol, 7
asparaginase, 26
Aspergillosis
  amphotericin B cholesteryl sulfate complex for, 20
  itraconazole for, 182
aspirin, 27
Asthma
  aminophylline for, 16
  beclomethasone for, 35
  budesonide for, 43
  cromolyn sodium for, 90
  epinephrine for, 124
  flunisolide for, 145
  fluticasone for, 149-150
  hydroxyzine for, 169
  isoproterenol for, 180
  metaproterenol for, 207-208

Asthma *(continued)*
  montelukast for, 221
  nedocromil for, 227
  pirbuterol for, 254
  salmeterol for, 278
  triamcinolone for, 305
  zafirlukast for, 314
  zileuton for, 316
AsthmaHaler Mist, 124
Asthma-Nefrin, 124
Asthma PF, 221
Atacand, 49
Atarax, 169
Atelectasis, acetylcysteine for, 5
atenolol, 27
Atherectomy, abciximab for, 2
Atherosclerosis, clopidogrel for, 85
AT-III, 24
Ativan, 195
ATnativ, 24
atorvastatin calcium, 28
atovaquone, 28
atropine sulfate, 28, 29
Atropisol, 29
Atropt, 29
Atrovent, 178
attapulgite, 29
Attention deficit hyperactivity disorder
  dextroamphetamine for, 103
  methamphetamine for, 209
  methylphenidate for, 211
  pemoline for, 243
Attenuvax, 201
Augmentin, 18
auranofin, 29
aurothioglucose, 30
Avapro, 179
Aventyl, 234
Avirax, 6
Avlosulfon, 98

Avomine, 263
Avonex, 177
Axid, 233
Axid AR, 233
Axsain, 52
Ayercillin, 245
Aygestin, 234
Azactam, 32
azathioprine, 30-31
azidothymidine, 315-316
azithromycin, 31
Azmacort, 305
Azo-Standard, 248
AZT, 315-316
aztreonam, 32
Azulfidine, 287

B

Baciguent, 32, 33
Baci-IM, 33
Bacitin, 32, 33
bacitracin, 32, 33
baclofen, 33
Bacteremia
    cefoperazone for, 62
    cefotaxime for, 62-63
    ceftazidime for, 65
    ceftizoxime for, 66
    ceftriaxone for, 67
Bacterial vaginosis
    clindamycin for, 83
    metronidazole for, 215
Bactocill, 239
Bactrim DS, 89
Bactroban, 222
Barbita, 249
Baridium, 248
Basal cell carcinoma, fluo-
    rouracil for, 146
Basaljel, 12
basiliximab, 34
Baycol, 70
Bayer Select Maximum
    Strength Backache
    Pain Relief
    Formula, 199

Bayer Timed-Release, 27
BCNU, 55
becaplermin, 34-35
Becloforte Inhaler, 35
beclomethasone dipropi-
    onate, 35
Beclovent, 35
Beconase AQ Nasal Spray,
    35
Beconase Nasal Inhaler,
    35
Bedoz, 91
Beesix, 268
Behavior disorders,
    haloperidol for, 164
Bell/ans, 283
Bellaspaz, 169
Benadryl, 110
benazepril hydrochloride,
    36
Benemid, 260
Benign prostatic hyperpla-
    sia
    finasteride for, 142
    tamsulosin for, 290
    terazosin for, 291
Bentyl, 106
Benuryl, 260
Benzodiazepine overdose,
    flumazenil for,
    144-145
benzonatate, 36
benztropine mesylate, 36
benzylpenicillin benza-
    thine, 244
benzylpenicillin potassi-
    um, 244-245
benzylpenicillin procaine,
    245
benzylpenicillin sodium,
    245
Bepadin, 37
bepridil hydrochloride, 37
beractant, 37
Beriberi, thiamine for, 295

Betagan, 189
betamethasone, 38
betamethasone acetate
    and betamethasone
    sodium phosphate,
    38
betamethasone dipropi-
    onate, 38
betamethasone sodium
    phosphate, 38
betamethasone valerate,
    38
Betamin, 295
Betapace, 285
Betaseron, 177
Betatrex, 38
Beta-Val, 38
betaxolol hydrochloride,
    39
bethanechol chloride, 39
Betimol, 298
Betnesol, 38
Betnovate, 38
Betoptic, 39
Betoptic S, 39
Biamine, 295
Biavax II, 278
Biaxin, 81
Bicillin L-A, 244
BiCNU, 55
Bile obstruction,
    cholestyramine for,
    75
Biliary tract infection, ce-
    fazolin for, 59
Biocef, 69
biperiden hydrochloride,
    40
biperiden lactate, 40
Bisac-Evac, 40
bisacodyl, 40
Bisacodyl Uniserts, 40
Bismatrol, 40
bismuth subsalicylate, 40
bisoprolol fumarate, 41

Bladder atony, postopera-
    tive, neostigmine
    bromide/neostig-
    mine methylsulfate
    for, 229
Bladder cancer
    cisplatin for, 79-80
    doxorubicin for, 119
Blastomycosis, itracona-
    zole for, 182
Bleeding. *See also* Uterine
    bleeding, abnor-
    mal.
    excessive, aminocaproic
    acid for, 15
    superficial, epinephrine
    for, 125
Blenoxane, 41
bleomycin sulfate, 41
Blocadren, 298
Blood pressure, maintain-
    ing, norepinephrine
    for, 233
Bonamine, 202
Bone disease, metabolic,
    calcifediol for, 46
Bone infection
    cefazolin for, 59
    cefonicid for, 61
    cefotaxime for, 62-63
    cefotetan for, 63
    cefoxitin for, 63-64
    ceftizoxime for, 66
    ceftriaxone for, 67
    cephalexin for, 69
    cephradine for, 69
    ciprofloxacin for, 78
    imipenem and cilastatin
    for, 172
    ticarcillin/clavulanate
    for, 297
Bone marrow transplanta-
    tion complications
    filgrastim for, 141
    sargramostim for, 279

Bowel evacuation, magnesium salts for, 198
Bowel examination preparation
    bisacodyl for, 40
    cascara sagrada for, 57
    senna for, 281
Bowel management, psyllium for, 267
Brain tumor
    carmustine for, 55
    lomustine for, 194
Breast cancer
    anastrozole for, 22
    capecitabine for, 50-51
    cyclophosphamide for, 92
    docetaxel for, 115
    doxorubicin for, 119
    esterified estrogens for, 130
    estradiol for, 131
    ethinyl estradiol for, 133
    fluorouracil for, 146
    fluoxymesterone for, 147
    goserelin for, 162
    letrozole for, 187
    megestrol for, 203
    methyltestosterone for, 212
    paclitaxel for, 241
    tamoxifen for, 289
    testosterone for, 292
    thiotepa for, 295
    toremifene for, 302
    trastuzumab for, 303-304
    vinblastine for, 313
Brethaire, 291
Brethine, 291
Bretylate, 41
bretylium tosylate, 41-42
Bretylol, 41
Brevibloc, 129
Bricanyl, 291

bromocriptine mesylate, 42
Bromphen, 42
brompheniramine maleate, 42-43
Bronchitis
    acetylcysteine for, 5
    cefdinir for, 59
    cefpodoxime for, 64
    ceftibuten for, 66
    co-trimoxazole for, 89
    dirithromycin for, 113
    grepafloxacin for, 162-163
    levofloxacin for, 189
    lomefloxacin for, 193-194
    loracarbef for, 194-195
    sparfloxacin for, 285
    trovafloxacin for, 309
Bronchospasm
    albuterol for, 7
    aminophylline for, 16
    cromolyn sodium for, 90
    epinephrine for, 124
    ipratropium for, 178
    isoproterenol for, 180, 181
    levalbuterol for, 188
    metaproterenol for, 207-208
    pirbuterol for, 254
    salmeterol for, 278-279
    terbutaline for, 291-292
    theophylline for, 293-294
Bronitin Mist, 124
Bronkaid Mist, 124
Bronkaid Mistometer, 124
Bronkaid Suspension Mist, 124
Bronkodyl, 293
Brucellosis, tetracycline for, 293
budesonide, 43
Bufferin, 27

BufOpto Atropine, 29
Bulimia nervosa, fluoxetine for, 147
bumetanide, 44
Bumex, 44
bupropion hydrochloride, 44
Burinex, 44
Burns
    bacitracin for, 32
    nitrofurazone for, 232
    silver sulfadiazine for, 282-283
Bursitis
    indomethacin for, 173
    naproxen for, 226
    sulindac for, 288
Buscopan, 280
BuSpar, 45
buspirone hydrochloride, 45
busulfan, 45
butoconazole nitrate, 45
butorphanol tartrate, 46

C

Calan, 312
Calan SR, 312
Calcarb 600, 49
CalCarb-HD, 49
Calci-Chew, 49
calcifediol, 46
Calciject, 48
Calcijex, 47
Calcilean, 165
Calcimar, 47
Calciparine, 165
calcipotriene, 46
calcitonin (human), 47
calcitonin (salmon), 47
calcitriol, 47
calcium acetate, 48
calcium carbonate, 49
calcium chloride, 48
calcium citrate, 48
calcium glubionate, 48

calcium gluceptate, 48
calcium gluconate, 48
calcium lactate, 48
calcium phosphate, tribasic, 48
calcium polycarbophil, 49
Calcium Rich Tums, 49
CaldeCort, 168
Calderol, 46
Camptosar, 179
Cancer. *See specific type.*
candesartan cilexetil, 49-50
Candidal infections. *See also* Candidiasis.
    amphotericin B for, 19
    butoconazole for, 45
    clotrimazole for, 86
Candidiasis
    clotrimazole for, 86
    econazole for, 122
    fluconazole for, 143
    itraconazole for, 182
    ketoconazole for, 183
    miconazole for, 216
    nystatin for, 235
    terconazole for, 292
    tioconazole for, 299
Canesten, 86
capecitabine, 50-51
Capoten, 52
capsaicin, 52
captopril, 52
Carafate, 287
carbachol, 52-53
carbamazepine, 53
carbamide peroxide, 53
carbidopa-levodopa, 54
Carbolith, 193
carboplatin, 54-55
Cardene, 229
Cardene IV, 229
Cardene SR, 229
Cardiac arrest
    calcium salts for, 48

Cardiac arrest *(continued)*
epinephrine for,
124-125
sodium bicarbonate for,
283
Cardiac output, increasing
dobutamine for, 115
dopamine for, 117
Cardiac surgery
acetylcysteine for complications of, 5
dobutamine as adjunct
in, 115
Cardiac vagal reflexes,
blocking
atropine for, 28
hyoscyamine for,
169-170
Cardizem, 109
Cardizem CD, 109
Cardizem SR, 109
carisoprodol, 55
carmustine, 55
carteolol hydrochloride,
56
Carter's Little Pills, 40
Cartrol, 56
carvedilol, 56-57
cascara sagrada, 57
Cataflam, 105
Catapres, 84
Catapres-TTS, 84
Caverject, 10
CCNU, 194
CdA, 81
CDDP, 79-80
Ceclor, 58
Cedax, 66
CeeNU, 194
cefaclor, 58
cefadroxil monohydrate,
58
Cefanex, 69
cefazolin sodium, 58-59
cefdinir, 59-60

cefepime hydrochloride,
60
Cefizox, 66
cefmetazole sodium, 61
cefmetazone, 61
Cefobid, 62
cefonicid sodium, 61
cefoperazone sodium, 62
Cefotan, 63
cefotaxime, 62-63
cefotetan disodium, 63
cefoxitin sodium, 63-64
cefpodoxime proxetil, 64
cefprozil, 65
ceftazidime, 65
ceftibuten, 66
Ceftin, 67
ceftizoxime sodium, 66
ceftriaxone sodium, 66
cefuroxime axetil, 67-68
cefuroxime sodium, 67-68
Cefzil, 65
Celebrex, 68
celecoxib, 68-69
Celestone, 38
Celestone Phosphate, 38
Celestone Soluspan, 38
Celexa, 80
CellCept, 222
CellCept Intravenous, 223
Cephalac, 185
cephalexin hydrochloride,
69
cephalexin monohydrate,
69
cephradine, 69-70
Ceptaz, 65
Cerebral edema, dexamethasone for, 101
Cerebral palsy, dantrolene
for, 98
Cerebrovascular accident,
dantrolene for, 98
Cerebyx, 153
cerivastatin sodium, 70
Cerubidine, 99

Cerumen impaction, carbamide peroxide
for, 53
Cervical ripening, dinoprostone for, 110
Cervicitis
azithromycin for, 31
grepafloxacin for, 163
ofloxacin for, 236
trovafloxacin for, 308
C.E.S., 132
cetirizine hydrochloride,
71
Charcoaid, 5
Charcocaps, 5
Cheilosis, riboflavin for,
274
Chemotherapy complications
amifostine for, 13
dolasetron for, 116
dronabinol for, 121
epoetin alfa for, 126
granisetron for, 162
metoclopramide for, 213
ondansetron for,
237-238
oprelvekin for, 238
Chickenpox, acyclovir
sodium for, 6
Chlamydial infection
sulfamethoxazole for,
287
sulfisoxazole for, 288
tetracycline for, 293
chloral hydrate, 71
chlorambucil, 72
chloramphenicol, 72
chlordiazepoxide, 73
chlordiazepoxide hydrochloride, 73

2-chlorodeoxyadenosine,
81
Chloromycetin
Ophthalmic, 72
Chloromycetin Otic, 72
Chloroptic, 72
Chloroptic S.O.P., 72
chloroquine hydrochloride, 73
chloroquine phosphate,
73
Chlorphed, 42
chlorpheniramine
maleate, 74
Chlorpromanyl-5, 74
Chlorpromanyl-20, 74
Chlorpromanyl-40, 74
chlorpromazine hydrochloride, 74-75
Chlorquin, 73
Chlorsig, 72
chlorthalidone, 75
Chlor-Trimeton, 74
cholestyramine, 75
choline magnesium trisalicylate, 75-76
choline salicylate and
magnesium salicylate, 75-76
Chooz, 49
Choriocarcinoma,
methotrexate for,
210
Chronic granulomatous
disease, interferon
gamma-1b for, 178
Chronic obstructive pulmonary disease,
azithromycin for,
31
Chronulac, 185
Cibacalcin, 47
Cibalith-S, 193
cidofovir, 76
Cidomycin, 157
Cilamox, 18

cilostazol, 76-77
Ciloxan, 79
cimetidine, 77-78
Cin-Quin, 270
Cipro, 78
ciprofloxacin, 78
ciprofloxacin hydrochloride, 79
Cipro I.V., 78
Ciproxin, 78
cisapride, 79
cisplatin, 79-80
cis-platinum, 79-80
citalopram hydrobromide, 80
Citracal, 48
citrate of magnesia, 198
Citrocarbonate, 283
Citroma, 198
Citro-Mag, 198
Citro-Nesia, 198
citrovorum factor, 188
Citrucel, 210
cladribine, 81
Claforan, 62
Claratyne, 195
clarithromycin, 81
Claritin, 195
Clavulin, 18
Clear Eyes, 225
clemastine fumarate, 82
Cleocin HCl, 82
Cleocin Pediatric, 82
Cleocin Phosphate, 82
Cleocin T, 82
Cleocin T Gel, Lotion, Solution, 83
Cleocin Vaginal Cream, 83
Climara, 130
Climara Patch, 131
clindamycin hydrochloride, 82-83
clindamycin palmitate hydrochloride, 82-83
clindamycin phosphate, 82-83

Clinoril, 288
Clofen, 33
clomipramine hydrochloride, 83
clonazepam, 84
clonidine, 84
clonidine hydrochloride, 84
clopidogrel bisulfate, 85
Clopra, 213
clorazepate dipotassium, 85
clotrimazole, 86
clozapine, 86-87
Clozaril, 86
CMV disease
    cytomegalovirus immune globulin (human), intravenous, for, 94
    ganciclovir for prevention of, 155-156
CMV-IGIV, 94
CMV retinitis
    cidofovir for, 76
    fomivirsen for, 152-153
    foscarnet for, 153
    ganciclovir for, 155
CNS infection
    cefotaxime for, 62-63
    ceftazidime for, 65
codeine phosphate, 87
codeine sulfate, 87
Codimal-A, 42
Codroxomin, 91
Cogentin, 36
Cognex, 289
Colace, 116
colchicine, 87
Colestid, 88
colestipol hydrochloride, 88
Colgout, 87
Cologel, 210

Colorectal cancer
    fluorouracil for, 146
    irinotecan for, 179-180
Colsalide, 87
CombiPatch, 131
Combivir, 186
Compa-Z, 262
Compazine, 261, 262
conjugated estrogens, 132
Conjunctivitis
    bacitracin for, 32
    chloramphenicol for, 72
    ciprofloxacin for, 79
    cromolyn sodium for, 90
    dexamethasone for, 102-103
    erythromycin for, 128-129
    ketorolac for, 184
Constipation
    bisacodyl for, 40
    calcium polycarbophil for, 49
    cascara sagrada for, 57
    glycerin for, 161
    lactulose for, 185
    magnesium salts for, 198
    methylcellulose for, 210
    psyllium for, 267
    senna for, 281
    sodium phosphates for, 284
Constulose, 185
Consumptive coagulopathy, heparin for, 166
Contraception
    ethinyl estradiol combinations for, 134-135
    levonorgestrel for, 190
    medroxyprogesterone for, 203

Contraception (continued)
    mestranol with norethindrone for, 135
    norethindrone for, 234
    norgestrel for, 234
Copaxone, 158
copolymer 1, 158
Cordarone, 17
Cordarone X, 17
Coreg, 56
Corgard, 223
Corlopam, 138
Corneal infections
    bacitracin for, 32
    chloramphenicol for, 72
Corneal injury, dexamethasone for, 102-103
Corneal ulcers, ciprofloxacin for, 79
Coronary artery bypass surgery, aprotinin for, 25
Coronary artery occlusion, alteplase for, 11
Coronary artery thrombosis, urokinase for, 309
Coronary insufficiency, dipyridamole for, 113
Coronary syndrome, acute
    eptifibatide for, 126-127
    tirofiban for, 298-299
CortaGel, 168
Cortaid, 168
Cortamed, 168
Cortate, 89
Cortef, 167, 168
Corticosteroid-responsive dermatoses
    betamethasone dipropionate for, 38
    dexamethasone for, 102

Corticosteroid responsive
dermatoses *(continued)*
fluocinonide for, 145
fluticasone for, 150
hydrocortisone for, 168
triamcinolone for, 305
corticotropin, 88
Cortifoam, 167
cortisone, 89
Cortizone 5, 168
Cortone Acetate, 89
Corvert, 170
Cosmegen, 96
Cotranzine, 262
co-trimoxazole, 89-90
Cough
benzonatate for, 36
codeine for, 87
diphenhydramine for,
110
hydromorphone for, 169
Coumadin, 314
Covera HS, 312
Cozaar, 196
Cretinism, liothyronine
for, 192
Crixivan, 173
Crohn's disease
infliximab for, 174
sulfasalazine for, 287
Crolom, 90
cromolyn sodium, 90
Crushing drugs, 321
Cryptococcal meningitis,
fluconazole for, 143
crystalline zinc insulin,
174-175
Crystamine, 91
Crystapen, 245
Crysticillin 300 A.S., 245
Crysti-12, 91
Cuprimine, 243
Curretab, 203

Cushing's syndrome,
aminoglutethimide
for, 15
Cutivate, 150
Cuts, bacitracin for, 32
cyanocobalamin, 91
Cyanoject, 91
Cyclidox, 120
cyclobenzaprine hy-
drochloride, 91
Cycloblastin, 92
Cyclogyl, 92
Cyclomen, 98
cyclopentolate hydrochlo-
ride, 92
cyclophosphamide, 92
Cycloplegia
atropine for, 29
cyclopentolate for, 92
scopolamine for, 280
cycloserine, 93
cyclosporin, 93
cyclosporine, 93
Cycrin, 203
Cylert, 243
Cylert Chewable, 243
Cyronine, 192
Cystic fibrosis, acetylcysteine for, 5
Cystinuria, penicillamine
for, 243-244
Cystitis
lomefloxacin for,
193-194
mesna for, 206-207
ofloxacin for, 236
Cystospaz, 169
Cytadren, 15
cytarabine, 94
CytoGam, 94
cytomegalovirus immune
globulin (human),
intravenous, 94
Cytomel, 192
Cytosar, 94
Cytosar-U, 94

cytosine arabinoside, 94
Cytotec, 219
Cytovene, 155
Cytoxan, 92
Cytoxan Lyophilized, 92

D

dacarbazine, 95
daclizumab, 95-96
Dacodyl, 40
dactinomycin, 96
Dalacin C, 82
Dalalone, 101
Dalalone D.P., 101
Dalmane, 148
dalteparin sodium, 97
danaparoid sodium, 97
danazol, 98
Danocrine, 98
Danptrium, 98
dantrolene sodium, 98
Dapacin, 3
dapsone, 98-99
Dapsone 100, 98
Daraprim, 268
Daypro, 239
Dazamide, 4
DDAVP, 101
ddC, 314-315
ddI, 106
Debrox, 53
Decaderm, 102
Decadron, 101
Decadron-LA, 101
Decadron Phosphate, 101
Decadron Phosphate
Ophthalmic, 102
Decaspray, 102
Declomycin, 100
Deep vein thrombosis
dalteparin for, 97
danaparoid for, 97

Deep vein thromboosis
(continued)
enoxaparin for, 123
heparin for, 165-166
Deficol, 40
delavirdine mesylate, 100
Delayed puberty, flu-
oxymesterone for,
147
Delestrogen, 131
Delirium, scopolamine for,
279-280
Delivery preparation,
bisacodyl for, 40
Delta-Cortef, 258
Delta D, 47
Demadex, 302
demeclocycline hy-
drochloride, 100
Dementia
donepezil for, 117
tacrine for, 289
Demerol, 205
Demulen 1/35, 134
Demulen 1/35, 134
Depakene, 310
Depakene Syrup, 310
Depakote, 310
Depakote Sprinkle, 310
Depen, 243
depGynogen, 130
depMedalone 40, 212
Depo-Estradiol, 130
Depoject-40, 212
Depo-Medrol, 212
Depopred-40, 212
Depo-Predate 40, 212
Depo-Provera, 203
Depo-Testosterone, 292
Depression
amitriptyline for, 17
amoxapine for, 18
bupropion for, 44
citalopram for, 80
desipramine for, 105
fluoxetine for, 146-147
imipramine for, 172

Depression *(continued)*
  mirtazapine for, 219
  nefazodone for, 227
  nortriptyline for,
    234-235
  paroxetine for, 242-243
  sertraline for, 281
  thioridazine for, 295
  trazodone for, 304
  trimipramine for, 307
  venlafaxine for, 312
Deralin, 265
Dermatitis herpetiformis,
  dapsone for, 99
Deseril, 213
desipramine hydrochlo-
  ride, 101
desmopressin acetate,
  101
Desogen, 134
Desoxyn, 209
Desyrel, 304
Detensol, 265
Detrol, 301
dexamethasone, 101-102,
  102, 102-103
dexamethasone acetate,
  101-102
dexamethasone sodium
  phosphate,
  101-103
Dexasone, 101
Dexasone-L.A., 101
Dexedrine, 103
Dexedrine Spansule, 103
dextroamphetamine sul-
  fate, 103
dextrose, 104
Dey-Dose Isoproterenol,
  180
Dey-Dose Metaproterenol,
  207
Dey-Lute Metaproterenol,
  207
d4T, 286
d-glucose, 104

D.H.E. 45, 108
DiaBeta, 160
Diabetes insipidus
  desmopressin for, 101
  vasopressin for, 311
Diabetes mellitus
  acarbose for, 2
  glimepiride for, 159
  glipizide for, 159-160
  glyburide for, 160-161
  insulin for, 175
  metformin for, 208
  repaglinide for, 272-273
  troglitazone for,
    307-308
Diabetic ketoacidosis, insulin for, 174-175
Diagnostic procedures,
  droperidol for,
  121-122
Dialume, 12
Diamox, 4
Diamox Parenteral, 4
Diamox Sequels, 4
Diaqua, 167
Diarrhea
  attapulgite for, 29
  bismuth for, 40
  calcium polycarbophil
    for, 49
  diphenoxylate and at-
    ropine for, 111
  loperamide for, 194
  neomycin for, 228
  opium tincture for, 238
Diasorb, 29
diazepam, 104-105
Diazepam Intensol, 104
diazoxide, 105
Dichlotride, 167
diclofenac potassium, 105
diclofenac sodium, 105
dicyclomine hydrochlo-
  ride, 106
didanosine, 106
dideoxycytidine, 314-315

Didronel, 135
Dietary supplement
  calcium carbonate for,
    49
  dextrose for, 104
Diflucan, 143
diflunisal, 106
Digibind, 108
Digitoxin intoxication,
  digoxin immune
  Fab (ovine) for, 108
digoxin, 107
Digoxin, 107
digoxin immune Fab
  (ovine), 108
Digoxin intoxication,
  digoxin immune
  Fab (ovine) for, 108
Dihydergot, 108
dihydroergotamine mesy-
  late, 108
dihydromorphinone hy-
  drochloride,
  168-169
1,25-dihydroxycholecal-
  ciferol, 47
Dilacor-XR, 109
Dilantin, 251
Dilantin Infatabs, 251
Dilantin Kapseals, 251
Dilatrate-SR, 181
Dilaudid, 168
Dilaudid-HP, 168
diltiazem hydrochloride,
  109
dimenhydrinate, 109
Dimetabs, 109
Dimetane, 42
Dinate, 109
dinoprostone, 110
Dioval, 131
Diovan, 311
Dipentum, 236
diphenhydramine hy-
  drochloride, 110

diphenoxylate hydrochlo-
  ride and atropine
  sulfate, 111
diphenylhydantoin,
  251-252
diphtheria and tetanus
  toxoids, adsorbed,
  111
diphtheria and tetanus
  toxoids and acellu-
  lar pertussis vac-
  cine, 112
diphtheria and tetanus
  toxoids and
  whole-cell pertus-
  sis vaccine, 112
dipivefrin, 112
Diprivan, 264
Diprolene, 38
Diprolene AF, 38
Diprosone, 38
dipyridamole, 113
dirithromycin, 113
disopyramide, 113-114
disopyramide phosphate,
  113-114
Disseminated intravascu-
  lar coagulation, he-
  parin for, 166
Disseminated MAC dis-
  ease
  azithromycin for, 31
  clarithromycin for, 81
  rifabutin for, 274
disulfiram, 114
divalproex sodium, 310
Dixarit, 84
Doan's, 199
dobutamine hydrochlo-
  ride, 115
Dobutrex, 115
docetaxel, 115
docusate calcium, 116
docusate sodium, 116
dolasetron mesylate,
  116-117

Dolobid, 106
Doloxene, 264
donepezil hydrochloride, 117
Donnagel, 29
Dopamet, 210
dopamine hydrochloride, 117
Dopar, 189
Doryx, 120
dorzolamide hydrochloride, 118
Dovonex, 46
doxorubicin hydrochloride, 119
Doxy-Caps, 120
Doxycin, 120
doxycycline calcium, 120
doxycycline hyclate, 120
doxycycline hydrochloride, 120
doxycycline monohydrate, 120
Doxylin, 120
D-Penamine, 243
DPT, 112
Dramamine, 109
Drixoral, 266
Dromitexan, 206
dronabinol, 121
droperidol, 121-122
Drug interactions, dangerous, 325
DTaP, 112
DTIC, 95
DTIC-Dome, 95
DTP, 112
DTwP, 112
Dulcagen, 40
Dulcolax, 40
Duodenal ulcers
cimetidine for, 77
famotidine for, 137
nizatidine for, 233
omeprazole for, 237
ranitidine for, 271-272

Duodenal ulcers (continued)
ranitidine bismuth citrate for, 272
sucralfate for, 287
lansoprazole for, 186
Duphalac, 185
Duragesic, 139
Duralone-40, 212
Duramorph, 221
Dura-Tabs, 270
Duricef, 58
Durolax, 40
Duvoid, 39
D-Vert, 202
Dynabac, 113
Dynacin, 217
DynaCirc, 182
Dyrenium, 306
Dyslipidemia
atorvastatin for, 28
cerivastatin for, 70
Dysmenorrhea
diclofenac for, 105
ibuprofen for, 170
ketoprofen for, 183
naproxen for, 226
Dyspepsia, activated charcoal for, 5
Dystonic reaction, benztropine for, 36

E

Ear infection, chloramphenicol for, 72
Eclampsia, magnesium sulfate for, 199
econazole nitrate, 122
Econopred Plus, 259
Ecostatin, 122
Ecotrin, 27
E-Cypionate, 130
Edecrin, 133
Edecrin Sodium, 133
Edema
acetazolamide for, 4

Edema (continued)
amiloride for, 14
bumetanide for, 44
chlorthalidone for, 75
ethacrynate for, 133
ethacrynic acid for, 133
hydrochlorothiazide for, 167
indapamide for, 173
metolazone for, 213
spironolactone for, 285
triamterene for, 306
EEG premedication, chloral hydrate for, 71
efavirenz, 122-123
Effexor, 312
Effexor XR, 312
Efidac-24, 266
Efudex, 146
Elavil, 17
Eldepryl, 281
Elspar, 26
Eltroxin, 190
Emphysema, acetylcysteine for, 5
Empyema, bacitracin for, 33
E-Mycin, 127
enalaprilat, 123
enalapril maleate, 123
Enbrel, 132
Endocarditis
cefazolin for, 59
cephradine for, 69
imipenem and cilastatin for, 172
Endocarditis prophylaxis
amoxicillin trihydrate for, 19
clindamycin for, 82
gentamicin for, 157
vancomycin for, 311
Endocervical infections
doxycycline for, 120
minocycline for, 218

Endometrial cancer
medroxyprogesterone for, 203
megestrol for, 203
Endometriosis
danazol for, 98
goserelin for, 162
norethindrone for, 234
Endometritis, piperacillin and tazobactam for, 253-254
Endoxan-Asta, 92
enoxaparin sodium, 123
EN-tab, 287
Enterocolitis, vancomycin for, 311
Enulose, 185
Enuresis, imipramine for, 172
Epifrin, 125
Epilim, 310
Epimorph, 221
Epinal, 125
epinephrine, 124-125
epinephrine bitartrate, 124-125
epinephrine hydrochloride, 124-125, 125
epinephryl borate, 125
EpiPen, 124
EpiPen Jr., 124
Epitol, 53
Epival, 310
Epivir, 185
epoetin alfa, 125-126
Epogen, 125
Eppy/N, 125
epsom salts, 198
eptastatin, 258
eptifibatide, 126-127
Equalactin, 49
Equivalents, table of, 328
Eramycin, 127
Erectile dysfunction
alprostadil for, 10-11
sildenafil for, 282

Ergodryl Mono, 127
Ergomar, 127
Ergostat, 127
ergotamine tartrate, 127
Eryc, 127
Erycette, 128
Ery-Derm, 128
Erygel, 128
EryPed, 128
EryPed 200, 128
Ery-Sol, 128
Erythrocin, 128
Erythrocin Stearate, 128
erythromycin, 127, 128
erythromycin base, 128
erythromycin estolate, 128
erythromycin ethylsuccinate, 128
erythromycin lactobionate, 128
erythromycin stearate, 128
erythropoietin, 125-126
Esidrix, 167
Eskalith CR, 193
esmolol hydrochloride, 129
Esophagitis
  lansoprazole for, 186
  omeprazole for, 237
Essential tremor, propranolol for, 265
estazolam, 130
esterified estrogens, 130
Estinyl, 134
Estrace, 130
Estraderm, 130
estradiol, 130-131
estradiol cypionate, 130-131
Estradiol L.A., 131
estradiol/norethindrone acetate transdermal system, 131

estradiol valerate, 130-131
Estra-L 20, 131
Estra-L 40, 131
Estratab, 130
Estrofem, 130
estrogenic substances, conjugated, 132
estrogens, conjugated, 132
estrogens, esterified, 130
estropipate, 132
etanercept, 132-133
ethacrynate sodium, 133
ethacrynic acid, 133
ethambutol hydrochloride, 133
ethinyl estradiol, 133-134
ethinyl estradiol with desogestrel, 134-135
ethinyl estradiol with ethynodiol diacetate, 134-135
ethinyl estradiol with levonorgestrel, 134-135
ethinyl estradiol with norethindrone, 134-135
ethinyl estradiol with norethindrone acetate and ferrous fumarate, 134-135
ethinyl estradiol with norgestimate, 134-135
ethinyl estradiol with norgestrel, 134-135
ethinyloestradiol, 133-134
Ethmozine, 221
Ethyol, 13
Etibi, 133
etidronate disodium, 135
etodolac, 135-136
Etopophos, 136

etoposide, 136
etoposide phosphate, 136
Euflex, 149
Euglucon, 160
Eulexin, 149
Eustachian tube congestion, pseudoephedrine for, 266-267
Evac-Q-Mag, 198
Evacuation of uterus, dinoprostone for, 110
Evista, 271
Ewing's sarcoma, dactinomycin for, 96
Exchange transfusion, calcium salts for, 48
Expectoration, promoting, guaifenesin for, 164
Extrapyramidal disorders, drug-induced
  benztropine for, 36
  biperiden for, 40
Eye infections
  bacitracin for, 32
  erythromycin for, 128-129
  gentamicin for, 158
  polymyxin B sulfate for, 255-256
  tobramycin for, 299
Eye inflammation, dexamethasone for, 102-103
Eye surgery
  acetylcholine for, 4
  carbachol for, 52

5-FC, 143
Feldene, 254
felodipine, 137-138
Female castration
  conjugated estrogens for, 132
  esterified estrogens for, 130
  estradiol for, 130-131
  estropipate for, 132
Female hypogonadism
  esterified estrogens for, 130
  estradiol for, 130-131
  estropipate for, 132
  ethinyl estradiol for, 134
Femara, 187
Femiron, 140
Femogex, 131
Femstat 3, 45
Fenac, 105
Fenicol, 72
fenofibrate (micronized), 138
fenoldopam mesylate, 138-139
fenoprofen calcium, 139
fentanyl citrate, 139
Fentanyl Oralet, 139
fentanyl transdermal system, 139
fentanyl transmucosal, 139
Feosol, 140, 141
Feostat, 140
Fergon, 140
ferrous fumarate, 140
ferrous gluconate, 140
ferrous sulfate, 140-141
ferrous sulfate, dried, 141
Fever
  acetaminophen for, 3
  aspirin for, 27
  choline magnesium trisalicylate for, 76
  fenoprofen for, 139

F
famciclovir, 136-137
famotidine, 137
Famvir, 136
Fansidar, 268
Fareston, 302
Fastin, 249

Fever *(continued)*
  ibuprofen for, 170
  ketoprofen for, 183
  magnesium salicylate
    for, 199
Feverall, 3
fexofenadine, 141
Fiberall, 49, 267
Fiber-Con, 49
Fiber-Lax, 49
FiberNorm, 49
Fibrocystic breast disease,
  danazol for, 98
filgrastim, 141-142
finasteride, 142
Flagyl, 214
Flagyl I.V. RTU, 214
Flamazine, 282
Flatulence
  activated charcoal for, 5
  simethicone for, 283
flecainide acetate, 142
Fleet Babylax, 161
Fleet Bisacodyl, 40
Fleet Bisacodyl Prep, 40
Fleet Enema, 284
Fleet Laxative, 40
Fletcher's Castoria, 281
Flexeril, 91
Flint SSD, 282
Flixotide, 149
Flomax, 290
Flonase, 150
Florinef, 143
Flovent Inhalation
  Aerosol, 149
Flovent Rotadisk, 149
Floxin, 236
Floxin I.V., 236
fluconazole, 143
flucytosine, 143
fludrocortisone acetate,
  143-144
Fluid replacement therapy,
  dextrose for, 104
Flumadine, 275

flumazenil, 144-145
flunisolide, 145
fluocinonide, 145-146
5-fluorocytosine, 143
Fluoroplex, 146
fluorouracil, 146
5-fluorouracil, 146
fluoxetine hydrochloride,
  146-147
fluoxymesterone, 147
fluphenazine decanoate,
  147-148
fluphenazine enanthate,
  147-148
fluphenazine hydrochlo-
  ride, 147-148
flurazepam hydrochloride,
  148
flurbiprofen, 148
flurbiprofen sodium, 149
flutamide, 149
Flutex, 305
fluticasone propionate,
  149-150, 150-151
fluvastatin sodium, 151
fluvoxamine maleate, 151
Folex PFS, 210
folic acid, 151-152
Folic acid antagonist overdose, leucovorin
  for, 188
folinic acid, 188
Folvite, 151
fomivirsen sodium,
  152-153
Fortaz, 65
Fortovase, 279
Fortral, 246
Fosamax, 8
foscarnet sodium, 153
Foscavir, 153
fosinopril sodium, 153

fosphenytoin sodium,
  153-154
4-way Long Acting, 314
Fowler's, 29
Fragmin, 97
FreAmine III, 14
Froben, 148
Froben SR, 148
frusemide, 154
5-FU, 146
Fulcin, 163
Fulvicin P/G, 163
Fulvicin-U/F, 163
Fumasorb, 140
Fumerin, 140
Fungal infections. *See
  also specific type.*
  amphotericin B for, 19
  clotrimazole for, 86
  flucytosine for, 143
  ketoconazole for, 183
Fungilin Oral, 19
Fungizone Intravenous, 19
Furacin, 232
Furadantin, 232
furosemide, 154

G
gabapentin, 155
Gabitril, 296
Galactorrhea, bromocrip-
  tine for, 42
ganciclovir, 155-156
Gantanol, 287
Gantrisin, 288
Gantrisin Pediatric, 288
Garamycin, 157, 158
Garamycin Ophthalmic,
  158
Gastric bloating, simeth-
  icone for, 283
Gastric ulcers.
  cimetidine for, 78
  famotidine for, 137
  misoprostol for prevent-
    ing, 219

Gastric ulcers *(continued)*
  nizatidine for, 233
  omeprazole for, 237
  ranitidine for, 271-272
Gastroenteritis, rotavirus
  vaccine, live, oral,
  tetravalent, for, 277
Gastroesophageal reflux
  disease
  cimetidine for, 78
  cisapride for, 79
  metoclopramide for, 213
  nizatidine for, 233
  omeprazole for, 237
  ranitidine for, 272
Gas-X, 283
GBH, 191
G-CSF, 141-142
gemcitabine hydrochlo-
  ride, 156
gemfibrozil, 157
Gemzar, 156
Genasoft, 116
Genital herpes
  acyclovir for, 5
  acyclovir sodium for, 6
  famciclovir for, 136-137
  valacyclovir for, 310
Genitourinary infections
  cefazolin for, 59
  cefoxitin for, 63-64
  cephradine for, 69
Genoptic, 158
Genora 1/35, 134
Genora 1/50, 135
Gentacidin, 158
Gentak, 158
Gentamicin Sulfate, 157
gentamicin sulfate, 157,
  158
Gen-XENE, 85
Gesterol 50, 262
GI disorders
  dicyclomine for, 106
  hyoscyamine for,
    169-170

GI tract infections
amphotericin B for, 19
cephalexin for, 69
cephradine for, 69
glatiramer acetate for injection, 158
Glaucoma
acetazolamide for, 4
betaxolol for, 39
carbachol for, 53
carteolol for, 56
dipivefrin for, 112
dorzolamide for, 118
epinephrine for, 125
latanoprost for, 187
levobunolol for, 189
pilocarpine for, 252
timolol for, 298
Glaucon, 125
glibenclamide, 160-161
glimepiride, 159
glipizide, 159-160
glucagon, 160
Glucophage, 208
Glucotrol, 159
Glucotrol XL, 159
Glu-K, 257
glyburide, 160-161
glycerin, 161
glyceryl guaiacolate, 164
glyceryl trinitrate, 232-233
Glynase PresTab, 160-161
Glytuss, 164
GM-CSF, 279
G-Myticin, 158
Goiter, nontoxic, liothyronine for, 192
Gold-50, 30
gold sodium thiomalate, 30
Gonorrhea
amoxicillin trihydrate for, 19
demeclocycline for, 100
grepafloxacin for, 163

Gonorrhea (continued)
minocycline for, 218
norfloxacin for, 234
ofloxacin for, 236
penicillin G procaine for, 245
probenecid for, 260
trovafloxacin for, 309
goserelin acetate, 162
Gout
allopurinol for, 9
colchicine for, 87
naproxen for, 226
probenecid for, 260
Gouty arthritis
colchicine for, 87
probenecid for, 260
sulfinpyrazone for, 288
sulindac for, 288
granisetron hydrochloride, 162
granulocyte colony-stimulating factor, 141-142
granulocyte-macrophage colony-stimulating factor, 279
Granuloma inguinale
demeclocycline for, 100
doxycycline for, 120
grepafloxacin hydrochloride, 162-163
Grifulvin V, 163
Grisactin, 163
Grisactin Ultra, 163
griseofulvin microsize, 163-164
griseofulvin ultramicrosize, 163
Griseostatin, 163
Grisovin, 163
Grisovin 500, 163
Grisovin-FP, 163
Gris-PEG, 163
guaifenesin, 164
G-well, 191

Gynecologic infections
alatrofloxacin for, 308
ampicillin sodium/sulbactam sodium for, 20-21
aztreonam for, 32
cefoperazone for, 62
cefotaxime for, 62-63
cefotetan for, 63
ceftazidime for, 65
ceftizoxime for, 66
ceftriaxone for, 67
imipenem and cilastatin for, 172
trovafloxacin for, 308
Gyne-Lotrimin, 86
Gynergen, 127
Gynogen L.A., 131

H

Habitrol, 230
Halcion, 306
Haldol, 164
Haldol Decanoate, 164
Haldol LA, 164
haloperidol, 164-165
haloperidol decanoate, 164-165
haloperidol lactate, 165
Halotestin, 147
Halotussin, 164
Hansen's disease, dapsone for, 98-99
Heartburn
cisapride for, 79
famotidine for, 137
Heart failure
acetazolamide for, 4
amiloride for, 14
amrinone for, 21
bumetanide for, 44
captopril for, 52
carvedilol for, 57
digoxin for, 107
dobutamine for, 115

Heart failure (continued)
fosinopril for, 153
lisinopril for, 192-193
metolazone for, 213
milrinone for, 217
nitroglycerin for, 233
nitroprusside for, 233
quinapril for, 270
ramipril for, 271
torsemide for, 302
trandolapril for, 303
Heart transplantation, immunosuppression in
cyclosporine for, 93
mycophenolate for, 222-223
Heat cramp, sodium chloride for, 284
Helicobacter pylori infection
clarithromycin for, 81
omeprazole for, 237
ranitidine bismuth citrate for, 272
Hemodynamic imbalances, dopamine for, 117
Hemofil M, 22
Hemophilia, antihemophilic factor for, 22-23
Hepalean, 165
heparin calcium, 165-166
heparin cofactor I, 24
Heparin overdose, protamine sulfate for, 266
heparin sodium, 165-166
Hepat-Amine, 15
Hepatic disease, bumetanide for, 44
Hepatic encephalopathy, lactulose for, 185

Hepatitis
  interferon alfacon-1 for, 177
  interferon alfa-2b, recombinant, for, 176
Herceptin, 303
Hereditary AT-III deficiency, antithrombin III, human, for, 24
Herpes simplex virus infection
  acyclovir for, 5
  acyclovir sodium for, 6
  foscarnet for, 153
Herpes zoster infection
  capsaicin for, 52
  famciclovir for, 136
  valacyclovir for, 310
Hexadrol, 101
Histantil, 263
Hip replacement surgery
  danaparoid for, 97
  enoxaparin for, 123
  etidronate for, 135
Hivid, 314
HIV infection
  abacavir for, 2
  amprenavir for, 21
  azithromycin for, 31
  clarithromycin for, 81
  delavirdine for, 100
  didanosine for, 106
  efavirenz for, 122-123
  epoetin alfa for, 126
  indinavir for, 173
  lamivudine for, 185
  lamivudine/zidovudine for, 186
  nelfinavir for, 227
  nevirapine for, 229
  rifabutin for, 274
  ritonavir for, 276
  saquinavir for, 279
  stavudine for, 286
  zalcitabine for, 314-315

HIV infection (continued)
  zidovudine for, 315-316
Hodgkin's disease
  bleomycin for, 41
  carmustine for, 55
  chlorambucil for, 72
  cyclophosphamide for, 92
  dacarbazine for, 95
  doxorubicin for, 119
  lomustine for, 194
  mechlorethamine for, 202
  procarbazine for, 261
  thiotepa for, 295
  vinblastine for, 313
  vincristine for, 313
Hookworm, mebendazole for, 202
H.P. Acthar Gel, 88
Humate-P, 22
Humalog, 175
Humibid L.A., 164
Humulin 50/50, 175
Humulin 70/30, 175
Humulin L, 175
Humulin N, 175
Humulin NPH, 175
Humulin R, 174
Humulin U, 175
Hyate:C, 22
Hycamtin, 301
Hydatidiform mole, methotrexate for, 210
Hydeltrasol, 258
Hydeltra-T.B.A., 259
hydralazine hydrochloride, 166
Hydramine, 110
Hydrobexan, 91
hydrochlorothiazide, 167
Hydro-Cobex, 91

hydrocortisone, 167-168
hydrocortisone acetate, 167-168
Hydrocortisone Acetate, 168
hydrocortisone butyrate, 168
hydrocortisone sodium phosphate, 167
hydrocortisone sodium succinate, 167
hydrocortisone valerate, 168
Hydrocortone, 167
Hydrocortone Acetate, 167
Hydrocortone Phosphate, 167
Hydro-Crysti-12, 91
HydroDIURIL, 167
hydromorphone hydrochloride, 168-169
Hydrostat, 168
hydroxocobalamin, 91
hydroxyzine embonate, 169
hydroxyzine hydrochloride, 169
hydroxyzine pamoate, 169
Hygroton, 75
hyoscine, 279-280
hyoscine butylbromide, 279-280
hyoscine hydrobromide, 280
hyoscyamine, 169-170
hyoscyamine sulfate, 169-170
Hy-Pam, 169
Hyperbilirubinemia, albumin 25% for, 7
Hypercalcemia
  calcitonin for, 47
  etidronate for, 135

Hypercalcemia (continued)
  pamidronate for, 241-242
  plicamycin for, 254-255
Hypercalciuria, plicamycin for, 254-255
Hypercholesterolemia
  atorvastatin for, 28
  cerivastatin for, 70
  cholestyramine for, 75
  colestipol for, 88
  fluvastatin for, 151
  lovastatin for, 196
  niacin for, 229
  pravastatin for, 258
  simvastatin for, 283
Hyperfibrinolysis, aminocaproic acid for, 15
Hyperkalemia, sodium polystyrene sulfonate for, 284
Hyperkinesia, hydroxyzine for, 169
Hyperlipidemia
  cholestyramine for, 75
  fenofibrate for, 138
  gemfibrozil for, 157
  niacin for, 229
Hyperparathyroidism, paricalcitol for, 242
Hyperphosphatemia, calcium salts for, 48
Hyperprolactinemia, bromocriptine for, 42
Hypersecretory conditions
  famotidine for, 137
  lansoprazole for, 186
  omeprazole for, 237
  ranitidine for, 271
Hypersensitivity reactions. See Allergic reactions.
Hyperstat IV, 105

Hypertension
acebutolol for, 3
amiloride for, 14
amiodipine for, 17
atenolol for, 27
benazepril for, 36
bisoprolol for, 41
candesartan for, 49
captopril for, 52
carteolol for, 56
carvedilol for, 56
chlorthalidone for, 75
clonidine for, 84
diltiazem for, 109
enalapril for, 123
esmolol for, 129
felodipine for, 137-138
fenoldopam for,
138-139
fosinopril for, 153
furosemide for, 155
hydralazine for, 166
hydrochlorothiazide for,
167
indapamide for, 173
irbesartan for, 179
isradipine for, 182
labetalol for, 185
lisinopril for, 192
losartan for, 196
methyldopa for, 210-211
metolazone for, 213
metoprolol for, 214
minoxidil for, 218
moexipril for, 220
nadolol for, 223
nicardipine for, 229-230
nifedipine for, 231
nisoldipine for, 231
nitroglycerin for, 233
pindolol for, 253
prazosin for, 258
propranolol for, 265
quinapril for, 269-270
ramipril for, 271
spironolactone for, 285

Hypertension *(continued)*
telmisartan for, 290
terazosin for, 290-291
timolol for, 298
torsemide for, 302
trandolapril for, 303
valsartan for, 311
verapamil for, 312
Hypertensive crisis
diazoxide for, 105
methyldopa for, 210-211
Hypertensive emergency
labetalol for, 185
nitroprusside for, 233
Hyperthyroidism
methimazole for, 209
propylthiouracil for, 266
Hypertrophic subaortic
stenosis, propra-
nolol for, 265
Hyperuricemia
allopurinol for, 9
probenecid for, 260
Hypnovel, 216
Hypocalcemia
calcifediol for, 46
calcitriol for, 47
Hypocalcemic emergency,
calcium salts for, 48
Hypocalcemic tetany, cal-
cium salts for, 48
Hypoestrogenemia, estra-
diol/norethindrone
acetate transdermal
system for, 131
Hypoglycemia, glucagon
for, 160
Hypogonadism. *See*
Female hypogo-
nadism *and* Male
hypogonadism.
Hypokalemia
potassium bicarbonate
for, 256
potassium chloride for,
256

Hypokalemia *(continued)*
potassium gluconate
for, 257
spironolactone for, 285
Hypomagnesemia
magnesium chloride for,
198
magnesium oxide for,
199
magnesium sulfate for,
200
Hyponatremia, sodium
chloride for, 284
Hypoparathyroidism, cal-
citriol for, 47
Hypoproteinemia, albumin
25% for, 7
Hypoprothrombinemia,
phytonadione for,
252
Hypotension
fludrocortisone for, 144
midodrine for, 217
nitroglycerin for con-
trolled, 233
phenylephrine for, 250
Hypovolemic shock, albu-
min 5%/25% for, 7
Hytrin, 290
Hyzine-50, 169

I

ibuprofen, 170
ibutilide fumarate,
170-171
Idamycin, 171
idarubicin hydrochloride,
171
IFEX, 171
IFN-alpha 2, 176
ifosfamide, 171
Ilosone, 128
Ilotycin Ophthalmic
Ointment, 128-129
IL-2, 8
Imdur, 181

imipenem and cilastatin,
172
imipramine hydrochloride,
172
imipramine pamoate, 172
Imitrex, 289
Immunization
diphtheria and tetanus
toxoids, ad-
sorbed, for, 111
diphtheria and tetanus
toxoids and acel-
lular pertussis
vaccine for, 112
diphtheria and tetanus
toxoids and
whole-cell pertus-
sis vaccine for,
112
measles, mumps, and
rubella virus vac-
cine, live, for,
200-201
measles and rubella
virus vaccine, live
attenuated, for,
201
measles virus vaccine,
live attenuated,
for, 201
mumps virus vaccine,
live, for, 222
pneumococcal vaccine,
polyvalent, for,
255
poliovirus vaccine, inac-
tivated, for, 255
poliovirus vaccine, live,
oral, trivalent, for,
255
rubella and mumps
virus vaccine, live,
for, 278
rubella virus vaccine,
live attenuated,
for, 278

Immunosuppression
betamethasone for, 38
methylprednisolone for, 211-212
prednisolone for, 258-259
prednisone for, 259
triamcinolone for, 305
Imodium A-D, 194
Impetigo, mupirocin for, 222
Impril, 172
Imuran, 30
Inapsine, 121
indapamide, 173
Inderal, 265
Inderal LA, 265
indinavir sulfate, 173
Indochron E-R, 173
Indocid P.D.A., 173
Indocid SR, 173
Indocin, 173
Indocin I.V., 173
Indocin SR, 173
indomethacin, 173-174
indomethacin sodium trihydrate, 173-174
Infections. See also specific type.
amikacin for, 14
amoxicillin trihydrate for, 18-19
cefdinir for, 59
ceftriaxone for, 67
cefuroxime for, 67-68
clindamycin for, 82
demeclocycline for, 100
doxycycline for, 120
gentamicin for, 157
metronidazole for, 214-215
mezlocillin for, 215-216
minocycline for, 217-218
nafcillin for, 223-224
neomycin for, 228

Infections (continued)
oxacillin for, 239
penicillin G potassium for, 244-245
penicillin G procaine for, 245
penicillin G sodium for, 245
piperacillin for, 253
sulfamethoxazole for, 287
sulfisoxazole for, 288
tetracycline for, 293
ticarcillin for, 296-297
tobramycin for, 300
vancomycin for, 311
Infergen, 177
Infertility, bromocriptine for, 42
Inflamase Forte, 259
Inflammation
aspirin for, 27
betamethasone for, 38
choline magnesium trisalicylate for, 75
cortisone for, 89
dexamethasone for, 101, 102
fluocinonide for, 145
fluticasone for, 150
hydrocortisone for, 167, 168
methylprednisolone for, 211-212
prednisolone for, 258-259
prednisone for, 259
triamcinolone for, 305
infliximab, 174
Influenza
amantadine for, 13
rimantadine for, 275-276
Influenza prophylaxis, rifampin for, 275

Infumorph 200, 221
INH, 180
Inocor, 21
Insomnia
chloral hydrate for, 71
estazolam for, 130
flurazepam for, 148
lorazepam for, 195
pentobarbital for, 247
secobarbital for, 280
temazepam for, 290
triazolam for, 306
zolpidem for, 316
insulin, 174-175
Insulin therapy replacement
glipizide for, 159-160
glyburide for, 161
insulin zinc suspension (lente), 175
insulin zinc suspension, extended (ultralente), 175
insulin zinc suspension, prompt (semilente), 175
Intal, 90
Intal Aerosol Spray, 90
Intal Nebulizer Solution, 90
Integrilin, 126
interferon alfacon-1, 177
interferon alfa-2a, recombinant, 176
interferon alfa-2b, recombinant, 176
interferon beta-1a, 177
interferon beta-1b, recombinant, 177
interferon gamma-1b, 178
interleukin-2, 8
Intermittent claudication
cilostazol for, 76-77
pentoxifylline for, 247
Intra-abdominal infections
alatrofloxacin for, 308

Intra-abdominal infections (continued)
ampicillin sodium/sulbactam sodium for, 20-21
aztreonam for, 32
cefmetazole for, 61
cefoperazone for, 62
cefotaxime for, 62-63
cefotetan for, 63
ceftazidime for, 65
ceftizoxime for, 66
ceftriaxone for, 67
imipenem and cilastatin for, 172
trovafloxacin for, 308
Intraocular pressure, reducing
apraclonidine for, 25
carteolol for, 56
dipivefrin for, 112
dorzolamide for, 118
latanoprost for, 187
Intron A, 176
Intropin, 117
Invirase, 279
Inza 250, 226
Iopidine, 25
Iosopan, 197
ipecac syrup, 178
IPOL, 255
ipratropium bromide, 178-179
IPV, 255
irbesartan, 179
Iridocyclitis, dexamethasone for, 102-103
irinotecan hydrochloride, 179-180
Iritis
atropine for, 29
scopolamine for, 280
Iron deficiency
ferrous fumarate for, 140

Iron deficiency *(continued)*
  ferrous gluconate for, 140
  ferrous sulfate for, 140-141
Irritability, lorazepam for, 195
Irritable bowel syndrome
  calcium polycarbophil for, 49
  dicyclomine for, 106
Ischemic stroke, alteplase for, 11-12
ISMO, 181
Isonate, 181
isoniazid, 180
Isoniazid poisoning, pyridoxine for, 268
isonicotinic acid hydrazide, 180
isophane insulin suspension, 175
isophane insulin suspension with insulin injection, 175
isoprenaline, 180-181
isoproterenol, 180-181
isoproterenol hydrochloride, 180-181
isoproterenol sulfate, 180-181
Isoptin, 312
Isoptin SR, 312
Isopto Atropine, 29
Isopto Carbachol, 52
Isopto Carpine, 252
Isopto Frin, 250
Isopto Hyoscine, 279, 280
Isorbid, 181
Isordil, 181
Isordil Tembids, 181
isosorbide dinitrate, 181-182
isosorbide mononitrate, 181-182

Isotrate, 181
isotretinoin, 182
isradipine, 182
Isuprel, 180
itraconazole, 182-183
I.V. Persantine, 113

JKL

Janimine, 172
Jenamicin, 157
Jenest-28, 134
Joint infections
  cefazolin for, 59
  cefonicid for, 61
  cefotaxime for, 62-63
  cefotetan for, 63
  cefoxitin for, 63-64
  ceftizoxime for, 66
  ceftriaxone for, 67
  cephalexin for, 69
  cephradine for, 69
  ciprofloxacin for, 78
  imipenem and cilastatin for, 172
  ticarcillin/clavulanate for, 297
Juvenile rheumatoid arthritis
  choline magnesium trisalicylate for, 75
  ibuprofen for, 170
  naproxen for, 226
K + 10, 256
Kabikinase, 286
Kaluril, 14
Kaochlor 10%, 256
Kaon Liquid, 257
Kaopectate II Caplets, 194
Kaposi's sarcoma
  alitretinoin for, 9
  interferon alfa-2a, recombinant, for, 176

Kaposi's sarcoma *(continued)*
  interferon alfa-2b, recombinant, for, 176
Kayexalate, 284
K + Care ET, 256
K-Dur, 256
Keflex, 69
Keftab, 69
Kefurox, 67
Kefzol, 58
Kenalog, 305
Kenalog-10, 305
Kenalone, 305
Keratitis, vidarabine for, 312-313
Keratoconjunctivitis, vidarabine for, 312-313
Keratoplasty, graft rejection after, dexamethasone for, 102-103
Kerlone, 39
ketoconazole, 183
ketoprofen, 183
ketorolac tromethamine, 184
Key-Pred-SP, 258
K-Ide, 256
Kidney transplantation, immunosuppression in
  azathioprine for, 30
  basiliximab for, 34
  cyclosporine for, 93
  daclizumab for, 95
  mycophenolate for, 222-223
Kidrolase, 26
Klonopin, 84
Klor-Con/EF, 256
K-Lyte, 256
K-Lyte/Cl, 256

Knee replacement surgery
  ardeparin for, 26
  enoxaparin for, 123
Koate-HP, 22
Koate-HS, 22
Kristalose, 185
K-Tab, 256
Kwellada, 191
Kytril, 162
LA-12, 91
labetalol hydrochloride, 185
Labor induction, oxytocin, synthetic injection, for, 241
Labor pain, pentazocine for, 246
Lactulax, 185
lactulose, 185
Lamictal, 186
Lamisil, 291
lamivudine, 185
lamivudine/zidovudine, 186
lamotrigine, 186
Lanoxicaps, 107
Lanoxin, 107
lansoprazole, 186-187
Larodopa, 189
Larotid, 18
Lasix, 154
L-asparaginase, 26
latanoprost, 187
Laxative effect, magnesium oxide for, 198
Ledermycin, 100
leflunomide, 187
Leg ulcers, becaplermin for, 34-35
Lennox-Gastaut syndrome, clonazepam for, 84
Lente Insulin, 175
Leprosy, dapsone for, 98-99
Lescol, 151
letrozole, 187

leucovorin calcium, 188
Leucovorin rescue, 188
Leukemia
  asparaginase for, 26
  busulfan for, 45
  chlorambucil for, 72
  cladribine for, 81
  cyclophosphamide for, 92
  cytarabine for, 94
  daunorubicin for, 99
  doxorubicin for, 119
  idarubicin for, 171
  interferon alfa-2a, recombinant, for, 176
  interferon alfa-2b, recombinant, for, 176
  mechlorethamine for, 202
  mercaptopurine for, 205
  methotrexate for, 210
  pegaspargase for, 243
  tretinoin for, 304-305
  vincristine for, 313
Leukeran, 72
Leukine, 279
Leustatin, 81
levalbuterol, 188
Levaquin, 189
levobunolol hydrochloride, 189
levodopa, 189
levofloxacin, 189
levonorgestrel, 190
Levophed, 233
Levo-T, 190
Levothroid, 190
levothyroxine sodium, 190
Levoxine, 190
Levoxyl, 190
Levsin, 169
Levsin S/L, 169
Libritabs, 73

Librium, 73
Lidemol, 145
Lidex, 145
Lidex-E, 145
lidocaine hydrochloride, 190-191
LidoPen Auto-Injector, 191
lignocaine hydrochloride, 190-191
lindane, 191
Lioresal, 33
Lioresal Intrathecal, 33
liothyronine sodium, 192
Lipex, 283
Lipitor, 28
Liquaemin Sodium, 165
Liqui-Char, 5
Liquid Pred, 259
lisinopril, 192-193
Lithane, 193
Lithicarb, 193
lithium carbonate, 193
lithium citrate, 193
Lithobid, 193
Lithonate, 193
Lithotabs, 193
Liver transplantation, immunosuppression in, cyclosporine for, 93
Liver transplantation prophylaxis, tacrolimus for, 289
Locoid, 168
Lodine, 135
Loestrin Fe 1/20, 134
Loestrin 21 1/20, 134
Logen, 111
Lomanate, 111
lomefloxacin hydrochloride, 193-194
Lomotil, 111
lomustine, 194
Loniten, 218
Lonox, 111
loperamide, 194

Lopid, 157
Lopresor SR, 214
Lopressor, 214
Lopurin, 9
Lorabid, 194
loracarbef, 194-195
loratadine, 195
lorazepam, 195-196
Lorazepam Intensol, 195
losartan potassium, 196
Losec, 237
Lotensin, 36
Lotrimin, 86
lovastatin, 196
Lovenox, 123
Lowsium, 197
Loxapac, 197
loxapine hydrochloride, 197
loxapine succinate, 197
Loxitane, 197
Loxitane C, 197
Loxitane IM, 197
Lozide, 173
Lozol, 173
L-phenylalanine mustard, 203-204
L-thyroxine sodium, 190
Luminal Sodium, 249
Lung cancer
  doxorubicin for, 119
  etoposide for, 136
  mechlorethamine for, 202
  vinorelbine for, 313
Luvox, 151
Lyme disease
  ceftriaxone for, 67
  cefuroxime for, 68
  doxycycline for, 120
  vaccine for, 197
Lyme disease vaccine (recombinant OspA), 197
LYMErix, 197

Lymphoma
  carmustine for, 55
  chlorambucil for, 72
  cyclophosphamide for, 92
  doxorubicin for, 119
  rituximab for, 276-277
  thiotepa for, 295
  vinblastine for, 313
Lymphosarcoma
  bleomycin for, 41
  chlorambucil for, 72
Lyphocin, 311

M

Maalox Daily Fiber Therapy, 267
Macrobid, 231
Macrodantin, 231, 232
magaldrate, 197
magnesium chloride, 198
magnesium citrate, 198
magnesium hydroxide, 199
Magnesium intoxication, calcium salts for, 48
magnesium oxide, 199
magnesium salicylate, 199
magnesium sulfate, 198, 199-200
Magnesium supplementation, magnesium salts for, 198, 199, 200
Mag-Ox 400, 199
Malaria
  chloroquine for, 73
  primaquine for, 259-260
  pyrimethamine for, 268-269
  pyrimethamine with sulfadoxine for, 268-269

Malaria prophylaxis, chloroquine for, 73
Male hypogonadism
fluoxymesterone for, 147
methyltestosterone for, 212
testosterone for, 292, 292
Male-pattern baldness. *See* Alopecia.
Malignant lymphoma. *See* Lymphoma.
Malignant melanoma, dacarbazine for, 95
Mania
lithium for, 193
valproic acid for, 310
mannitol, 200
Maox 420, 199
Marinol, 121
Matulane, 261
Mavik, 303
Maxair, 254
Maxair Autohaler, 254
Maxalt, 277
Maxalt-MLT, 277
Maxaquin, 193
Maxidex Ophthalmic, 102
Maxidex Ophthalmic Suspension, 102
Maxipime, 60
Maxivate, 38
Maxolon, 213
measles, mumps, and rubella virus vaccine, live, 200-201
Measles outbreak control, measles virus vaccine, live attenuated, for, 201
measles and rubella virus vaccine, live attenuated, 201
measles virus vaccine, live attenuated, 201

mebendazole, 202
Mechanical ventilation, facilitating, propofol for, 264
mechlorethamine hydrochloride, 202
meclizine hydrochloride, 202
Medihaler-Epi, 124
Medihaler Ergotamine, 127
Medihaler-Iso, 180
Medralone-40, 212
Medrol, 211
medroxyprogesterone acetate, 203
Mefoxin, 63
Megace, 203
Megacillin, 245
megestrol acetate, 203
Megostat, 203
Melipramine, 172
Mellaril, 295
Mellaril Concentrate, 295
melphalan, 203-204
Menaval-20, 131
Menest, 130
Meni-D, 202
Meningitis
amphotericin B for, 19
ceftizoxime for, 66
ceftriaxone for, 67
cefuroxime for, 67-68
fluconazole for, 143
gentamicin for, 157
meropenem for, 206
Meningitis prophylaxis, meningococcal polysaccharide vaccine for, 204
Meningococcal carrier state
minocycline for, 218
rifampin for, 274-275

meningococcal polysaccharide vaccine, 204
Menomune-A/C/Y/W-135, 204
Menopausal symptoms
estradiol for, 130-131
estradiol/norethindrone acetate transdermal system for, 131
ethinyl estradiol for, 134
menotropins, 204-205
meperidine hydrochloride, 205
Mepron, 28
mercaptopurine, 205
6-mercaptopurine, 205
Meridia, 281
meropenem, 206
Merrem IV, 206
mesalamine, 206
mesna, 206-207
Mesnex, 206
mesoridazine besylate, 207
Mestinon, 267
Mestinon-SR, 267
Mestinon Timespans, 267
mestranol with norethindrone, 135
Metabolic acidosis, sodium bicarbonate for, 283
Metamucil, 267
Metaprel, 207
metaproterenol sulfate, 207-208
metformin hydrochloride, 208
methadone, 208
methamphetamine, 209
Methergine, 211
methimazole, 209
methocarbamol, 209
methotrexate, 210

methotrexate sodium, 210
methylcellulose, 210
methyldopa, 210-211
methyldopate hydrochloride, 210-211
methylergonovine maleate, 211
Methylmalonic aciduria, cyanocobalamin for, 91
methylphenidate hydrochloride, 211
methylprednisolone, 211-212
methylprednisolone acetate, 211-212
methylprednisolone sodium succinate, 212
methyltestosterone, 212
methysergide maleate, 212-213
Meticorten, 259
metoclopramide hydrochloride, 213
metolazone, 213
metoprolol succinate, 214
metoprolol tartrate, 214
MetroGel, 215
MetroGel-Vaginal, 215
Metro I.V., 214
metronidazole, 214-215, 215
metronidazole hydrochloride, 214-215
Metrozine, 214
Mevacor, 196
mevinolin, 196
Mexate-AQ, 210
mexiletine hydrochloride, 215
Mexitil, 215
Mezlin, 215
mezlocillin sodium, 215-216
Miacalcin, 47
Miacalcin Nasal Spray, 47

Micardis, 290
Micatin, 216
miconazole nitrate, 216
Micronase, 161
Micronor, 234
Midamor, 14
midazolam hydrochloride, 216
midodrine hydrochloride, 217
Migraine headache
dihydroergotamine for, 108
divalproex for, 310
ergotamine for, 127
methysergide for, 212-213
naratriptan for, 227
rizatriptan for, 277
sumatriptan for, 289
timolol for, 298
zolmitriptan for, 316
milk of magnesia, 198
Milk of Magnesia, 198
milrinone lactate, 217
Minax, 214
Minidiab, 159
Minipress, 258
Minirin, 101
Minocin, 217
minocycline hydrochloride, 217-218
minoxidil, 218, 218-219
Miocarpine, 252
Miochol, 4
Miosis
carbachol for, 52
flurbiprofen for intraoperative inhibition of, 149
Miostat, 52
Mirapex, 257
mirtazapine, 219
misoprostol, 219
Mithracin, 255
mithramycin, 254-255

mitomycin, 219
mitomycin-C, 219
M-M-R II, 201
Moban, 220
Mobidin, 199
modafinil, 219-220
Modecate, 147
Moditen HCl, 147
moexipril hydrochloride, 220
molindone hydrochloride, 220-221
Mol-Iron, 140
Monistat-Derm Cream/Lotion, 216
Monistat 7, 216
Monistat 3 Vaginal Suppository, 216
Monocid, 61
Monodox, 120
Monoket, 181
Monopril, 153
montelukast sodium, 221
moricizine hydrochloride, 221
Morphine H.P., 221
morphine hydrochloride, 221-222
morphine sulfate, 221-222
morphine tartrate, 221-222
Morphitec, 221
M.O.S., 221
Motion sickness
dimenhydrinate for, 109
diphenhydramine for, 110
meclizine for, 202
promethazine for, 263
scopolamine for, 280
Motrin, 170
Motrin-IB Caplets, 170
Motrin-IB Tablets, 170
6-MP, 205
M-R Vax II, 201

MS Contin, 221
MTX, 210
Mucomyst, 5
Mucomyst 10, 5
Mucosil-10, 5
Mucosil-20, 5
Multipax, 169
Multiple lymphoma, cyclophosphamide for, 92
Multiple myeloma
carmustine for, 55
melphalan for, 203-204
pamidronate for, 242
Multiple sclerosis
baclofen for, 33
dantrolene for, 98
glatiramer acetate for injection for, 158
interferon beta-1a for, 177
interferon beta-1b, recombinant, for, 177
methylprednisolone for, 211
Mumpsvax, 222
mumps virus vaccine, live, 222
mupirocin, 222
Muscle spasm
cyclobenzaprine for, 91
diazepam for, 104
Musculoskeletal conditions
carisoprodol for, 55
methocarbamol for, 209
Mustargen, 202
Mutamycin, 219
Myambutol, 133
Myasthenia gravis
neostigmine bromide/
neostigmine methylsulfate for, 228

Myasthenia gravis (continued)
pyridostigmine for, 267-268
Mycelex, 86
Mycelex-G, 86
Mycelex OTC, 86
Mycelex-7, 86
Mycifradin, 228
Myciguent, 228
Mycobutin, 274
mycophenolate mofetil, 222-223
mycophenolate mofetil hydrochloride, 222-223
Mycosis fungoides, cyclophosphamide for, 92
Mycostatin, 235
Mydfrin, 250
Mydriasis
cyclopentolate for, 92
phenylephrine for, 250-251
pilocarpine for, 252-253
Myelosuppressive therapy, filgrastim for, 141
Mykrox, 213
Mylanta Gas, 283
Mylanta Natural Fiber Supplement, 267
Mylanta, 45
Mylicon, 283
Myocardial infarction
alteplase for, 11
aspirin for, 27
atenolol for, 27
captopril for, 52
eptifibatide for, 126-127
heparin for, 165
lisinopril for, 193
metoprolol for, 214
propranolol for, 265

Myocardial infarction
(continued)
reteplase, recombinant,
for, 273
timolol for, 298
Myocardial infarction prophylaxis, aspirin
for, 27
Myocardial perfusion
scintigraphy,
dipyridamole for,
113
Myochrysine, 30
Myotonachol, 39
Myrosemide, 154
Mysoline, 260
Myxedema, liothyronine
for, 192
Myxedema coma
levothyroxine for, 190
liothyronine for, 192

N

nabumetone, 223
nadolol, 223
Nadostine, 235
nafcillin sodium, 223-224
nalbuphine hydrochloride,
224
Nalfon, 139
Nalfon 200, 139
Nallpen, 223
naloxone hydrochloride,
224-225
naltrexone hydrochloride,
225
naphazoline hydrochlo-
ride, 225-226
Naprelan, 226
Naprogesic, 226
Naprosyn, 226
Naprosyn SR, 226
naproxen, 226
naproxen sodium, 226
naratriptan hydrochloride,
227

Narcan, 224
Narcolepsy
dextroamphetamine for,
103
methylphenidate for,
211
modafinil for, 219-220
Narcotic depression,
naloxone for, 225
Narcotic withdrawal,
methadone for, 208
Nasacort, 305
Nasal congestion
epinephrine for, 125
naphazoline for,
225-226
oxymetazoline for, 240
phenylephrine for, 251
pseudoephedrine for,
266-267
xylometazoline for, 314
Nasalcrom, 90
Nasalide, 145
Nasal polyps, preventing
recurrence of, be-
clomethasone for,
35
Natrilix, 173
Natulan, 261
natural lung surfactant, 37
Nausea and vomiting
chlorpromazine for,
74-75
dolasetron for, 116-117
dronabinol for, 121
metoclopramide for, 213
ondansetron for,
237-238
perphenazine for, 248
prochlorperazine for,
261-262
promethazine for, 263
Navane, 296
Navelbine, 313

Nebcin, 300
NebuPent, 245
nedocromil sodium, 227
nefazodone hydrochlo-
ride, 227
nelfinavir mesylate, 227
Nembutal, 247
Nembutal Sodium, 247
Neo-Calglucon, 48
Neo-Estrone, 130
Neo-fradin, 228
Neo-Metric, 214
neomycin sulfate, 228
Neopap, 3
Neoplasias, dexametha-
sone for, 101
Neoquess, 106, 169
Neoral, 93
Neosar, 92
Neo-Spec, 164
neostigmine
bromide/neostig-
mine methylsulfate,
228-229
Neosulf, 228
Neo-Synephrine, 250, 251
Neo-Synephrine 12 Hr
Nasal Spray, 240
Neo-Synephrine II, 314
Neo-Tabs, 228
Nephrotic syndrome, cy-
clophosphamide
for, 92
Nephrox, 12
Nestrex, 268
Neumega, 238
Neupogen, 141
Neuroblastoma
cyclophosphamide for,
92
doxorubicin for, 119
Neurogenic bladder,
bethanechol for, 39
Neurontin, 155
Neutropenia, congenital,
filgrastim for, 142

nevirapine, 229
Niac, 229
niacin, 229
niacinamide, 229
Niacor, 229
nicardipine, 229-230
Nicobid, 229
Nicoderm, 230
Nico-400, 229
Nicolar, 229
Nicorette, 230
Nicorette DS, 230
nicotinamide, 229
nicotine polacrilex, 230
nicotine resin complex,
230
nicotine transdermal sys-
tem, 230-231
Nicotine withdrawal
nicotine polacrilex for,
230
nicotine transdermal
system for,
230-231
nicotinic acid, 229
Nicotrol, 230
nifedipine, 231
Nilandron, 231
Nilstat, 235
nilutamide, 231
nisoldipine, 231
Nitro-Bid, 232
Nitrocine, 232
Nitrodisc, 232
Nitro-Dur, 232
nitrofurantoin macrocrys-
tals, 231-232
nitrofurantoin microcrys-
tals, 231-232
nitrofurazone, 232
Nitrogard, 232
nitrogen mustard, 202
nitroglycerin, 232-233
Nitroglyn, 232
Nitrol, 232
Nitrolingual, 232

Nitropress, 233
nitroprusside sodium, 233
Nitrostat, 232
nizatidine, 233
Nizoral, 183
Noctec, 71
Nolvadex, 289
Nolvadex-D, 289
Nondepolarizing neuro-
  muscular blocker
  antidote
  neostigmine
    bromide/neostig-
    mine methylsul-
    fate for, 229
  pyridostigmine for, 267
Nordette, 134
norepinephrine bitartrate,
  233
Norepinephrine extravasa-
  tion, phentolamine
  for, 250
norethindrone, 234
norethindrone acetate,
  234
norfloxacin, 234
Norfranil, 172
norgestrel, 234
Norisodrine Aerotrol, 180
Norlutate, 234
Normiflo Injection, 26
Normodyne, 185
Noroxin, 234
Norpace, 113
Norpace CR, 113
Norplant System, 190
Norpramin, 101
Nor-Pred T.B.A., 259
Nor-Q.D., 234
nortriptyline hydrochlo-
  ride, 234-235
Norvasc, 17
Norvir, 276
Noten, 27
Nova Rectal, 247
Novo-Alprazol, 10

Novo-AZ, 315
Novo-Captoril, 52
Novo-Carbamaz, 53
Novo-Chlorhydrate, 71
Novoclopate, 85
Novocolchicine, 87
Novodigoxin, 107
Novoflupam, 148
Novofolacid, 151
Novofumar, 140
Novohexidyl, 307
Novo-Hylazin, 166
Novolin 70/30, 175
Novolin L, 175
Novolin N, 175
Novolin R, 174
Novo-Lorazem, 195
Novomedopa, 210
Novo-Methacin, 173
Novo-Naprox, 226
Novonidazol, 214
Novo-Peridol, 164
Novo-Pirocam, 254
Novo-Poxide, 73
Novopranol, 265
Novo-Ridazine, 295
Novosecobarb, 280
Novosemide, 154
Novo-Soxazole, 288
Novo-Spiroton, 285
Novo-Sundac, 288
Novo-Thalidone, 75
Novo-Veramil, 312
NPH insulin, 175
Nu-Alpraz, 10
Nu-Atenol, 27
Nubain, 224
Nu-Loraz, 195
Nu-Nifed, 231
Nuprin Caplets, 170
Nuprin Tablets, 170
Nutritional support, amino
  acid infusions for,
  15
Nu-Verap, 312
nystatin, 235

Nystex, 235
Nytol Maximum Strength,
  110

O

Obesity
  dextroamphetamine for,
    103
  methamphetamine for,
    209
  orlistat for, 238-239
  phentermine for, 249
  sibutramine for, 281
Obsessive-compulsive
  disorder
  clomipramine for, 83
  fluoxetine for, 146-147
  fluvoxamine for, 151
  sertraline for, 281
Obstetric amnesia, scopo-
  lamine for, 279-280
Octamide, 213
octreotide acetate, 235
OcuClear, 240
Ocufen Liquifilm, 149
Ocular congestion, napha-
  zoline for, 225
Ocular hypertension
  betaxolol for, 39
  dorzolamide for, 118
  latanoprost for, 187
  levobunolol for, 189
  timolol for, 298
Ocular irritation
  naphazoline for, 225
  oxymetazoline for,
    240-241
Ocu-Mycin, 158
Ocupress Ophthalmic
  Solution 1%, 56
Ocusert Pilo, 252
oestradiol, 130-131
oestradiol valerate,
  130-131
oestrogens, conjugated,
  132

Nystex, 235
ofloxacin, 236
Ogen, 132
olanzapine, 236
Oliguria, mannitol for, 200
olsalazine sodium,
  236-237
omeprazole, 237
Omnicef, 59
Oncaspar, 243
Oncovin, 313
ondansetron hydrochlo-
  ride, 237-238
Ophthalmic neonatorum,
  erythromycin for,
  129
Ophthoclor Ophthalmic, 72
Opioid dependence, nal-
  trexone for, 225
opium tincture, 238
opium tincture, camphor-
  ated, 238
oprelvekin, 238
Optazine, 225
Oral infections, nystatin
  for, 235
Orap, 253
Oretic, 167
Oreton Methyl, 212
Organ perfusion, improv-
  ing, dopamine for,
  117
Organ rejection prophy-
  laxis
  basiliximab for, 34
  cyclosporine for, 93
  daclizumab for, 95
  mycophenolate for,
    222-223
  tacrolimus for, 289
Orgaran, 97
Orimune, 255
orlistat, 238-239
Ormazine, 74
Ortho-Cyclen, 134
OrthoEST, 132

Ortho-Novum 7/7/7, 134-135
Ortho Tri-Cyclen, 135
Orudis, 183
Oruvail, 183
Os-Cal 500, 49
Osmitrol, 200
Osteitis deformans. *See* Paget's disease of bone.
Osteoarthritis
  capsaicin for, 52
  celecoxib for, 68, 69
  diclofenac, 105
  diflunisal for, 106
  fenoprofen for, 139
  flurbiprofen for, 148
  ibuprofen for, 170
  indomethacin for, 173
  ketoprofen for, 183
  nabumetone for, 223
  naproxen for, 226
  oxaprozin for, 239
  piroxicam for, 254
  sulindac for, 288
Osteocalcin, 47
Osteoporosis
  alendronate for, 8
  calcitonin for, 47
  conjugated estrogens for, 132
  estropipate for, 132
  raloxifene for, 271
Otitis media
  amoxicillin/clavulanate potassium for, 18
  azithromycin for, 31
  cefaclor for, 58
  cefdinir for, 59
  cefprozil for, 65
  ceftibuten for, 66
  cefuroxime for, 67-68
  cephalexin for, 69
  cephradine for, 69-70
  loracarbef for, 195
Otrivin, 314

Ovarian cancer
  carboplatin for, 54-55
  cisplatin for, 79
  cyclophosphamide for, 92
  doxorubicin for, 119
  melphalan for, 204
  paclitaxel for, 241
  thiotepa for, 295
  topotecan for, 301-302
Overactive bladder, tolterodine for, 301
Ovral, 134
Ovrette, 234
oxacillin sodium, 239
oxaprozin, 239
oxazepam, 239
oxycodone hydrochloride, 239-240
oxycodone pectinate, 240
OxyContin, 240
Oxydess II, 103
Oxy IR, 240
oxymetazoline hydrochloride, 240, 240-241
oxytocin, synthetic injection, 241

P

paclitaxel, 241
Paget's disease of bone
  alendronate for, 8
  calcitonin for, 47
  etidronate for, 135
  pamidronate for, 242
  tiludronate for, 297-298
Pain
  acetaminophen for, 3
  aspirin for, 27
  butorphanol for, 46
  capsaicin for, 52
  choline magnesium trisalicylate for, 76
  codeine for, 87

Pain *(continued)*
  diflunisal for, 106
  etodolac for, 135-136
  fenoprofen for, 139
  fentanyl for, 140
  hydromorphone for, 168
  ibuprofen for, 170
  ketoprofen for, 183
  ketorolac for, 184
  magnesium salicylate for, 199
  meperidine for, 205
  methadone for, 208
  morphine for, 221-222
  nalbuphine for, 224
  naproxen for, 226
  oxycodone for, 239
  pentazocine for, 246
  propoxyphene for, 264
  tramadol for, 302-303
Panadol, 3
Panasol, 259
Pancreatic cancer
  fluorouracil for, 146
  gemcitabine for, 156
  mitomycin for, 219
  streptozocin for, 286-287
Panic disorder
  alprazolam for, 10
  paroxetine for, 243
Panmycin P, 293
Panretin, 9
Panshape M, 249
Panwarfin, 314
Paraplatin, 54
Paraplatin-AQ, 54
Parasitic infestation, lindane for, 191
paregoric, 238
paricalcitol, 242

Parkinsonism
  amantadine for, 13
  benztropine for, 36
  biperiden for, 40
  bromocriptine for, 42
  carbidopa-levodopa for, 54
  diphenhydramine for, 110
  levodopa for, 189
  pergolide for, 247
  pramipexole for, 257-258
  ropinirole for, 277
  selegiline for, 281
  tolcapone for, 300
  trihexyphenidyl for, 306-307
Parlodel, 42
paroxetine hydrochloride, 242-243
Patent ductus arteriosus
  alprostadil for, 11
  indomethacin for, 173-174
Paveral, 87
Paxil, 242
Paxil CR, 242
Pedia Care Infant's Decongestant, 266
Pedia Profen, 170
Pediculosis, lindane for, 191
pegaspargase, 243
PEG-L-asparaginase, 243
Pellagra
  niacin for, 229
  riboflavin for, 274
Pelvic inflammatory disease
  clindamycin for, 82-83
  doxycycline for, 120
  erythromycin for, 127-128
  ofloxacin for, 236

Pelvic inflammatory disease (continued)
piperacillin and tazobactam for, 253-254
trovafloxacin for, 308
pemoline, 243
penicillamine, 243-244
penicillin G benzathine, 244
penicillin G potassium, 244-245
penicillin G procaine, 245
penicillin G sodium, 245
Pentacarinat, 245
Pentam 300, 246
pentamidine isethionate, 245-246
Pentamycetin, 72
Pentazine, 263
pentazocine hydrochloride, 246
pentazocine hydrochloride and naloxone hydrochloride, 246
pentazocine lactate, 246
pentobarbital, 247
pentobarbital sodium, 247
pentoxifylline, 247
Pepcid, 137
Pepcid AC, 137
Pepcidine, 137
Peptic ulcers
hyoscyamine for, 169-170
propantheline for, 264
Pepto-Bismol, 40
Percutaneous transluminal coronary angioplasty
abciximab for, 2
eptifibatide for, 126-127
pergolide mesylate, 247
Pergonal, 204
Peridol, 164
Peritonitis, meropenem for, 206

Permapen, 244
Permax, 247
Permitil Concentrate, 147
Pernicious anemia, cyanocobalamin for, 91
perphenazine, 247-248
Persantin, 113
Persantine, 113
Pertofran, 101
Pertofrane, 101
pethidine hydrochloride, 205
Pfizerpen, 245
Pharyngitis
azithromycin for, 31
cefadroxil for, 58
cefdinir for, 60
cefprozil for, 65
ceftibuten for, 66
cefuroxime for, 67-68
clarithromycin for, 81
loracarbef for, 195
Phenazine 25, 263
Phenazo, 248
phenazopyridine hydrochloride, 248
Phencen-50, 263
Phenergan, 263
Phenergan Fortis, 263
phenobarbital, 248-249
phenobarbital sodium, 249
phenobarbitone, 248-249
phenobarbitone sodium, 249
Phenoject-50, 263
Phentercot, 249
phentermine hydrochloride, 249
phentolamine mesylate, 249-250
Phentride, 249
phenylazo diamino pyridine hydrochloride, 248

phenylephrine hydrochloride, 250, 250-251
Phenytex, 251
phenytoin, 251-252
phenytoin sodium, 251-252
Pheochromocytoma
phentolamine for, 249-250
propranolol for, 265
Phillips' Milk of Magnesia, 198
Phos-Ex, 48
Phos-Lo, 48
phosphonoformic acid, 153
Phyllocontin, 16
phytonadione, 252
Pilagan, 252
Pilocar, 252
pilocarpine, 252-253
pilocarpine hydrochloride, 252-253
pilocarpine nitrate, 252-253
Pilopt, 252
pimozide, 253
pindolol, 253
Pink Bismuth, 40
Pinworm, mebendazole for, 202
piperacillin sodium, 253
piperacillin sodium and tazobactam sodium, 253-254
piperazine estrone sulfate, 132
Pipracil, 253
Pipril, 253
pirbuterol acetate, 254
piroxicam, 254
Pitocin, 241
Pitressin, 311
Pituitary trauma, desmopressin for, 101
Platamine, 79

Platelet adhesion, inhibiting, dipyridamole for, 113
Platinol, 79
Platinol AQ, 79
Plavix, 85
Pletal, 76
Pleural effusion, bleomycin for, 41
plicamycin, 254-255
PMS-Benztropine, 36
PMS-Methylphenidate, 211
PMS Metronidazole, 214
PMS Perphenazine, 247-248
PMS Primidone, 260
PMS Prochlorperazine, 261, 262
PMS-Promethazine, 263
PMS Thioridazine, 295
pneumococcal vaccine, polyvalent, 255
Pneumocystis carinii pneumonia
atovaquone for, 28
pentamidine for, 245-246
Pneumonia
acetylcysteine for, 5
alatrofloxacin for, 308
azithromycin for, 31
bacitracin for, 33
cefdinir for, 59
cefepime for, 60
cefpodoxime for, 64
dirithromycin for, 113
grepafloxacin for, 163
levofloxacin for, 189
loracarbef for, 195
penicillin G procaine for, 245
piperacillin and tazobactam for, 253-254
sparfloxacin for, 285
trovafloxacin for, 308

Pneumovax 23, 255
Pnu-Imune 23, 255
Poisoning. *See also specific type.*
  activated charcoal for, 5
  ipecac syrup for, 178
poliovirus vaccine, inactivated, 255
poliovirus vaccine, live, oral, trivalent, 255
Polymox, 18
polymyxin B sulfate, 255-256
Polyneuritis, riboflavin for, 274
Postoperative care, fentanyl for, 140
Postpartum bleeding
  methylergonovine for, 206
  oxytocin, synthetic injection, for, 241
Poststreptococcal rheumatic fever prophylaxis, penicillin G benzathine for, 244
Posture, 48
potassium bicarbonate, 256
potassium chloride, 256
potassium gluconate, 257
potassium iodide, 257
  saturated solution, 257
pramipexole dihydrochloride, 257-258
Prandin, 272
Pravachol, 258
pravastatin sodium, 258
prazosin hydrochloride, 258
Precose, 2
Pred-Forte, 259
Prednicen-M, 259
prednisolone, 258-259

prednisolone acetate (suspension), 259
prednisolone sodium phosphate, 258-259
prednisolone tebutate, 258-259
prednisone, 259
Prednisone Intensol, 259
Preeclampsia, magnesium sulfate for, 199
Premarin, 132
Premarin Intravenous, 132
Prepidil, 110
Presolol, 185
Prevacid, 186
Prevalite, 75
Priftin, 275
Prilosec, 237
Primacor, 217
primaquine phosphate, 259-260
Primary ovarian failure
  conjugated estrogens for, 132
  esterified estrogens for, 130
  estradiol for, 130-131
  estropipate for, 132
Primatene Mist, 124
Primaxin IM, 172
Primaxin IV, 172
primidone, 260
Primogyn Depot, 131
Prinivil, 192
Privine, 225
ProAmatine, 217
Pro-Banthine, 264
probenecid, 260-261
procainamide hydrochloride, 261
Procanbid, 261
procarbazine hydrochloride, 261
Procardia, 231

Procardia XL, 231
prochlorperazine, 261-262
prochlorperazine edisylate, 261-262
prochlorperazine maleate, 262
Procrit, 125
Proctitis
  hydrocortisone for, 168
  mesalamine for, 206
Proctosigmoiditis, mesalamine for, 206
Procytox, 92
Prodium, 248
progesterone, 262-263
Prograf, 289
Pro-Lax, 267
Proleukin, 8
Prolixin, 147
Prolixin Concentrate, 147-148
Prolixin Decanoate, 147
Prolixin Enanthate, 147
Proloprim, 307
promethazine hydrochloride, 263
promethazine theoclate, 263
Promine, 261
Pronestyl, 261
propafenone hydrochloride, 263
propantheline bromide, 264
Propecia, 142
Propine, 112
propofol, 264
propoxyphene hydrochloride, 264
propoxyphene napsylate, 264
propranolol hydrochloride, 265
Propulsid, 79

propylthiouracil, 266
Propyl-Thyracil, 266
Prorazin, 261, 262
Proscar, 142
ProSom, 130
Prostate cancer
  esterified estrogens for, 130
  estradiol for, 131
  ethinyl estradiol for, 134
  flutamide for, 149
  goserelin for, 162
  nilutamide for, 231
Prostatitis
  ciprofloxacin for, 78
  co-trimoxazole for, 90
  ofloxacin for, 236
  trovafloxacin for, 308
ProStep, 230
Prostigmin, 228
Prostin E2, 110
Prostin VR Pediatric, 110
protamine sulfate, 266
protamine zinc suspension, 175
Prothazine, 263
Protostat, 214
Proventil, 7
Proventil Repetabs, 7
Provera, 203
Provigil, 219
Prozac, 146
Prozac 20, 146
Pruritus due to allergies, hydroxyzine for, 169
pseudoephedrine hydrochloride, 266-267
pseudoephedrine sulfate, 266-267
Pseudohypoparathyroidism, calcitriol for, 47
Psittacosis
  demeclocycline for, 100
  doxycycline for, 120

Psoriasis, calcipotriene for, 46

Psychoneurotic manifestations, mesoridazine for, 207

Psychotic disorders
chlorpromazine for, 74
fluphenazine for, 147
haloperidol for, 164
loxapine for, 197
molindone for, 220-221
olanzapine for, 236
perphenazine for, 247-248
prochlorperazine for, 262
quetiapine for, 269
risperidone for, 276
thioridazine for, 295
thiothixene for, 296
trifluoperazine for, 306

psyllium, 267
PTU, 266
Pulmicort Turbuhaler, 43
Pulmonary edema
ethacrynate for, 133
ethacrynic acid for, 133
furosemide for, 154
Pulmonary embolism
alteplase for, 11
enoxaparin for, 123
heparin for, 165-166
streptokinase for, 286
urokinase for, 309
warfarin for, 314

Purinethol, 205
Purinol, 9
P.V. Carpine Liquifilm, 252
pyrazinamide, 267
Pyrazinamide, 267
Pyridium, 248
pyridostigmine bromide, 267-268
pyridoxine hydrochloride, 268

pyrimethamine, 268
pyrimethamine with sulfadoxine, 268
PZI insulin, 175

QR
Questran, 75
Questran Light, 75
quetiapine fumarate, 269
Quinaglute, 270
Quinalan, 270
quinapril hydrochloride, 269-270
Quinate, 270
Quinidex Extentabs, 270
quinidine gluconate, 270
quinidine sulfate, 270
RA 27/3, 278
Racepinephrine, 124
Radiation protection for thyroid gland, potassium iodide for, 257
Radiation therapy complications, ondansetron for, 238
Radiologic examination
glucagon as diagnostic aid for, 160
metoclopramide as diagnostic aid for, 213
raloxifene hydrochloride, 271
Ramace, 271
ramipril, 271
ranitidine bismuth citrate, 272
ranitidine hydrochloride, 271-272
Raxar, 162
Reclomide, 213

Recommended daily allowance, folic acid for, 151-152
Rectal examination preparation
bisacodyl for, 40
cascara sagrada for, 57
senna for, 281
Rectal infections
doxycycline for, 120
minocycline for, 218
Regitine, 249
Reglan, 213
Regonol, 267
Regranex Gel, 34
Regular (Conc.) Iletin II, 174
regular insulin, 174-175
Relafen, 223
Remeron, 219
Remicade, 174
Renal cancer, medroxyprogesterone for, 203
Renal cell carcinoma, aldesleukin for, 8
Renal disease, bumetanide for, 44
Renal failure
calcifediol for, 46
cidofovir-induced, probenecid for, 260
torsemide for, 302
Renal function, assessing, mannitol for, 200
Renitec, 123
ReoPro, 2
repaglinide, 272-273
repository corticotropin, 88
Requip, 277
Rescriptor, 100
Resonium A, 284
RespiGam, 273

Respiratory depression, narcotic-induced, naloxone for, 224-225
Respiratory distress syndrome, beractant for, 37
Respiratory syncytial virus
respiratory syncytial virus immune globulin intravenous, human, for, 273
ribavirin for, 273-274
respiratory syncytial virus immune globulin intravenous, human, 273
Respiratory tract illnesses, amantadine for, 13
Respiratory tract infections
amoxicillin/clavulanate potassium for, 18
aztreonam for, 32
cefaclor for, 58
cefazolin for, 59
cefmetazole for, 61
cefoperazone for, 62
cefotaxime for, 62-63
cefotetan for, 63
cefoxitin for, 63-64
ceftazidime for, 65
ceftizoxime for, 66
ceftriaxone for, 67
cefuroxime for, 67-68
cephalexin for, 69
cephradine for, 69
co-trimoxazole for, 89
erythromycin for, 128
imipenem and cilastatin for, 172
ofloxacin for, 236

Respiratory tract infections *(continued)*
  penicillin G benzathine for, 244
  respiratory syncytial virus immune globulin intravenous, human, for, 273
  ticarcillin/clavulanate for, 297
Respolin Inhaler, 7
Respolin Respirator Solution, 7
Restoril, 290
Retavase, 273
reteplase, recombinant, 273
Reticulum cell carcinoma, bleomycin for, 41
Retinoblastoma, cyclophosphamide for, 92
retinoic acid, 304
Retrovir, 315
ReVia, 225
Revimine, 117
Rezulin, 307
Rhabdomyosarcoma, dactinomycin for, 96
Rheaban Maximum Strength, 29
Rheumacin, 173
Rheumatoid arthritis
  aspirin for, 27
  auranofin for, 29
  aurothioglucose for, 30
  azathioprine for, 31
  capsaicin for, 52
  celecoxib for, 68-69
  choline magnesium trisalicylate for, 75
  diclofenac for, 105
  diflunisal for, 106
  etanercept for, 132-133

Rheumatoid arthritis *(continued)*
  fenoprofen for, 139
  flurbiprofen for, 148
  gold sodium thiomalate for, 30
  ibuprofen for, 170
  indomethacin for, 173
  ketoprofen for, 183
  leflunomide for, 187
  nabumetone for, 223
  naproxen for, 226
  oxaprozin for, 239
  penicillamine for, 244
  piroxicam for, 254
  sulfasalazine for, 287
  sulindac for, 288
Rheumatrex, 210
Rhinitis
  beclomethasone for, 35
  brompheniramine for, 42-43
  budesonide for, 43
  cetirizine for, 71
  chlorpheniramine for, 74
  clemastine for, 82
  cromolyn sodium for, 90
  diphenhydramine for, 110
  fexofenadine for, 141
  flunisolide for, 145
  fluticasone for, 150-151
  ipratropium for, 179
  loratadine for, 195
  promethazine for, 263
  triamcinolone for, 305
Rhinocort, 43
Rhinorrhea, cold-induced, ipratropium for, 179. *See also* Rhinitis.
ribavirin, 273-274
riboflavin, 274
Riboflavin deficiency, riboflavin for, 274
Ridaura, 29

rifabutin, 274
Rifadin, 274
Rifadin IV, 274
rifampicin, 274-275
rifampin, 274-275
rifapentine, 275
rIFN-A, 176
Rilutek, 275
riluzole, 275
Rimactane, 274
rimantadine hydrochloride, 275-276
Rimycin, 274
Ringworm. *See* Tinea infections.
Riopan, 197
Risperdal, 276
risperidone, 276
Ritalin, 211
Ritalin-SR, 211
ritonavir, 276
Rituxan, 276
rituximab, 276-277
rizatriptan benzoate, 277
Roaccutane, 182
Robaxin, 209
Robimycin, 127
Robitet, 293
Robitussin, 164
Rocaltrol, 47
Rocephin, 67
Rodex, 268
Rofact, 274
Roferon-A, 176
Rogaine, 218
Rogitine, 249
Rolaids, 49
Romazicon, 144
ropinirole hydrochloride, 277
RotaShield, 277
rotavirus vaccine live, oral, tetravalent, 277
Roundworm, mebendazole for, 202

Rowasa, 206
Roxanol, 221
Roxicodone, 240
Roxicodone Intensol, 240
RSV-IGIV, 273
rubella and mumps virus vaccine, live, 278
rubella virus vaccine, live attenuated, 278
Rubex, 119
Rythmodan, 113
Rythmodan-LA, 113
Rythmol, 263

S

salazosulfapyridine, 287
salbutamol, 7-8
salbutamol sulfate, 7-8
salmeterol xinafoate, 278-279
Salmonine, 93
Salt-losing adrenogenital syndrome, fludrocortisone for, 143-144
Sandimmun, 93
Sandimmune, 93
Sandostatin, 235
Sandostatin LAR, 235
Sani-Supp, 161
Sansert, 213
saquinavir, 279
saquinavir mesylate, 279
Sarcoma
  cyclophosphamide for, 92
  dactinomycin for, 96
  doxorubicin for, 119
sargramostim, 279
Scabene, 191
Scabies, lindane for, 191
SCF, 287
Schizophrenia
  clozapine for, 86-87
  mesoridazine for, 207
  trifluoperazine for, 306

scopolamine, 279-280
scopolamine butylbro-
mide, 279-280
scopolamine hydrobro-
mide, 280
Seborrheic dermatitis
hydrocortisone for, 168
ketoconazole for, 183
secobarbital sodium,
280-281
Seconal Sodium, 280
Secretions, diminishing
atropine for, 28
hyoscyamine for,
169-170
Sectral, 3
Sedation
chloral hydrate for, 71
diphenhydramine for,
110
hydroxyzine for, 169
lorazepam for, 196
midazolam for, 216
pentobarbital for, 247
phenobarbital for, 249
promethazine for, 263
propofol for, 264
scopolamine for,
279-280
secobarbital for, 280
Sedative effects, revers-
ing, flumazenil for,
144
Seizures
carbamazepine for, 53
clonazepam for, 84
clorazepate for, 85
diazepam for, 105
fosphenytoin for, 154
gabapentin for, 155
lamotrigine for, 186
magnesium sulfate for,
200
phenobarbital for,
248-249
phenytoin for, 251

Seizures (continued)
primidone for, 260
pyridoxine for, 268
tiagabine for, 296
topiramate for, 301
valproic acid for, 310
selegiline hydrochloride,
281
Semilente, 175
Senexon, 281
senna, 281
Senokot, 281
Septicemia
aztreonam for, 32
cefazolin for, 59
cefonicid for, 61
cefoperazone for, 62
cefotaxime for, 62-63
ceftazidime for, 65
ceftizoxime for, 66
ceftriaxone for, 67
cephradine for, 69
imipenem and cilastatin
for, 172
ticarcillin/clavulanate
for, 297
Septra, 89
Serax, 239
Serenace, 164
Serentil, 207
Serentil Concentrate, 207
Serevent, 278
Serevent Diskus, 278
Seromycin, 93
Seroquel, 269
Sertan, 260
sertraline hydrochloride,
281
Serzone, 227
Shigellosis, co-
trimoxazole for, 89
Shingles. See Herpes
zoster infection.
Shock. See also specific
type.
dexamethasone for, 102

Shock (continued)
dopamine for, 117
hydrocortisone for, 167
isoproterenol for, 180
methylprednisolone for,
212
phenylephrine for, 250
sibutramine hydrochloride
monohydrate,
281-282
sildenafil citrate, 282
Silvadene, 282
silver sulfadiazine,
282-283
simethicone, 283
Simron, 140
Simulect, 34
simvastatin, 283
Sinemet, 54
Sinemet CR, 54
Sinex, 251
Singulair, 221
Sinusitis
amoxicillin/clavulanate
potassium for, 18
cefdinir for, 59
cefprozil for, 65
clarithromycin for, 81
levofloxacin for, 189
loracarbef for, 195
trovafloxacin for, 308
692, 264
Skelid, 297
Skin graft rejection, preventing, nitrofura-
zone for, 232
Skin infections
amoxicillin/clavulanate
potassium for, 18
ampicillin sodium/sul-
bactam sodium
for, 20-21
aztreonam for, 32
cefaclor for, 58
cefadroxil for, 58
cefazolin for, 59

Skin infections (continued)
cefdinir for, 59
cefmetazole for, 61
cefonicid for, 61
cefoperazone for, 62
cefotaxime for, 62-63
cefotetan for, 63
cefoxitin for, 63-64
ceftazidime for, 65
ceftizoxime for, 66
ceftriaxone for, 67
cefuroxime for, 67-68
cephalexin for, 69
cephradine for, 69
ciprofloxacin for, 78
dirithromycin for, 113
erythromycin for, 128
gentamicin for, 158
imipenem and cilastatin
for, 172
levofloxacin for, 189
ofloxacin for, 236
piperacillin and tazobac-
tam for, 253-254
tetracycline for, 293
ticarcillin/clavulanate
for, 297
trovafloxacin for, 308,
309
Slo-Phyllin, 293
Slow-K, 256
Slow-Mag, 198
Small-bowel intubation,
facilitating, meto-
clopramide for, 213
Smoking cessation,
bupropion for, 44
SMZ-TMP, 89
Soda Mint, 283
sodium bicarbonate, 283
sodium chloride, 283
sodium cromoglycate, 90
sodium phosphates, 284
sodium polystyrene sul-
fonate, 284
Sodol, 55

Sofarin, 314
Soft-tissue infections
cefaclor for, 58
cefadroxil for, 58
cefazolin for, 59
cefoxitin for, 63-64
cephalexin for, 69
cephradine for, 69
erythromycin for, 128
imipenem and cilastatin for, 172
Solazine, 306
Solfoton, 249
Solganal, 30
Solu-Cortef, 167
Solu-Medrol, 212
Soma, 55
Sominex, 110
Sopamycetin, 72
Sorbitrate, 181
Sotacor, 285
sotalol, 285
Spancap #1, 103
sparfloxacin, 285
Spasmoban, 106
Spasticity
baclofen for, 33
dantrolene for, 98
scopolamine for, 279
Spectazole, 122
Spermatogenesis, stimu-
lating, menotropins for, 205
Spinal cord injury
baclofen for, 33
dantrolene for, 98
spironolactone, 285
Sporanox, 182
SPS, 284
Squamous cell carcinoma,
bleomycin for, 41
Squibb-HC, 168
SSKI, 257
Stadol, 46
Stadol NS, 46

Status epilepticus
diazepam for, 105
fosphenytoin for, 153-154
phenobarbital for, 249
phenytoin for, 251-252
secobarbital for, 280-281
stavudine, 286
Stelazine, 306
Stemetil, 262
Stimate, 101
Stomach acid, neutralizing
aluminum carbonate for, 12
aluminum hydroxide for, 12
calcium carbonate for, 49
magaldrate for, 197
magnesium oxide for, 199
magnesium salts for, 199
Stomach cancer
doxorubicin for, 119
fluorouracil for, 146
mitomycin for, 219
Stool softening, docusate for, 116
Streptase, 286
streptokinase, 286
streptozocin, 286-287
Stroke, ischemic. See
Ischemic stroke.
thrombotic. See
Thrombotic stroke.
strong iodine solution, 257
Sublimaze, 139
sucralfate, 287
Sudafed, 266
Sular, 231
Sulcrate, 287
sulfamethoxazole, 287

sulfasalazine, 287
Sulfate ADD-Vantage, 157
Sulfatrim, 89
sulfinpyrazone, 288
sulfisoxazole, 288
sulfisoxazole acetyl, 288
sulindac, 288
sulphasalazine, 287
sumatriptan succinate, 289
Sumycin, 293
Supeudol, 240
Suppression therapy, ni-
trofurantoin for, 231-232
Surfactant deficiency, beractant for, 37
Surfak, 116
Surgery preparation
alatrofloxacin for, 308
bisacodyl for, 40
butorphanol for, 46
chloral hydrate for, 71
droperidol for, 121
fentanyl for, 139
lorazepam for, 196
meperidine for, 205
midazolam for, 216
neomycin for, 228
pentobarbital for, 247
phenobarbital for, 249
piperacillin for, 253
promethazine for, 263
scopolamine for, 279-280
secobarbital for, 280
trovafloxacin for, 308
Surgery prophylaxis
cefazolin for, 58-59
cefonicid for, 61
cefotaxime for, 62
cefotetan for, 63
cefoxitin for, 63-64
cefuroxime for, 67-68
cephradine for, 69

Surgical infections, aztre-
onam for, 32
Surmontil, 307
Survanta, 37
Sus-Phrine, 124
Sustiva, 122
Symadine, 13
Symmetrel, 13
Synflex, 226
Synthroid, 190
Syphilis
minocycline for, 218
penicillin G benzathine for, 244
syvinolin, 283

T
T_3, 192
T_4, 190
tacrine hydrochloride, 289
tacrolimus, 289
Tagamet, 77
Tagamet HB, 77
Talwin, 246
Talwin-Nx, 246
Tambocor, 142
tamoxifen citrate, 289
tamsulosin hydrochloride, 290
Tapazole, 209
Tasmar, 300
Tavist, 82
Tavist-1, 82
Taxol, 241
Taxotere, 115
Tazac, 233
Tazicef, 65
Tazidime, 65
Tebrazid, 267
Tegretol, 53
Teldrin, 74
telmisartan, 290
temazepam, 290

Tempra, 3
Tendinitis
  indomethacin for, 173
  naproxen for, 226
  sulindac for, 288
Tenormin, 27
Tension, hydroxyzine for, 169
Terazol 3 Vaginal Ovules, 292
Terazol 7 Vaginal Ovules Cream, 292
terazosin hydrochloride, 290-291
terbinafine hydrochloride, 291
terbutaline sulfate, 291-292
terconazole, 292
Terfluzine, 306
Tertroxin, 192
TESPA, 295
Tessalon, 36
Testamone 100, 292
Testex, 292
Testicular cancer
  bleomycin for, 41
  cisplatin for, 79
  dactinomycin for, 96
  etoposide for, 136
  ifosfamide for, 171
  plicamycin for, 255
  vinblastine for, 313
Testicular deficiency, fluoxymesterone for, 147
Testoderm, 292
testosterone, 292-293
testosterone cypionate, 292-293
testosterone propionate, 292-293
testosterone transdermal system, 292-293
Testred, 212

Tetanus management, methocarbamol for, 209
tetracycline hydrochloride, 293
Tetracyn, 293
Theo-Dur, 293
theophylline, 293-294
theophylline ethylenediamine, 16
theophylline sodium glycinate, 293-294
Theralax, 40
Thermazene, 282
thiamine hydrochloride, 295
Thioplex, 295
Thioprine, 30
thioridazine hydrochloride, 295
thiotepa, 295
thiothixene, 296
thiothixene hydrochloride, 296
Thoracic surgery complications, acetylcysteine for, 5
Thorazine, 74
Thrombate III, 24
Thrombocytopenia, anagrelide for, 22
Thromboembolism, antithrombin III, human, for, 24
Thrombotic stroke, ticlopidine for, 297
Thyroid cancer, doxorubicin for, 119
Thyroidectomy preparation, potassium iodide for, 257
Thyroid hormone replacement
  levothyroxine for, 190
  liothyronine for, 192

Thyrotoxic crisis
  potassium iodide for, 257
  propylthiouracil for, 266
tiagabine hydrochloride, 296
Tiazac, 109
Ticar, 296
ticarcillin disodium, 296-297
ticarcillin disodium/clavulanate potassium, 297
Ticillin, 296
Ticlid, 297
ticlopidine hydrochloride, 297
Tilade, 227
tiludronate disodium, 297-298
Timentin, 297
timolol maleate, 298
Timoptic Solution, 298
Timoptic-XE, 298
Tinea infections
  econazole for, 122
  griseofulvin for, 163-164
  ketoconazole for, 183
  miconazole for, 216
  terbinafine for, 291
  tioconazole, 299
Tipramine, 172
tirofiban hydrochloride, 298-299
tissue plasminogen activator, recombinant, 11-12
tobramycin, 299
tobramycin sulfate, 300
Tobrex, 299
tocainide hydrochloride, 300
Tofranil, 172
Tofranil-PM, 172
tolcapone, 300

tolterodine tartrate, 301
Tonocard, 300
Tonsillitis
  azithromycin for, 31
  cefadroxil for, 58
  cefdinir for, 60
  cefprozil for, 65
  ceftibuten for, 66
  cefuroxime for, 67-68
  clarithromycin for, 81
  loracarbef for, 195
Topamax, 301
Topical infections, bacitracin for, 32
Topicycline, 293
topiramate, 301
topotecan hydrochloride, 301-302
Toprol XL, 214
Topsyn, 145
TOPV, 255
Toradol, 184
toremifene citrate, 302
torsemide, 302
Total parenteral nutrition, amino acid infusions for, 14
Tourette syndrome, pimozide for, 253
Toxoplasmosis, pyrimethamine for, 269
t-PA, 11-12
Trachoma, erythromycin for, 128-129
tramadol hydrochloride, 302-303
Trandate, 185
trandolapril, 303
Transderm-Nitro, 232
Transderm-Scop, 279
Transderm-V, 279
Tranxene, 85
Tranxene-SD, 85
Tranxene-T-Tab, 85
trastuzumab, 303-304
Trasylol, 25

Travasol with Electrolytes, 14

trazodone hydrochloride, 304

Trazon, 304

Trental, 247

tretinoin, 304-305

Triacet, 305

Trialodine, 304

triamcinolone acetonide, 305

Triamonide 40, 305

triamterene, 306

triazolam, 306

Trichomoniasis, metronidazole for, 214

Tricor, 138

Tricosal, 75

Tridil, 232

triethylenethiophosphoramide, 295

trifluoperazine hydrochloride, 306

Trihexane, 307

trihexyphenidyl hydrochloride, 306-307

Tri-Immunol, 112

Trikacide, 214

Trilafon, 248

Trilafon Concentrate, 248

Trilisate, 75

Trilog, 305

trimethoprim, 307

trimethoprim-sulfamethoxazole, 89-90

trimipramine maleate, 307

Trimox, 18

Trimpex, 307

Triostat, 192

Tripedia, 112

Triphasil, 134

Triprim, 307

Tritace, 271

Tritec, 272

troglitazone, 307-308

Trophoblastic tumors
dactinomycin for, 96
methotrexate for, 210

trovafloxacin mesylate, 308-309

Trovan I.V., 308

Trovan Tablets, 308

Truphylline, 16

Trusopt, 118

TSPA, 295

Tuberculosis
acetylcysteine for, 5
cycloserine for, 93
ethambutol for, 133
isoniazid for, 180
pyrazinamide for, 267
rifampin for, 274
rifapentine for, 275

Tumor complications, octreotide for, 235

Tylenol, 3

UV

Ukidan, 309

Ulcerative colitis
mesalamine for, 206
olsalazine for, 236
sulfasalazine for, 287

Ulcers. *See specific type.*

Ultracef, 58

Ultralente Insulin, 175

Ultram, 302

Ultrazine-10, 262

Unasyn, 62

Uniparin, 165

Unipen, 223

Univasc, 220

Urabeth, 39

Urecholine, 39

Urethral infections
doxycycline for, 120
minocycline for, 218

Urethritis
azithromycin for, 31
grepafloxacin for, 163
ofloxacin for, 236

Urex, 154

Urge incontinence, tolterodine for, 301

Uridon, 75

Urinary alkalinization, sodium bicarbonate for, 283

Urinary phosphate stones, preventing, aluminum carbonate for, 12

Urinary tract infections
amikacin for, 14
amoxicillin/clavulanate potassium for, 18
amoxicillin trihydrate for, 18-19
aztreonam for, 32
cefaclor for, 58
cefadroxil for, 58
cefepime for, 60
cefmetazole for, 61
cefonicid for, 61
cefotaxime for, 62-63
cefotetan for, 63
cefpodoxime for, 64
ceftazidime for, 65
ceftizoxime for, 66
ceftriaxone for, 67
cefuroxime for, 67-68
ciprofloxacin for, 78
co-trimoxazole for, 89, 90
imipenem and cilastatin for, 172
levofloxacin for, 189
lomefloxacin for, 193-194
nitrofurantoin for, 231
norfloxacin for, 234
ofloxacin for, 236
phenazopyridine for, 248
sulfamethoxazole for, 287
sulfisoxazole for, 288

Urinary tract infections *(continued)*
ticarcillin/clavulanate for, 297
trimethoprim for, 307
trovafloxacin for, 309

Urine retention, bethanechol for, 39

Urocarb Tablets, 39

urokinase, 309

Uro-Mag, 199

Urticaria
cetirizine for, 71
clemastine for, 82

Uterine bleeding, abnormal
conjugated estrogens for, 132
medroxyprogesterone for, 203
norethindrone for, 234
progesterone for, 263

Uveitis
atropine for, 29
dexamethasone for, 102-103
scopolamine for, 280

Vaginal atrophy, estradiol/norethindrone acetate transdermal system for, 131

Vaginal infections, nystatin for, 235

Vagistat-1, 299

valacyclovir hydrochloride, 310

Valisone, 38

Valium, 104

valproate sodium, 310

valproic acid, 310

valsartan, 311

Valtrex, 310

Vamate, 169

Vancenase AQ Double Strength, 35

Vancenase AQ Nasal Spray, 35
Vancenase Nasal Inhaler, 35
Vanceril, 35
Vancocin, 311
Vancoled, 311
vancomycin hydrochloride, 311
Vantin, 64
Vapo-Iso, 180
Vaponefrin, 124
Varicella infections, acyclovir sodium for, 6
Vascor, 37
Vascular headache
    dihydroergotamine for, 108
    ergotamine for, 127
    methysergide for, 212-213
VasoClear, 225
vasopressin, 311
Vasotec, 123
Vasotec I.V., 123
VCR, 313
Velban, 313
Velbe, 313
Velosef, 69
Veltane, 42
venlafaxine hydrochloride, 312
Venous thrombosis, streptokinase for, 286
Venous thrombosis prophylaxis, heparin for, 165-166
Ventolin, 7
VePesid, 136
verapamil, 312
verapamil hydrochloride, 312
Verelan, 312
Vergon, 202
Vermox, 202

Versed, 216
Vertigo, meclizine for, 202
Vesanoid, 304
V-Gan-25, 263
Viagra, 282
Vibramycin, 120
Vibra-Tabs 50, 120
vidarabine, 312-313
Videx, 106
vinblastine sulfate, 313
Vincasar PFS, 313
vincristine sulfate, 313
vinorelbine tartrate, 313
Vira-A, 312
Viracept, 227
Viramune, 229
Virazole, 273
Visine L.R., 240
Visken, 253
Vistaquel, 169
Vistaril, 169
Vistazine 50, 169
Vistide, 76
vitamin A acid, 304
vitamin B$_1$, 295
vitamin B$_2$, 274
vitamin B$_3$, 229
vitamin B$_6$, 268
Vitamin B$_6$ deficiency, pyridoxine for, 268
vitamin B$_{12}$, 91
Vitamin B$_{12}$ deficiency, cyanocobalamin for, 91
Vitamin B$_{12}$ malabsorption, cyanocobalamin for, 91
vitamin K$_1$, 252
Vitravene, 152
VLB, 313
Voltaren, 105
Voltaren SR, 105
Vomiting. *See* Nausea and vomiting.
VP-16, 136

Vulvar atrophy, estradiol/norethindrone acetate transdermal system for, 131
Vulvovaginal mycotic infections, butoconazole for, 45

WXYZ

warfarin sodium, 314
Warfilone Sodium, 314
Weight loss, unexplained, megestrol for, 203
Wellbutrin, 44
Wellcovorin, 188
Wernicke's encephalopathy, thiamine for, 295
Westcort Cream, 168
Whipworm, mebendazole for, 202
Wilms' tumor
    dactinomycin for, 96
    doxorubicin for, 119
Wilson's disease, penicillamine for, 243
Wounds, bacitracin for, 32
Wycillin, 245
Wymox, 18
Xalatan, 187
Xanax, 10
Xeloda, 50
Xenical, 238
Xopenex, 188
Xylocaine, 191
xylometazoline hydrochloride, 314
zafirlukast, 314
Zagam, 285
zalcitabine, 314-315
Zanosar, 286
Zantac, 271
Zantac-C, 271
Zantac 75, 271
Zapex, 239

Zaroxolyn, 213
Zebeta, 41
Zefazone, 61
Zemplar, 242
Zenapax, 95
Zerit, 286
Zestril, 192
Zetran, 104
Ziagen, 2
zidovudine, 315-316
zileuton, 316
Zinacef, 67
Zithromax, 31
Zocor, 283
Zofran, 237
Zoladex, 162
Zolicef, 58
Zollinger-Ellison syndrome, lansoprazole for, 186. *See also* Hypersecretory conditions.
zolmitriptan, 316
Zoloft, 281
zolpidem tartrate, 316
Zomig, 316
Zostrix, 52
Zostrix-HP 0.075%, 52
Zosyn, 253
Zovirax, 5, 6
Zyban, 44
Zyflo, 316
Zyloprim, 9
Zyprexa, 236
Zyrtec, 71